BEYOND NATURE–NURTURE

Essays in Honor
of Elizabeth Bates

BEYOND NATURE–NURTURE

Essays in Honor
of Elizabeth Bates

Edited by

Michael Tomasello
Max Planck Institute for Evolutionary Anthropology
Leipzig, Germany

Dan Isaac Slobin
University of California, Berkeley

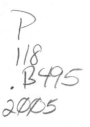

LEA LAWRENCE ERLBAUM ASSOCIATES, PUBLISHERS
2005 Mahwah, New Jersey   London

Lawrence Erlbaum Associates, Inc., Publishers
10 Industrial Avenue
Mahwah, New Jersey 07430

Cover design by Kathryn Houghtaling Lacey

Two daughter–mother photographs: Elizabeth Bates and
Kathleen Bates (taken by Dan Slobin, Berkeley, 1977),
Julia Catherine Carnevale and Elizabeth Bates
(taken by George Carnevale, San Francisco, 1995).

Library of Congress Cataloging-in-Publication Data

Beyond nature–nurture : essays in honor of Elizabeth Bates / edited by
Michael Tomasello, Dan I. Slobin.
    p. cm.
Includes bibliographical references and index.
ISBN 0-8058-5027-9 (pbk. : alk. paper)
1. Language acquisition. 2. Language development. 3. Psycholinguistics.
4. Nature and nurture. 5. Culture and cognition. 6. Language and culture.
7. Communication and culture. 8. Bates, Elizabeth. I. Bates, Elizabeth.
II. Tomasello, Michael. III. Slobin, Dan Isaac.

P118.B495 2004
401'.93—dc22

                                 2004042516
                                     CIP

Books published by Lawrence Erlbaum Associates are printed on acid-free paper,
and their bindings are chosen for strength and durability.

Printed in the United States of America
10 9 8 7 6 5 4 3 2 1

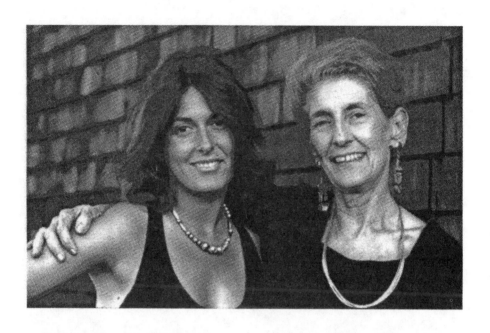

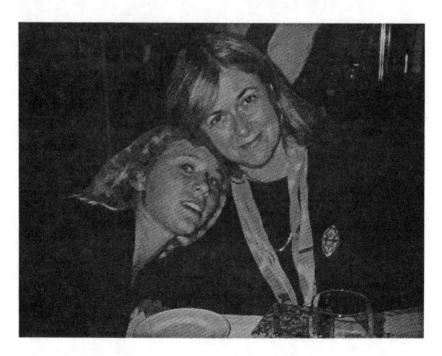

This book is an all-too-early tribute to Liz Bates
from many colleagues and friends
who have learned so much from her
and have been deeply touched
by her participation in our lives and work.

Contents

Contributors

Jennifer Aydelott
University of London
London, UK

Olga Capirci
Consiglio Nazionale delle Ricerche
(CNR)
Rome, Italy

Maria Cristina Caselli
Consiglio Nazionale delle Ricerche
(CNR)
Rome, Italy

Philip S. Dale
University of Missouri–Columbia
USA

Simonetta D'Amico
Università La Sapienza
Rome, Italy

Antonella Devescovi
Università La Sapienza
Rome, Italy

Frederic Dick
University of California, San Diego
and
University of Chicago
USA

Nina F. Dronkers
University of California, San Diego
and
University of California, Davis
USA

Jeffrey L. Elman
University of California, San Diego
USA

Kara D. Federmeier
University of Illinois at
Champaign–Urbana
USA

Barbara L. Finlay
Cornell University
Ithaca, NY
USA

Judith C. Goodman
University of Missouri–Columbia
USA

Mary Hare
Bowling Green State University
Bowling Green, Ohio
USA

Annette Karmiloff-Smith
Institute of Child Health
London, UK

Marta Kutas
University of California, San Diego
USA

Brian MacWhinney
Carnegie Mellon University
Pittsburgh, Pennsylvania
USA

Virginia A. Marchman
The University of Texas at Dallas
USA

William D. Marslen-Wilson
MRC Cognition and Brain Sciences
   Unit
Cambridge, UK

Ken McRae
University of Western Ontario
London, Ontario
Canada

Luigi Pizzamiglio
Università La Sapienza
Rome, Italy

Elena Pizzuto
Consiglio Nazionale delle Ricerche
   (CNR)
Rome, Italy

Ayse Pinar Saygin
University of California, San Diego
USA

Dan I. Slobin
University of California, Berkeley
USA

Steven L. Small
University of Chicago
USA

Donna J. Thal
San Diego State University
and
University of California, San Diego
USA

Michael Tomasello
Max Planck Institute for Evolutionary
   Anthropology
Leipzig, Germany

Lorraine K. Tyler
University of Cambridge, UK

Virginia Volterra
Consiglio Nazionale delle Ricerche
   (CNR)
Rome, Italy

Stephen Wilson
University of California, San Diego
and
University of California, Los Angeles
   (UCLA)
USA

Introduction

Dan I. Slobin
University of California, Berkeley

Michael Tomasello
Max Planck Institute for Evolutionary Anthropology
Leipzig

This book is dedicated to Elizabeth Bates by her many colleagues and friends. Her bibliography spans three decades of intense activity in the sciences of the mind: 1973–2003. Through this period, Liz was a pioneer in so many different areas of developmental psycholinguistics it is difficult to know where to start. She took a "many-perspectives" view of children's acquisition of language and made significant contributions from virtually all of these perspectives.

- **Pragmatics.** She initiated some of the first modern studies of children's use of different kinds of communicative devices—from prelinguistic gestures to linguistic markers of politeness—to achieve pragmatics ends.
- **Crosslinguistic Comparisons.** She initiated some of the first modern studies of children's language—from first words to complex grammar—in which systematic crosslinguistic comparisons were used to make inferences about the human capacity for language.
- **Lexical Development.** She originated the idea for the MacArthur Communicative Development Inventory—now the most widely used instrument in the field for measuring children's vocabulary development—and applied it to answer many specific questions.
- **Grammatical Development.** She was one of the originators of the Competition Model and its application to children learning many different

languages in an effort to identify the grammatical devices—from word order to complex morphology—that children use at different stages of development to identify important grammatical relations in their language.

- **Individual Differences.** She was among the first to systematically study individual differences in language acquisition, and also to focus attention on the theoretical importance of the fact that different children learn language in different ways.

- **Connectionism.** She was a collaborator and contributor in some of the most important work applying principles of connectionist modeling to problems of child language acquisition.

- **Neurophysiology and Evolution.** She was among the first to systematically study children with various kinds of brain damage and to apply insights from this research to basic questions of child language development. She was also innovative in crosslinguistic studies of language capacity in neurologically critical adult populations, including various sorts of aphasia and aging. Her theoretical insights on the relation of phylogeny and ontogeny in language development have been extremely influential.

- **Processing.** She was a collaborator and contributor in important work studying online language processing in adults, as well as in some of the most important work applying principles of online processing to problems of child language acquisition.

In this volume some of Elizabeth Bates's colleagues and collaborators provide up-to-date reviews of these and other areas of research in an attempt to continue in the directions in which she pointed us. The volume also contains a list of her many important publications, as well as some personal reflections of some of the contributors, noting ways in which she made a difference in their lives. In this introduction we provide a brief overview of Bates's scientific history by focusing on the major books she produced, either singly or, as is most often the case, with many important coauthors.

Language and Context: The Acquisition of Pragmatics (1976)

Language is a tool. We use it to do things.

With these words, the just-graduated, 29-year-old Elizabeth Bates begins her first book and thereby throws down the theoretical gauntlet. She wants to explore how young children learn to use language to accomplish social ends, but she will not let this be considered a peripheral enterprise, as was customary in the 1970s. Language is not a formal object that can be used in some informal ways; its essence is use. Tools such as hammers and compasses and linguistic symbols are what they do, and their form is in the service of their function. This way of viewing things was fairly heretical at the time in linguistics—with the theoretical scene being dominated by Chomskian approaches—but it has now gained much wider acceptance under the rubric of "usage-based linguistics." Not the last time Elizabeth Bates turns out to be ahead of her time.

The empirical work reported in this initial book covers a wide range of phenomena in child language acquisition, from prelinguistic gestures to grammar, and is surprisingly modern and still useful in many ways. First is the justly famous work with Camaioni and Volterra on early gestures, such as pointing, and their protoimperative and protodeclarative functions. Bates et al. argue that protoimperatives are communicative procedures in which the child uses the adult as a tool to gain access to an object, whereas protodeclaratives are communicative procedures in which the child uses an object to manipulate adult attention. The distinction between these two functions of early communicative devices has been adopted by virtually all researchers in the field, and indeed it turns out to be crucial in several unanticipated ways. For example, it turns out that apes raised by humans often learn to point imperatively but not declaratively. Children with autism also point only imperatively, and indeed it turns out that the absence of declarative pointing is a key clinical marker for identifying very young children with autism. Other developments of this work concern the interrelations of language and gesture in early development, a topic represented in the current volume by Volterra, Caselli, and Capirici.

The other empirical work reported in this book concerns Italian-speaking children's developing skills with such things as (a) politeness forms, (b) counterfactual conditionals, and (c) topic-focus structures. One thing these studies accomplished when they were first published was to help to make the English-speaking world aware of some of the ways in which crosslinguistic differences are important in language acquisition. Of special interest is the study of topic-comment structure (often called, more generally, information structure), and its expression in various languages by grammatical devices such as word order, stress, and special morphology. This work set the stage for her later collaborative activities with Brian MacWhinney, in which they systematically compared children's acquisition of such devices across languages that work rather differently from one another. Perhaps presaging the competition model:

> In all languages, there is interaction and competition between the pragmatic system for highlighting important information, and the semantic system for expressing reference, case relations, and other propositional structures. (p. 161)

She goes on to enumerate the four kinds of signals of which all languages are composed (lexical items, word order, morphological markers, intonation contours) and the ways these forms compete for the expression of particular functions. She also enumerates some of the many devices used crosslinguistically for expressing topic and focus. These points were crucial in the influential collaborative papers outlining the competition model (Bates & MacWhinney, 1979, 1982, 1987, 1989), discussed in the current volume by MacWhinney and by Devescovi and d'Amico.

Finally, this book of youth also presaged the later focus on online processing. The overall theoretical framework of the book is explicitly Piagetian. But this is not orthodox Piaget. Instead, the focus is on Piaget's distinction between figurative and operative cognitive structures, and what these might mean for processing. Briefly, the idea is that figurative refers to the creation of mental objects for some higher system, and operative refers to the subject's mental manipulation of those figurative products—a kind of recursion. Some ideas from the newly emerging field of artificial intelligence are also included, so that what we get is the first glimmerings of a concern with the actual online processes by means of which children learn and use linguistic symbols and structures.

The Emergence of Symbols: Cognition and Communication in Infancy (1979), From First Words to Grammar: Individual Differences and Dissociable Mechanisms (1988)

The first chapter of the 1979 book is entitled "The Evolution and Development of Symbols" and the last chapter is entitled "The Biology of Symbols." This indicates quite nicely its primary theoretical concern: to develop a way of thinking about the biological bases of language that is more sophisticated than the kind of simplistic nativism permeating the linguistics of the time. The general orientation is indicated by the opening sentences of the book (p. 1):

> Nature is a miser. She clothes her children in hand-me-downs, builds new machinery in makeshift fashion from sundry old parts, and saves genetic expenditures whenever she can by relying on high-probability world events to ensure and stabilize outcomes.

And a few pages later in somewhat different metaphorical terms (p. 6):

> In our search for prerequisites to language . . . . we are suggesting that there is a Great Borrowing going on, in which language is viewed as a parasitic system that builds its structures by raiding the software packages of prior or parallel cognitive capacities.

Drawing on modern biology in a way that philosophical nativists never do, the arguments of this book repeatedly invoke the concept of *heterochrony,* by means of which the behavioral and cognitive capacities of a species may change dramatically simply as a result of changes in the timing of ontogenetic processes. Also, it is repeatedly pointed out that many stable and universal outcomes in human behavior are produced by the interaction of general skills and strong task constraints in the environment. Bates's famous question about human behavior is: "Is eating with the hands innate?" Everyone in all cultures does it (either with or without implements) and needs basically no training to learn to do it. But is there a gene for eating with the hands? Of course not. The answer is that hands are excellent means for transporting objects in manipulative space, and here is an environmental problem—the same for everyone in all cultures—of transporting food from somewhere else into the mouth. And it just turns out that everyone comes up with very similar solutions. In these and other ways the book argues against an innate module for language and argues instead for language as "a new system made up of old parts." These are of course themes that will be addressed more fully and with new theoretical tools in the 1996 book, *Rethinking innateness.*

The empirical part of the book is a search for the prerequisites of language—the old parts that are its components—in other cognitive skills that emerge either just before or along with early language from 9 to 13 months of age. The main candidates are tool use (means-ends analysis), imitation, communicative intention, and symbolic play. The model developed on the basis of the correlational results is the Local Homology model, in which specific skills form the basis for specific aspects of linguistic competence. In the final chapter the model is spelled out ontogenetically in what may be the first dynamic systems model of language development (Figure 7.4, Bates et al., 1979, p. 368; see Figure 7, Marchman & Thal, this volume). The idea is that each of the different components has its own developmental trajectory, and the use of symbols cannot begin until all of them have reached some critical threshold. And it may even happen all of them are "ready" but language still awaits the development of one last control parameter, for example, imitation skills or vocal-auditory processing skills. This model has important implications for understanding why some children are late talkers and why there are so many different ways to be atypical in language development.

The model also has important implications for individual differences in language acquisition, implications that are spelled out more fully in the 1988 book *From first words to grammar: Individual differences and dissociable mechanisms.* This book reports a series of 12 studies with a longitudinal sample of children, taking over at the age where the 1979 book left off (13 to 28 months of age). The main finding was that there may be three partially dissociable language acquisition mechanisms during this age span, dealing with comprehension, rote production, and analyzed production. No differences were found between processes of lexical and grammatical development. This is a finding that has been replicated in a number of different ways in subsequent studies, reviewed in the current volume by Marchman and Thal.

An outgrowth of these two large-scale longitudinal studies was the MacArthur Communicative Development Inventory (MCDI). It began as a structured interview of mothers' knowledge of their children's vocabulary, and has now grown into a standardized measure with very good validity and reliability. Its advantages are many, its disadvantages relatively few. It has now become a mainstay of work in lexical development. For this volume Dale and Goodman review some recent work on lexical and grammatical development using the MCDI.

The Crosslinguistic Study of Sentence Processing (1989)

This book is a collaborative volume with Brian MacWhinney and the international group of psycholinguists who worked together in refining and testing the Competition Model.[1] It provides a strong exposition of the model, supported by studies of child language acquisition, adult sentence processing, aphasia, second-language acquisition, and computer simulation in an impressive array of languages: Cantonese, Finnish, French, German, Hungarian, Hebrew, Italian, Japanese, Kannada, Mandarin, Serbo-Croatian, Slovenian, Spanish, Taiwanese, Turkish, and Warlpiri. Collaborative and crosslinguistic research has always been a hallmark of Bates's way of working, and nowhere more impressively demonstrated than in this remarkable collection of studies. In the preface, the editors set forth a strong set of criteria for psycholinguistics—admirably instantiated by the work presented in the volume (p. xi):

> A good psycholinguistic theory ought to account for many different aspects of natural language use, including comprehension and production of meaningful speech, first language acquisition, second language acquisition, the deterioration of language under pathological conditions, normal speech errors, error monitoring, and judgments of well-formedness. While accounting for this dazzling range of performance phenomena, a good psycholinguistic theory must also be so general that it will work for any natural language. If the theory can explain facts about English but cannot account for sentence processing in

---

[1]The collaborators are Edith Bavin, Antonella Devescovi, Takehiko Ito, Michèle Kail, Kerry Kilborn, Wolfgang Klein, Janet McDonald, Clive Perdue, Csaba Pléh, Tim Shopen, Jeffrey Sokolov, S. N. Sridhar, and Beverly Wulfeck.

Italian, Hungarian, or Warlpiri, then the theory ought to be rejected out of hand.

The great contribution of this volume is to provide a specific definition of linguistic factors that explain different patterns of sentence processing across languages. This is accomplished by a model in which various types of "cues" compete in acquisition and online processing. Based on the perceptual psychology of Brunwsik and Gibson, the model introduces the construct of *cue validity*—that is, the extent to which a formal feature of a language provides reliable information about form-function mapping. Cue validity is analyzed into three components: (1) *availability*, essentially determined by frequency of occurrence, (2) *reliability*, defined in terms of the degree to which a cue leads to correct interpretation across instances, and (3) *conflict validity*, reflecting the strength of a cue in resolving conflicts with other cues. The Competition Model provides precise definitions of the cues in a particular language, with predictions about how the three components interact to influence sentence processing. For example, the Model explains why articles tend to be missing in Broca's aphasia in English, whereas they are retained better in Italian and even better in German. This is due to the cue validity of articles in the three languages, based on the information that they convey: only definiteness in English; definiteness, gender, and number in Italian; definiteness, gender, number, and case in German.

In this book we find tools for the precise study of components of sentence processing—tests that have become standard in study of the various populations listed above. The methods include comprehension of sentences that relate to pictures (e.g., point to who is "pushing" in a picture described as "The cow the horse pushes") and production of sentences to describe a series of pictures. These production tasks tap syntax, pragmatics, and semantics—what can be said, what must be said, and what it means. For example, if the first picture shows a rabbit and the second a rabbit that is jumping, the first picture calls for some kind of presentational sentence, such as "There's a rabbit," whereas the second picture might allow for a pronominal or zero subject, depending on the language. On the basis of careful norming of preferred strategies of production and comprehension in adult speakers of various language, the authors are able to examine the relative strengths of various cues in language development and breakdown. The findings point to the need to relativize claims about what is specific to the human language capacity in general to the demands of using a particular type of language.

The studies in this volume demonstrate the applicability of Bates's overall approach not only to issues of acquisition, but also adult language processing, breakdown, bilingualism, and second-language acquisition. In addition, we see the beginnings of attempts at computer modeling that became significant in the collaborations of the following decade. In the current volume, Devescovi and d'Amico provide a detailed assessment of the Competition Model, reviewing a large body of continuing research that has been stimulated by the model. And Elman's chapter gives an update on successful attempts to implement the model, reviewing research on experiments, corpus analysis, and simulation. The chapters by Tyler, and by Aydelott and Kutas, bring these issues to the modern arenas of theories of language processing and their neurological bases.

Rethinking Innateness: A Connectionist Perspective on Development (1996)

This book carries on the interdisciplinary and international tradition of Bates's work. It puts together psychology, biology, and computer science to make what may well be the most significant contemporary contribution to the vexed debates about innate components in the development and behavior of higher-order cognition and language. Bates's coauthors in this monumental endeavor are Jeffry Elman, Mark Johnson, Annette Karmiloff-Smith, Domenico Parisi, and Kim Plunkett. Elman and Karmiloff-Smith provide thoughtful updates in the current volume, along with Finlay and Dick, Dronkers, Small, Saygin, and Wilson. *Rethinking innateness* provides scientific and theoretical substance to the major challenges to nativism in Bates's writings of the seventies and eighties.

The central question is: "Where does knowledge come from?" And the answers lie in *epigenesis*—that is, the interaction between genes, bodies, and environments, unfolding over time, and *emergence*—that is, the ways in which structures can arise without being prespecified, given material and temporal constraints. The key word is *time*—time in the evolution of the species, the development of the embryo and child, and the microdevelopmental processes that can be carried out by computers. The earlier keyword, *heterochrony*, is united with *plasiticty*, in the framework of neuroscience.

Emergentism becomes the framework for a new approach, set forth to the scientific world in a volume edited by Brian MacWhinney (1999), *The emergence of language*, with many of the same contributors. In the Preface to that book, MacWhinney offers some of Bates's most compelling examples of emergence. For example, there is nothing in the behavior or genes of individual bees that accounts for the hexagonal shapes of the holes in a honeycomb. Rather, if hundreds of round little bodies are at work burrowing into a compact substance with the molecular structure of honey, the hexagon is the only possible solution—and it is an emergent solution. This emerging approach to cognitive science provides a way out of unresolvable dichotomies and oppositions that we have inherited from formalist and modular theories of mind.

After careful study of *Rethinking innateness,* one can never read about "genetic determinism" in the same way. Nor can one rely on traditional ideas of "learning" and "maturation." And one is taught how to critically understand beautiful graphs of linear and nonlinear change—what to believe and what not to believe about the temporal events that might underlie such graphs. Finally, regardless of one's previous attitudes toward connectionism, the authors show why this approach to the central question must be taken seriously.

Bates and her coauthors end with a caveat about how to use and interpret the much-abused term "innate." They are neither nativists or empiricists, but something much more subtle and much more interesting. They end with a ringing plea for more careful attention to the social questions for uncritical use of scientific terms (p. 391):

> If scientists use words like "instinct" and "innateness" in reference to human abilities, then we have a moral responsibility to be very clear and explicit about what we mean, to avoid our conclusions being interpreted in rigid nativist ways by political institutions. Throughout we have stressed that we are not anti-nativist, but that we deem it essential to specify at precisely what level we are talking when we use terms like "innate." If our careless, underspecified choice of words inadvertently does damage to future generations of children, we cannot turn with innocent outrage to the judge and say "But your Honor, I didn't realize the word was loaded."

The very last sentence of *Rethinking innateness* echoes the excitement we feel in reviewing the scientific career of Elizabeth Bates, and the excitement that we are sure the reader will find in the present collection of papers dedicated to her (p. 396).

> We hope that you, the reader, may feel some part of the excitement which we feel at the new prospects for understanding just what it is that makes us human, and how we get to be that way.

REFERENCES

Bates, E. (1976). *Language and context: The acquisition of pragmatics.* New York: Academic Press.

Bates, E. (1979). *The emergence of symbols: Cognition and communication in infancy.* New York: Academic Press.

Bates, E., & MacWhinney, B. (1979). The functionalist approach to the acquisition of grammar. In E. Ochs & B. Schieffelin (Eds.), *Developmental pragmatics.* New York: Academic Press.

Bates, E., & MacWhinney, B. (1982). A functionalist approach to grammatical development. In E. Wanner & L. Gleitman (Eds.), *Language acquisition: The state of the art.* Cambridge: Cambridge University Press.

Bates, E., & MacWhinney, B. (1987). Competition, variation, and language learning. In B. MacWhinney (Ed.), *Mechanisms of language acquisition*. Hillsdale, NJ: Erlbaum.

Bates, E., & MacWhinney, B. (1989). Functionalism and the competition model. In B. MacWhinney and E. Bates (Eds.), *The crosslinguistic study of sentence processing*. Cambridge: Cambridge University Press.

Bates, E., & MacWhinney, B. (1989). (Eds.), *The crosslinguistic study of sentence processing*. Cambridge: Cambridge University Press.

Bates, E., Bretherton, I., & Snyder, L. (1988). *From first words to grammar: Individual differences and dissociable mechanisms*. Cambridge: Cambridge University Press.

Elman, J. L., Bates, E., Johnson, M., Karmiloff-Smith, A., Parisi, D., & Plunkett, K. (1996). *Rethinking innateness: A connectionist perspective on development*. Cambridge MA: MIT Press.

MacWhinney, B. (1999). (Ed.), *The emergence of language*. Mahwah, NJ: Erlbaum.

Elizabeth Bates's Aphorisms for the Study of Language, Cognition, Development, Biology, and Evolution

In reading through the works of Elizabeth Bates and her coauthors one finds luminous guideposts for the conduct of science and the conceptualization of language in its biological, developmental, and evolutionary frameworks. We have extracted a collection of "Bates's Aphorisms" here. Given the intensely collaborative nature of her work, almost all of these gems have coauthors, but Bates's genius shines through all of them. The kernel for most of these ideas can be found in her early work.

—Dan Slobin and Michael Tomasello

How to Conceptualize and Carry Out Science

"[I]t is better scientific policy to assume that any phenomenon can be shown to belong to a more general family of facts. This approach is particularly wise when we are dealing with biological processes that had to evolve from simpler beginnings." (Bates, Bretherton, & Snyder, 1988, p. 298)

"A good psycholinguistic theory ought to account for many different aspects of natural language use, including comprehension and production of meaningful speech, first language acquisition, second language acquisition, the deterioration of language under pathological conditions, normal speech errors, error monitoring, and judgments of well-formedness. While accounting for this dazzling range of performance phenomena, a good psycholinguistic theory must also be so general that it will work for any natural language." (MacWhinney & Bates, 1989, p. xi)

"[T]he field of child language has reached a new level of precision and sophistication in the way that we code and quantify linguistic data. Single-case studies, qualitative descriptions, and compelling anecdotes will continue to play an important role. But they cannot and will not be forced to bear the full weight of theory building in our field." (Bates & Carnevale, 1993)

"If one sincerely believes in the social–experiential bases of language and change, then there is no reason to fear quantification or precision. Indeed, the increased precision offered by these new models make it impossible to hide from the contributions of social and contextual factors." (Bates & Carnevale, 1993, p. 463)

"Connectionism provides a useful conceptual framework for understanding emergent form and the interaction of constraints at multiple levels. . . (p. 359) Connectionism is not a theory of development as such. Rather, it is a tool for modeling and testing developmental hypotheses (p. 392)" (Elman, Bates, Johnson, Karmiloff-Smith, Parisi, & Plunkett, 1996).

"[I]ndividual differences can provide evidence about the biological substrates of language." (Bates, Bretherton, & Snyder, 1988, p. 275)

How to Think About the Structure of the Mind and Its Evolution

"[T]he form of the solution [to the problem of behavioral universals] is determined by the interaction of *three* sources of structure: genes, environment, and the critical structure of the task. Genes and environment provide material and efficient causal inputs to the solution; the task structure produces the rest of the solution via the operation of logico-mathematical formal causal principles." (Bates, 1979, pp. 17–18)

"Modules are not born, they are made." (Bates, Bretherton, & Snyder, 1988, p. 284)

"[L]ocalization and innateness are not the same thing." (Elman, Bates, Johnson, Karmiloff-Smith, Parisi, & Plunkett, 1996, p. 378)

"[S]tructural relationships between language and nonlinguistic capacities exist at the level of underlying software that permits various behaviors to occur." (p. 14) . . . "[C]ertain behaviors are correlated because the 'software' that is needed to carry out those behaviors is the same. (p. 19)" (Bates, 1979)

"The problem space itself constrains what are likely outcomes." (Elman, Bates, Johnson, Karmiloff-Smith, Parisi, & Plunkett, 1996, p. 353)

"The relationship between mechanisms and behaviors is frequently nonlinear. Dramatic effects can be produced by small changes." (Elman, Bates, Johnson, Karmiloff-Smith, Parisi, & Plunkett, 1996, p. 359)

"Time is a powerful mechanism for developmental change, and dramatic changes in species or individuals can result from small changes in the timing of developmental sequences." (Elman, Bates, Johnson, Karmiloff-Smith, Parisi, & Plunkett, 1996, p. 360)

"Discontinuous outcomes can emerge from continuous change within a single system." (Bates & Carnevale, 1993, p. 461)

"[C]omplex [individual] differences in strategy and style might be the result of rather simple differences in the relative timing of component skills." (Bates, 1979, p. 370)

How to Think About Evolution and the Nature of Language

"[T]he human capacity for language could be both innate and species-specific, and yet involve no mechanisms that evolved specifically and uniquely for language itself. Language could be viewed as a new machine constructed entirely out of old parts." (Bates & MacWhinney, 1989, p. 10)

"Language may have evolved through 'heterochrony,' or changes in the timing and growth curves for old capacities. The emergence of symbols in human children may reflect the resulting interaction of old parts in the creation of a new system." (Bates, 1979, p. 21)

"Language can be viewed as a new machine created out of various cognitive and social components that evolved initially in the service of completely different functions." (Bates, 1979, p. 31)

How to Think About Language Acquisition

"An adequate account of language development will necessarily involve a mixture of function-driven and form-driven learning." (Bates & MacWhinney, 1989, p. 27)

"[E]arly lexical and grammatical development are paced by the same mechanisms." (Bates, Bretherton, & Snyder, 1988, p. 264)

"Both arbitrary and analyzed learning are necessary for rapid and efficient acquisition of language." (Bates, 1979, p. 361)

"Development is a process of emergence." (Elman, Bates, Johnson, Karmiloff-Smith, Parisi, & Plunkett, 1996, p. 359)

"[S]emantics is derived ontogenetically from pragmatics. . . . Insofar as the content of early utterances is built out of the child's early procedures or action schemes, semantics is derived from efforts to do things with words." (Bates, 1976, p. 354)

"Language acquisition is a perceptual-motor problem. The child is trying to extract patterns . . . Once patterns have been isolated, the child will also try to reproduce them . . ." (Bates & MacWhinney, 1989, p. 31)

How to Think About Language Processing

"[T]he language processor can make use of compound cues that cross traditional boundaries (e.g., segmental phonology, suprasegmental phonology, morphology, the lexicon, and positional frames)." (Bates & MacWhinney, 1989, p. 41)

"Mechanisms responsible for rote reproduction of forms can be separated from mechanisms for segmenting and analyzing the internal structure of those forms. Mechanisms responsible for comprehension can be dissociated from the mechanisms responsible for production. However, these partially dissociable mechanisms seem to cut across the traditional linguistic levels of grammar and semantics." (Bates, Bretherton, & Snyder, 1988, p. 8)

How to Think About Linguistics

"[W]e must be careful not to take various formal linguistic models too literally when we apply them to psychological functioning. (p. 346) . . . [T]he description of conventions . . . is a separate enterprise from psychological explanations of how people acquire and use these conventions. (p. 353)" (Bates, 1976)

"Grammars can be viewed as a class of solutions to the problem of mapping nonlinear meanings onto a highly constrained linear medium whose only devices are word order, lexical marking, and suprasegmentals. The universal and culture-specific contents of cognition interact with universal constraints on human information processing, creating a complex multivectorial problem space." (Bates & MacWhinney, 1989, p. 8)

"Language differences are most theoretically interesting when considered against the backdrop of crosslinguistic similarities." (MacWhinney & Bates, 1989, p. xii)

"[I]t is useful to handle *all* lexical items (closed- and open-class, bound and free) within a single lexicon . . ." (Bates & Wulfeck, 1989, p. 351)

"In all languages, there is interaction and competition between the pragmatic system for highlighting important information, and the semantic system for expressing reference, case relations, and other propositional structures." (Bates, 1976, p. 161)

How to Think About Language Breakdown and Atypical Development

"By looking at the way that things come apart, under normal or abnormal conditions, we can see more clearly how they were put together in the first place." (Bates, Bretherton, & Snyder, 1988, p. 299)

"At least some forms of language deficiency may result from a deficit in one or more of the nonlinguistic components that underlie the capacity for symbols." (Bates, 1979, p. 31)

"The best way to characterize the breakdown of morphology is in terms of *accessing* rather than *loss.*" (Bates & Wulfeck, 1989, p. 329)

"[G]rammatical morphology is selectively vulnerable under a wide range of conditions, genetic and environmental. A parsimonious account of all these findings would be that grammatical morphology is a weak link in the processing chain of auditory input, one that is highly likely to be impaired when things go awry. None of these examples points necessarily to specific genes for grammar." (Elman, Bates, Johnson, Karmiloff-Smith, Parisi, & Plunkett, 1996, p. 377)

REFERENCES

Bates, E. (1976). *Language and context: The acquisition of pragmatics.* New York: Academic Press.

Bates, E., Benigni, L., Bretherton, I., Camaioni, L., & Volterra, V. (1979). *The emergence of symbols: Cognition and communication in infancy.* New York: Academic Press.

Bates, E., Bretherton, I., & Snyder, L. (1988). *From first words to grammar: Individual differences and dissociable mechanisms.* Cambridge: Cambridge University Press.

Bates, E., & Carnevale, G. F. (1993). New directions in research on language development. *Developmental Review, 13,* 436–470.

Bates, E., & MacWhinney, B. (1989). Functionalism and the Competition Model. In B. MacWhinney & E. Bates (Eds.), *The crosslinguistic study of sentence processing* (pp. 3–76). Cambridge: Cambridge University Press.

Bates, E., & Wulfeck, B. (1989). Crosslinguistic studies of aphasia. In B. MacWhinney & E. Bates (Eds.), *The crosslinguistic study of sentence processing* (pp. 328–371). Cambridge: Cambridge University Press.

Elman, J. L., Bates, E. A., Johnson, M. H., Karmiloff-Smith, A., Parisi, D., & Plunkett, K. (1996). *Rethinking innateness: A connectionist perspective on development.* Cambridge, MA: MIT Press.

MacWhinney, B., & Bates, E. (Eds.). (1989). *The crosslinguistic study of sentence processing.* Cambridge: Cambridge University Press.

Vita of Elizabeth Bates

Born: July 27, 1947 in Wichita, Kansas
Died: December 13, 2003 in La Jolla, California

Education:

- Ph.D., Human Development, University of Chicago, 1974
- M.A., Human Development, University of Chicago, 1971
- B.A., Psychology, St. Louis University, 1968

Honors and Awards:

- Phi Beta Kappa, Saint Louis University   1968
- Keynote Address, Stanford Child Language Research Forum   1978
- Boyd R. McCandless Distinguished Young Scientist Award, Division 7, Psychological Association   1979
- John Simon Guggenheim Memorial Fellowship   1981
- Fellow-Elect, Center for Advanced Study in the Behavioral Sciences   1983
- M.D. Steer Distinguished Lecture, Purdue University   1991
- Ida & Cecil Green Visiting Professor/Lecturer, Texas Christian University   1991
- Honorary Doctorate, University of Paris V "René Descartes"   1992

- University Lecture, University of Wisconsin, Madison   1992
- Abbey Grunewald Lecture, University of Arizona   1992
- James Mark Baldwin Lecture, University of Alabama,
  Birmingham   1994
- Boyd McCandless Lecture, Emory University, Atlanta, Georgia 1994
- Otto Koerner Lecture, University of British Columbia,
  Vancouver, B.C.   1994
- Master Lecture, Society for Research in Child Development   1995
- Keynote Address, Academy of Aphasia   1997
- Honorary Doctorate, New Bulgarian University, Sofia   1997

Professional Positions:

- Professor of Cognitive Science, University of California,
  San Diego   1988–2003
- Professor of Psychology, University of California,
  San Diego   1983–2002
- Director, UCSD Project in Cognitive & Neural
  Development   1989–2003
- Director, UCSD Center for Research in Language   1995–2003
- Co-Director SDSU/UCSD Joint Doctoral Program
  in Language & Communicative Disorders   1996–2003
- Associate Professor of Psychology, University
  of California, San Diego   1981–1983
- Assistant/Associate Professor of Psychology,
  University of Colorado, Boulder   1974–1981
- Visiting Assistant Professor of Psychology,
  University of California, Berkeley   1976–1977

Publications (as of November 2003):
- **10 books and monographs**
- **172 journal articles**
- **64 chapters and conference proceedings**

Books and Monographs

1. Bates, E. (1976). *Language and context: The acquisition of pragmatics.* New York: Academic Press. [Paperback edition issued 1980].
2. Camaioni, L., Volterra, V., & Bates, E. (1976). *La comunicazione nel primo anno di vita.* Rome: Boringhieri.

3. Bates, E., with L. Benigni, I. Bretherton, L. Camaioni, & V. Volterra. (1979). *The emergence of symbols: Cognition & communication in infancy.* New York: Academic Press.

4. Bates, E., Bretherton, I., & Snyder, L. (1988). *From first words to grammar: Individual differences and dissociable mechanisms.* New York: Cambridge University Press. [Paperback edition issued 1991].

5. MacWhinney, B., & Bates, E. (Eds.). (1989). *The crosslinguistic study of sentence processing.* New York: Cambridge University Press.

6. Bates, E. (Ed.). (1991). Special issue: Cross-linguistic studies of aphasia. *Brain & Language,* 41(2).

7. Fenson, L., Dale, P., Reznick, J. S., Thal, D., Bates, E., Hartung, J., Pethick, S., & Reilly, J. (1993). *The MacArthur Communicative Development Inventories: User's guide & technical manual.* San Diego: Singular Press.

8. Fenson, L., Dale, P., Reznick, J., Bates, E., Thal, D., & Pethick, S. (1994). Variability in early communicative development. *Monographs of the Society for Research in Child Development, Serial No. 242, Vol. 59,* No. 5.

9. Elman, J., Bates, E., Johnson, M., Karmiloff-Smith, A., Parisi, D., & Plunkett, K. (1996). *Rethinking innateness: A connectionist perspective on development.* Cambridge, MA: MIT Press/Bradford Books. [Paperback edition issued 1998; Japanese translation 1998].

10. Tomasello, M., & Bates, E., (Eds.). (2001). *Language development: The essential readings.* Oxford: Basil Blackwell.

Journal Articles

1. Bates, E. (1973). Il paradigma linguistico e la psicologia evolutiva. *Critica Sociologica,* 3, 8–24.

2. Bates, E. (1974). The acquisition of pragmatic competence. *Journal of Child Language, 1(2),* 277–282.

3. Bates, E., Camaioni, L., & Volterra, V. (1975). The acquisition of performatives prior to speech. *Merrill-Palmer Quarterly, 21(3),* 205–226. [Reprinted in E. Ochs & B. Schieffelin, Eds., *Developmental pragmatics.* New York: Academic Press, 1979, 111–128; Reprinted in A. Kasher, Ed., *Pragmatics: Critical concepts.* London: Routledge, 1998, 274–295].

4. Bates, E. (1977). Review of Marcato, Ursini & Politi, "Dialetto e italiano". *Language in Society.*

5. Bates, E., & Silvern, L. (1977). Social adjustment and politeness in preschoolers. *Journal of Communication, 27(2),* 104–111.

6. Cremona, C., & Bates, E. (1977). The development of attitudes toward dialect in Italian children. *Journal of Psycholinguistic Research, 6(3),* 223–232.

7. Bates, E., & Benigni, L. (1978). Rules of address in Italy: A sociological survey. *Language in Society, 4,* 271–288.

8. Kintsch, W., & Bates, E. (1977). Recognition memory for statements from a classroom lecture. *Journal of Experimental Psychology: Human Learning and Memory,*

3:2, 187–197. [Reprinted in J. G. Seamon, Ed., *Human memory: Contemporary readings*. New York: Oxford University Press, 1980].

9. MacWhinney, B., & Bates, E. (1978). Sentential devices for conveying giveness and newness. *Journal of Verbal Learning & Verbal Behavior, 17*, 539–558.

10. Bates, E., Masling, M., & Kintsch, W. (1978). Recognition memory for aspects of dialogue. *Journal of Experimental Psychology: Human Learning and Memory, 4(3)*, 187–197.

11. Bates, E. (1979). In the beginning, before the word: Review of S. Harnad, H. Steklis, & T. Lancaster, "Origins of Language and Speech". In *Contemporary Psychology, 24(3)*, 169–171.

12. Bates, E. (1979). Piaget and Brainerd with Aristotle looking on: Response to Brainerd's critique of Piaget. In *Behavioral and Brain Sciences*.

13. Bates, E., & Rankin, J. (1979). Morphological development in Italian: Connotation and denotation. *Journal of Child Language, 6*, 29–52.

14. Camaioni, L., Volterra, V., & Bates, E. (1979). Dal gesto alla prima parola: lo sviluppo comunicativo e cognitivo tra i 9 e i 13 mesi. *Età evolutiva, 2*, 55–75.

15. Bates, E. (1980). Review of D. McNeill "Conceptual basis of language". *American Scientist.*

16. Bates, E., Carlson-Luden, V., & Bretherton, I. (1980). Perceptual aspects of tool use in infancy. *Infant Behavior and Development, 3*, 127–141.

17. Bates, E., Bretherton, I., Snyder, L., Shore, C., & Volterra, V. (1980). Vocal and gestural symbols at 13 months. *Merrill-Palmer Quarterly, 26:4*, 407–423.

18. Bates, E., Kintsch, W., Fletcher, C., & Giuliani, V. (1980). On the role of pronominalization and ellipsis in texts: Some memory experiments. *Journal of Experimental Psychology: Human Learning and Memory, 6*, 676–691.

19. Snyder, L., Bates, E., & Bretherton, I. (1981). Content and context in early lexical development. *Journal of Child Language, 8*, 565–582.

20. Bretherton, I., Bates, E., McNew, S., Shore, C., Williamson, C., & Beeghly-Smith, M. (1981). Comprehension and production of symbols in infancy: An experimental study. *Developmental Psychology, 17(6)*, 728–737.

21. Bates, E., McNew, S., MacWhinney, B., Devescovi, A., & Smith, S. (1982). Functional constraints on sentence comprehension: A cross-linguistic study. *Cognition, 11*, 245–299.

22. Bretherton, I., McNew, S., Snyder, L., & Bates, E. (1983). Individual differences at 20 months. *Journal of Child Language, 10*, 293–320.

23. Bates, E., Hamby, S., & Zurif, E. (1983). The effects of focal brain damage on pragmatic expression. Special Issue on Brain and Language (Doreen Kimura, Ed.), *Canadian Journal of Psychology, 37(1)*, 59–83.

24. Bates, E. (1984). Bioprograms and the innateness hypothesis: Response to D. Bickerton. *Behavioral and Brain Sciences, 7(2)*, 188–190.

25. Bates, E., & Volterra, V. (1984). On the invention of language: An alternative view. Response to S. Goldin-Meadow & C. Mylander, Gestural communication in deaf children: The effects and noneffects of parental input on early language development. *Monographs of the Society for Research in Child Development, Serial No. 207, Vol. 49, Nos. 3–4.*

26. Bates, E., MacWhinney, B., Caselli, C., Devescovi, A., Natale, F., & Venza, V. (1984). A cross-linguistic study of the development of sentence interpretation strategies. *Child Development, 55*, 341–354.

27. Shore, C., O'Connell, B., & Bates, E. (1984). First sentences in language and symbolic play. *Developmental Psychology, 20(5)*, 872–880.

28. MacWhinney, B., Bates, E., & Kliegl, R. (1984). Cue validity and sentence interpretation in English, Italian and German. *Journal of Verbal Learning and Verbal Behavior, 23*, 127–150.

29. MacWhinney, B., Pléh, C., & Bates, E. (1985) The development of sentence interpretation in Hungarian. *Cognitive Psychology, 17*, 178–209.

30. Bates, E., O'Connell, B., Vaid, J., Sledge, P., & Oakes, L. (1986). Language and hand preference in early development. *Developmental Neuropsychology, 2(1)*, 1–15.

31. Smith, S., & Bates, E. (1987). Accessibility of case and gender contrasts for assignment of agent-object relations in Broca's aphasics and fluent anomics. *Brain and Language, 30*, 8–32.

32. Giuliani, V., Bates, E., O'Connell, B., & Pelliccia, M. (1987). Recognition memory for forms of reference: The effects of text and language type. *Discourse Processes, 10(1)*, 43–62.

33. Bates, E., Friederici, A., & Wulfeck, B. (1987). Comprehension in aphasia: A cross-linguistic study. *Brain and Language, 32*(1), 19–68.

34. Bates, E., Friederici, A., & Wulfeck, B. (1987). Grammatical morphology in aphasia: Evidence from three languages. *Cortex, 23*, 545–574.

35. Bates, E., Friederici, A., Wulfeck, B., & Juarez, L. (1988). On the preservation of word order in aphasia. *Brain and Language, 33*(2), 323–364.

36. Thal, D., & Bates, E. (1988). Language and gesture in late talkers. *Journal of Speech and Hearing Research, 31*, 115–123.

37. Bates, E., Friederici, A., & Wulfeck, B. (1988). Grammatical morphology in aphasia: A reply to Niemi et al. *Cortex, 24*, 583–588.

38. Bates, E. (1989). La psicolinguistica. *Sistemi Intelligenti, 1:3*, 305–325.

39. Bates, E. (1989). Review of F. Kessel (Ed.), "The development of language and language researchers". *American Scientist.*

40. Bates, E., Thal, D., Whitesell, K., Oakes, L., & Fenson, L. (1989). Integrating language and gesture in infancy. *Developmental Psychology, 25*(6), 1004–1019.

41. Bates, E., & Wulfeck, B. (1989), Comparative aphasiology: A cross-linguistic approach to language breakdown. Invited review article with peer commentary. *Aphasiology, 3*(2), 111–142.

42. Dale, P., Bates, E., Reznick, S., & Morisset, C. (1989). The validity of a parent report instrument of child language at 20 months. *Journal of Child Language, 16*, 239–249.

43. Thal, D., & Bates, E. (1989). Language and communication in early childhood. *Pediatric Annals, 18*(5), 299–306.

44. Thal, D., Bates, E., & Bellugi, U. (1989). Language and cognition in two children with Williams' Syndrome. *Journal of Speech and Hearing Research, 32*, 489–500.

45. Volterra, V., & Bates, E. (1989). Selective impairment of Italian grammatical morphology in the congenitally deaf: A case study. *Cognitive Neuropsychology, 6*(3), 273–308.

46. Wulfeck, B., Bates, E., Juarez, L., Opie, M., Friederici, A., MacWhinney, B., & Zurif, E. (1989). The pragmatics of reference in aphasia: Cross-linguistic evidence. *Language and Speech, 32*(4), 315–336.

47. MacWhinney, B., & Bates, E. (1990). Welcome to functionalism: Comment on S. Pinker & P. Bloom "Natural language and natural selection." *Behavioral and Brain Sciences, 13*(4), 727–728.

48. Bates, E., MacDonald, J., MacWhinney, B., & Appelbaum, M. (1991). A maximum likelihood procedure for the analysis of group and individual data in aphasia research. *Brain and Language, 40*(2), 231–265.

49. Bates, E., Appelbaum, M., & Allard, L. (1991). Statistical constraints on the use of single cases in neuropsychological research. *Brain and Language, 40*(3), 295–329.

50. Marchman, V., Bates, E., Burkhardt, A., & Good, A. (1991). Functional constraints on the acquisition of the passive: Toward a model of the competence to perform. *First Language, 11*, 65–92.

51. Marchman, V., Miller, R., & Bates, E. (1991). Babble and first words in infants with focal brain injury. *Applied Psycholinguistics, 12*(1), 1–22.

52. Thal, D., Marchman, V., Stiles, J., Aram, D., Trauner, D., Nass, R., & Bates, E. (1991). Early lexical development in children with focal brain injury. *Brain and Language, 40*(4), 491–527.

53. Bates, E., Wulfeck, B., & MacWhinney, B. (1991). Cross-linguistic studies of aphasia: An overview. Special issue on cross-linguistic studies of aphasia (E. Bates, Ed.). *Brain and Language, 41*(2), 123–148.

54. Bates, E., Chen, S., Tzeng, O., Li, P., & Opie, M. (1991). The noun-verb problem in Chinese aphasia. Special issue on cross-linguistic studies of aphasia (E. Bates, Ed.). *Brain and Language, 41*(2), 203–233.

55. Wulfeck B., Bates, E., & Capasso, R. (1991). A cross-linguistic study of grammaticality judgments in Broca's aphasia. Special issue on cross-linguistic studies of aphasia. *Brain and Language, 41*(2), 311–346.

56. Wulfeck, B., & Bates, E. (1991). Differential sensitivity to errors of agreement and word order in Broca's aphasia. *Journal of Cognitive Neuroscience, 3*(3), 254–272.

57. Bates, E. (1992). Language development. In E. Kandel & L. Squire (Eds.), Special Issue on Cognitive Neuroscience. *Current Opinion in Neurobiology, 2*, 180–185.

58. Liu, H., Bates, E., & Li, P. (1992). Sentence interpretation in bilingual speakers of English and Chinese. *Applied Psycholinguistics, 13*, 451–484.

59. Bates, E., & Carnevale, G. F. (1993). New directions in research on language development. *Developmental Review, 13*, 436–470.

60. Bates, E., Chen, S., Li, P., Opie, M., & Tzeng, O. (1993). Where is the boundary between compounds and phrases in Chinese?: A reply to Zhou et al. *Brain and Language, 45*, 94–107.

61. Jackson-Maldonado, D., Thal, D., Marchman, V., Bates, E., & Gutierrez-Clellen, V. (1993). Early lexical development in Spanish-speaking infants and toddlers. *Journal of Child Language, 20*(3), 523–549.

62. Li, P., Bates, E., & MacWhinney, B. (1993). Processing a language without inflections: A reaction time study of sentence interpretation in Chinese. *Journal of Memory and Language, 32,* 169–192.

63. Bates, E. (1993). Comprehension and production in early language development: Comments on Savage-Rumbaugh, S., Murphy, J., Sevcik, R., Brakke, K., Williams, S., & Rumbaugh, D., Language comprehension in ape and child. *Monographs of the Society for Research in Child Development, Serial No. 233, Vol. 58,* Nos. 3–4, 222–242.

64. Bates, E. (1994). Modularity, domain specificity and the development of language. In D. C. Gajdusek, G. M. McKhann, & C. L. Bolis (Eds.), Evolution and neurology of language. *Discussions in Neuroscience, 10*(1–2), 136–149. [Reprinted in W. Bechtel, P. Mandik, J. Mundale, & R. Stufflebeam (Eds.). *Philosophy and the neurosciences: A reader.* Oxford: Blackwell, 134–151].

65. Bates, E., Devescovi, A., Dronkers, N., Pizzamiglio, L., Wulfeck, B., Hernandez, A., Juarez, L., & Marangolo, P. (1994). Grammatical deficits in patients without agrammatism: Sentence interpretation under stress in English and Italian. *Brain and Language, 47*(3), 400–402.

66. Bates, E., Marchman, V., Thal, D., Fenson, L., Dale, P., Reznick, S., Reilly, J., & Hartung, J. (1994). Developmental and stylistic variation in the composition of early vocabulary. *Journal of Child Language, 21*(1), 85–124. [Reprinted in K. Perera, Ed., Growing points in child language. Cambridge: Cambridge University Press, 1997].

67. Dall'Oglio, A., Bates, E., Volterra, V., Di Capua, M., & Pezzini, G. (1994). Early cognition, communication and language in children with focal brain injury. *Developmental Medicine and Child Neurology, 36,* 1076–1098.

68. Devescovi, A., Pizzamiglio, L., Bates, E., Hernandez, A., & Marangolo, P. (1994). Grammatical deficits in patients without agrammatism: Detection of agreement errors by Italian aphasics and controls. *Brain and Language, 47*(3), 449–452.

69. Hernandez, A., & Bates, E. (1994). Interactive activation in normal and brain-damaged individuals: Can context penetrate the lexical 'module'? In D. Hillert (Ed.), Special edition: Linguistics and Cognitive Neuroscience. *Linguistische Berichte, 6,* 145–167.

70. Hernandez, A., Bates, E., & Avila, L. (1994). On-line sentence interpretation in Spanish-English bilinguals: What does it mean to be "in between"? *Applied Psycholinguistics, 15,* 417–446.

71. Marchman, V., & Bates, E. (1994). Continuity in lexical and morphological development: A test of the critical mass hypothesis. *Journal of Child Language, 21,* 339–366.

72. Bates, E., Devescovi, A., Hernandez, A., & Pizzamiglio, L. (1995). Gender and lexical access in Italian. *Perception & Psychophysics, 57*(6), 847–862.

73. Bates, E., Marchman, V., Harris, C., Wulfeck, B., & Kritchevsky, M. (1995). Production of complex syntax in normal aging and Alzheimer's Disease. *Language & Cognitive Processes, 10*(5), 487–539.

74. Blackwell, A., & Bates, E. (1995). Inducing agrammatic profiles in normals: Evidence for the selective vulnerability of morphology under cognitive resource limitation. *Journal of Cognitive Neuroscience, 7*(2), 228–257.

75. Caselli, M. C., Bates, C., Casadio, P., Fenson, L., Fenson, J., Sanderl, L., & Weir, J. (1995). A cross-linguistic study of early lexical development. *Cognitive Development, 10,* 159–199. [redacted version published in M. Tomasello & E. Bates (Eds.), *Language development: The essential readings.* Oxford: Basil Blackwell, 2001].

76. Bates, E., Devescovi, A., & Hernandez, A., & Pizzamiglio, L. (1996). Gender priming in Italian. *Perception & Psychophysics, 58*(7), 992–1004.

77. Bates, E., & Elman, J. (1996). Learning rediscovered. *Science, 274*(5294), 1849–1850.

78. Bates, L., & Liu, H. (1996). Cued shadowing. In F. Grosjean & U. Frauenfelder (Eds.), A guide to spoken word recognition paradigms. Special issue of *Language & Cognitive Processes, 11*(6), 577–581.

79. Bates, E., Pizzamiglio, L., Devescovi, A., Marangolo, P., Ciurli, P., & Razzano, C. (1996). Gender priming and gender processing in aphasia (Abstract). *Brain and Language, 55*(1), 104–106.

80. Blackwell, A., Bates, E., & Fisher, D. (1996). The time course of grammaticality judgment. *Language & Cognitive Processes, 11*(4), 337–406.

81. Hernandez, A., Bates, E., & Avila, L. X. (1996). Processing across the language boundary: A cross-modal priming study of Spanish-English bilinguals. *Journal of Experimental Psychology: Learning, Memory and Cognition, 22*(4), 846–864.

82. Kempler, D., Van Lancker, D., Marchman, V., & Bates, E. (1996). The effects of childhood vs. adult brain damage on literal and idiomatic language comprehension (Abstract). *Brain and Language, 55*(1), 167–169.

83. Thal, D., Bates, E., Zappia, M. J., & Oroz, M. (1996). Ties between lexical and grammatical development: Evidence from early talkers. *Journal of Child Language, 23*(2), 349–368.

84. Von Berger, E., Wulfeck, B., Bates, E., & Fink, N. (1996). Developmental changes in real-time sentence processing. *First Language, 16,* 192–222.

85. Bates, E. (1997). Origins of language disorders: A comparative approach. In D. Thal & J. Reilly, (Eds.), Special issue on Origins of Communication Disorders, *Developmental Neuropsychology, 13*(3), 275–343.

86. Bates, E. (1997). On language savants and the structure of the mind: A review of Neil Smith and Ianthi-Maria Tsimpli, "The mind of a savant: Language learning and modularity". *International Journal of Bilingualism,* 1(2), 163–186.

87. Bates, E., & Goodman, J. (1997). On the inseparability of grammar and the lexicon: Evidence from acquisition, aphasia and real-time processing. *Language and Cognitive Processes, 12*(5/6), 507–586. [redacted version reprinted in M. Tomasello & E. Bates (Eds.), *Essential readings in language development.* Oxford: Basil Blackwell, 2000].

88. Bates, E., Thal, D., Trauner, D., Fenson, J., Aram, D., Eisele, J., & Nass, R. (1997). From first words to grammar in children with focal brain injury. In D. Thal & J. Reilly, (Eds.), Special issue on Origins of Communication Disorders. *Developmental Neuropsychology, 13*(3), 447–476.

89. Devescovi, A., Bates, E., D'Amico, S., Hernandez, A., Marangolo, P., Pizza-miglio, L., & Razzano, C. (1997). An on-line study of grammaticality judgments in normal and aphasic speakers of Italian. *Aphasiology, 11*(6), 543–579.

90. Elman, J., & Bates, E. (1997). Acquiring language: Response. *Science (Letters), 276*, 1180.

91. Federmeier, K. D., & Bates, E. (1997). Contexts that pack a punch: Lexical class priming of picture naming. *Center for Research in Language Newsletter, 11*(2). La Jolla: University of California, San Diego.

92. Herron, D., & Bates, E. (1997). Sentential and acoustic factors in the recognition of open- and closed-class words. *Journal of Memory and Language*, 217–239.

93. Johnson, M. H., Bates, E., Elman, J. L., Karmiloff-Smith, A., & Plunkett, K. (1997). Constraints on the construction of cognition (peer commentary on Quartz & Sejnowski). *Behavioral and Brain Sciences, 20*(4), 569–570.

94. Liu, H., Bates, E., Powell, T., & Wulfeck, B. (1997). Single-word shadowing and the study of lexical access: A life span study. *Applied Psycholinguistics, 18*(2), 157–180.

95. Plunkett, K., Karmiloff-Smith, A., Bates, E., Elman, J., & Johnson, M. (1997). Connectionism and developmental psychology. *Annual Review of the Journal of Child Psychology and Psychiatry, 38*, 53–80.

96. Singer-Harris, N., Bellugi, U., Bates, E., Rossen, M., & Jones, W. (1997). Emerging language in two genetically based neurodevelopmental disorders. In D. Thal & J. Reilly, (Eds.), Special issue on Origins of Communication Disorders, *Developmental Neuropsychology, 13*(3), 345–370.

97. Thal, D., Bates, E., Goodman, J., & Jahn-Samilo, J. (1997). Continuity of language abilities in late- and early-talking toddlers. In D. Thal & J. Reilly (Eds.), Special issue on Origins of Communication Disorders, *Developmental Neuropsychology, 13*(3), 239–273.

98. Zaroff, L., Wulfeck, B., Bates, E., & Reilly, J. (1997). Morphosyntactic production abilities in anomic aphasia (Abstract). *Brain and Language, 60*, 84–86.

99. Bates, E. (1998). Construction grammar and its implications for child language: Comment on Tomasello. *Journal of Child Language, 25*(2), 462–466.

100. Bates, E. (1998). Recovery and development after trauma. Review of S. Broman & M. E. Michel (Eds.), "Traumatic head injury in children". *Contemporary Psychology, 43*(1), 39–40.

101. Chen, S., & Bates, E. (1998). The dissociation between nouns and verbs in Broca's and Wernicke's aphasia: Findings from Chinese. *Aphasiology, 12*(1), 5–36.

102. Dick, F., Bates, E., Wulfeck, B., & Dronkers, N. (1998). Simulating deficits in the interpretation of complex sentences in normals under adverse processing conditions (Abstract). *Brain and Language, 65*(1), 57–59.

103. Karmiloff-Smith, A., Plunkett, K., Johnson, M., Elman, J., & Bates, E. (1998). What does it mean to claim that something is "innate"? Response to Clark, Harris, Lightfoot and Samuels. *Mind & Language, 13*(4), 588–597.

104. Kohnert, K., Hernandez, A., & Bates, E. (1998). Bilingual performance on the Boston Naming Test: Preliminary norms in Spanish and English. *Brain and Language, 65*, 422–440.

105. Lu, C.-C., Tzeng, O., Bates, E., & Wulfeck, B. (1998). Sensitivity to agrammaticality in Chinese aphasics (Abstract). *Brain and Language, 65*(1), 63–64.

106. Reilly, J., Bates, E., & Marchman, V. (1998). Narrative discourse in children with early focal brain injury. M. Dennis (Ed.), Special issue, Discourse in children with anomalous brain development or acquired brain injury. *Brain and Language, 61*(3), 335–375.

107. Utman, J., & Bates, E. (1998). Effects of acoustic degradation and semantic context on lexical access: Implications for aphasic deficits (Abstract). *Brain and Language, 65*(1), 217–218.

108. Akhutina, T., Kurgansky, A., Polinsky, M., & Bates, E. (1999). Processing of grammatical gender in a three-gender system: Experimental evidence from Russian. *Journal of Psycholinguistic Research, 28*(6), 695–713.

109. Appelbaum, M., Bates, E., Pizzamiglio, L., & Marangolo, P. (1999). Quantifying dissociations in aphasia (Abstract). *Brain and Language, 69*(3), 313–316.

110. Bates, E. (1999). Nativism vs. development: Comments on Baillargeon & Smith. *Developmental Science, 2*(2), 148–149.

111. Bates, E. (1999). Language and the infant brain. *Journal of Communication Disorders, 32*, 195–205.

112. Bates, E., Devescovi, A., & D'Amico, S. (1999). Processing complex sentences: A cross-linguistic study. *Language and Cognitive Processes, 14*(1), 69–123.

113. Bates, E., Reilly, J., Wulfeck, B., Dronkers, N., Opie, M., Miller, L., Fenson, J., Herbst, K., & Kriz, S. (1999). Comparing free speech in children and adults with left- vs. right-hemisphere injury (Abstract). *Brain and Language, 39*(3), 377–379.

114. Bentrovato, S., Devescovi, A, D'Amico, S., & Bates, E. (1999). The effect of grammatical gender and semantic context on lexical access in Italian. *Journal of Psycholinguistic Research, 28*(6), 677–693.

115. Bates, E., Dick, F., & Wulfeck, B. (1999). Not so fast: Domain-general factors can account for domain-specific deficits in grammatical processing. *Behavioral & Brain Sciences, 22*(1), 96–97.

116. Bates, E., & Dronkers, N. (1999). Comparing lesion studies with functional imaging in normal subjects (Abstract). *Brain and Language, 69*(3), 251–252.

117. Caselli, M. C., Casadio, P., & Bates, E. (1999). A comparison of the transition from first words to grammar in English and Italian. *Journal of Child Language, 26*, 69–111. [redacted version published in M. Tomasello & E. Bates (Eds.), *Essential readings in language development.* Oxford: Basil Blackwell, 2000].

118. Dick, F., Bates, E., Ferstl, E., & Friederici, A. (1999). Receptive agrammatism in English- and German-speaking college students processing under stress. *Journal of Cognitive Neuroscience. Supplement, 1*, 48.

119. Dick, F., Wulfeck, B., Bates, E., Naucler, N., & Dronkers, N. (1999). Interpretation of complex syntax by aphasic adults and children with focal lesions or specific language impairment. *Brain and Language, 69*(3), 335–337.

120. Kempler, D., Van Lancker, D., Marchman, V., & Bates, E. (1999). Idiom comprehension in children and adults with unilateral brain damage. *Developmental Neuropsychology, 15*(3), 327–349.

121. Kohnert, K., Bates, E., & Hernandez, A. (1999). Balancing bilinguals: Lexical-semantic production and cognitive processing in children learning Spanish and English. *Journal of Speech, Language, and Hearing Research, 42*, 1400–1413.

122. Plunkett, K., Elman, J. L., & Bates, E. (1999) Understanding the modelling endeavour. *Journal of Child Language, 26*(1), 253–260.

123. Akhutina, T., Kurgansky, A., Kurganskaya, M., Polinsky, M., & Bates, E. (2000). Processing of grammatical gender in Russian-speaking aphasics (Abstract). *Brain and Language, 74*(3), 512–514.

124. Bates, E., Federmeier, K., Herron, D., Iyer, G., Jacobsen, T., Pechmann, T., D'Amico, S., Devescovi, A., Wicha, N., Orozco-Figueroa, A., Kohnert, K., Gutierrez, G., Lu, C.-C., Hung, D., Hsu, J., Tzeng, O., Andonova, E., Gerdjikova, G., Mehotcheva, T., Székely, A., & Pléh, C. (2000). Introducing the CRL International Picture-Naming Project (CRL-IPNP). *Center for Research in Language Newsletter, 12*(1). La Jolla: University of California, San Diego.

125. Bates, E., & Dick, F. (2000). Beyond phrenology: Brain and language in the next millennium. *Brain and Language, 71*(1), 18–21.

126. Dick, F., & Bates, E. (2000). Grodzinsky's Latest Stand—or, just how specific are "lesion-specific" deficits? *Behavioral and Brain Sciences, 23*(1), 29.

127. Fenson, L., Bates, E., Dale, P., Goodman, J., Reznick, J. S., & Thal, D. (2000). Measuring variability in early child language: Don't shoot the messenger. Comment on Feldman et al. *Child Development, 71*(2), 323–328.

128. Hernandez, A. E., Sierra, I., & Bates, E. (2000). Sentence interpretation in bilingual and monolingual Spanish speakers: Grammatical processing in a monolingual mode. *Spanish Applied Linguistics, 4*:2, 179–213.

129. Lu, C.-C., Bates, E., Li, P., Tzeng, O., Hung, D., Tsai, C.-H., Lee, S.-E., & Chung, Y.-M. (2000). Judgments of grammaticality in aphasia: The special case of Chinese. *Aphasiology, 14*(10), 1021–1054.

130. Roe, K., Jahn-Samilo, J., Juarez, L., Mickel, N., Royer, I., & Bates, E. (2000). Contextual effects on word production: A life-span study. *Memory & Cognition, 28*, 756–765.

131. Székely, A., & Bates, E. (2000). Objective visual complexity as a variable in studies of picture naming. *Center for Research in Language Newsletter, 12*(2). La Jolla: University of California, San Diego.

132. Vicari, S., Albertoni, A., Chilosi, A., Cipriani, P., Cioni, G., & Bates, E. (2000). Plasticity and reorganization during early language learning in children with congenital brain injury. *Cortex, 36*, 31–46.

133. Wicha, N., Bates, E., Moreno, E., & Kutas, M. (2000). Grammatical gender modulates semantic integration of a picture in a Spanish sentence. *Journal of Cognitive Neuroscience, Supplement.*

134. Akhutina, T., Kurgansky, A., Kurganskaya, M., Polinsky, M., Polonskaya, N., Larina, O., Bates, E., & Appelbaum, M. (2001). Gender priming in normal and aphasic speakers of Russian. *Cortex, 37*:3, 295–326.

135. Bates, E. (2001). Brain evolution and development: Passing through the eye of the needle. Commentary on M. Kingsbury & B. Finlay, 'The cortex in multidimensional space'. *Developmental Science, 4*:2, 143–144.

136. Bates, E. (2001). Tailoring the emperor's new clothes: Commentary on D. Van Lancker's "Is your syntactic component really necessary?" *Aphasiology, 15*(4), 391–395.

137. Bates, E., Burani, C., D'Amico, S., & Barca, L. (2001). Word reading and picture naming in Italian. *Memory & Cognition, 29*(7), 986–999.

138. Bates, E., Devescovi, A., & Wulfeck, B. (2001). Psycholinguistics: A cross-language perspective. *Annual Review of Psychology, 52,* 369–398.

139. Bates, E., F., Moineau, S., Miller, L., Ludy, C., & Dronkers, N. (2001). Processing the component parts of active and passive sentences: Why are passives hard? *Brain and Language, 79(1),* 115–116.

140. Bates, E., Marangolo, P., Pizzamiglio, L., & Dick, F. (2001). Linguistic and non-linguistic priming in aphasia. *Brain and* Language, *76*(1), 62–69.

141. Bates, E., Tager-Flusberg, H., Vicari, S., & Volterra, V. (2001). Brief Correspondence: Debate over language's link with intelligence. *Nature, 413,* 565–566.

142. D'Amico, S., Devescovi, A., & Bates, E. (2001). Picture naming and lexical access in Italian-speaking children and adults. *Journal of Cognition and Development, 2(1),* 71–105.

143. Dick, F., Bates, E., Wulfeck, B., Utman, J., Dronkers, N., & Gernsbacher, M. (2001). Language deficits, localization and grammar: Evidence for a distributive model of language breakdown in aphasics and normals. *Psychological Review, 108*(4), 759–788.

144. Dick, F., Saccuman, C., Wulfeck, B., Mueller, R.-A., Bates, E., & Sereno, M. (2001). Language production and comprehension in fMRI: Consistency and variability over individuals and group averages. *Journal of Cognitive Science, Supplement,* p. 55.

145. Hernandez, A. E., Fennema-Notestine, C., Udell, C., & Bates, E. (2001). Lexical and sentential priming in competition: Implications for two-stage theories of lexical access. *Applied Psycholinguistics, 22*(2), 191–215.

146. Iyer, G., Saccuman, C., Bates, E., & Wulfeck, B. (2001). A study of age-of-acquisition (AoA) ratings in adults. *Center for Research in Language Newsletter 12(2).*

147. Saygin, A., Dick. F., & Bates, E. (2001). Linguistic and non-linguistic auditory processing in aphasia. *Brain and Language, 79(1),* 143–145.

148. Wicha, N., Bates, E., Moreno, E., & Kutas, M. (2001). Grammatical gender modulates semantic integration of a picture in a Spanish sentence context. *Journal of Cognitive Science, Supplement,* p. 14.

149. Arévalo, A., Wulfeck, B., & Bates, E. (2002). Teasing apart actions and objects: A picture-naming study. *Center for Research in Language Newsletter. 14*(2). La Jolla, University of California, San Diego.

150. Bates, E. (2002). Specific language impairment: Why it is NOT specific. *Developmental Medicine and Child Neurology, 44,* 4. (Supplement No. 92).

151. Bates, E., & Dick, F. (2002). Language, gesture and the developing brain. In B. J. Casey & Y. Munakata (Eds)., Special issue: Converging method approach to the study of developmental science. *Developmental Psychobiology, 40*(3), 293–310.

152. Bates, E., Reilly, J., Wulfeck, B., Dronkers, N., Opie, M., Fenson, J., Kriz, S., Jeffries, R., Miller, L., & Herbst, K. (2002). Differential effects of unilateral lesions on language production in children and adults. *Brain and Language, 79*(2), 223–265.

153. Harris, C., & Bates, E. (2002). Clausal backgrounding and pronominal reference: A functionalist approach to C-command. *Language and Cognitive Processes,* 17, 237–269.

154. Kohnert, K., & Bates, E. (2002). Balancing bilinguals II: Lexical comprehension and cognitive processing in children learning Spanish and English. *Journal of Speech, Language and Hearing Research, 45*(2), 347–359.

155. Lu, C.-C., Bates, E., Hung, D., Tzeng, O., Hsu, J., Tsai, C.-H., & Roe, K. (2002). Syntactic priming of nouns and verbs in Chinese. *Language and Speech, 44*(4), 437–471.

156. Saccuman, C., Dick, F., Bates, E., Mueller, R.-A., Bussiere, J., Krupa-Kwiatkowski, M., & Wulfeck, B. (2002). Lexical access and sentence processing: A developmental fMRI study of language processing (Abstract). *Journal of the Cognitive Neuroscience Society, Supplement.* p. 47.

157. Stiles, J, Bates, E., Thal, D., Trauner, D., & Reilly, J. (2002). Linguistic and spatial cognitive development in children with pre- and perinatal focal brain injury: A ten-year overview of the San Diego longitudinal project. In M. H. Johnson, Y. Munakata, & R. O. Gilmore (Eds.), *Brain development and cognition: A reader.* London: Blackwell; 2nd ed., pp. 272–291.

158. Dick, F., Bates, E., & Ferstl, E. C. (2003). Spectral and temporal degradation of speech as a simulation of morphosyntactic deficits in English and German. *Brain and Language, 85*(3), 535–542.

159. Saygin, A., Dick, F., Wilson, S., Dronkers, N., & Bates, E. (2003). Neural resources for processing language and environmental sounds: Evidence from aphasia. *Brain, 126*(4), 928–945.

160. Aydelott, J., & Bates, E. (in press). Effects of acoustic distortion and semantic context on lexical access. *Language and Cognitive Processes.*

161. Bates, E. (in press). Explaining and interpreting deficits in language development across clinical groups: Where do we go from here? In B. Wulfeck & J. Reilly, J., (Eds.), Plasticity and development: Language in atypical children. Special issue, *Brain and Language.*

162. Bates, E., Appelbaum, M., Salcedo, J., Saygin, A., & Pizzamiglio, L. (in press). Quantifying dissociations in neuropsychological research. *Journal of Clinical and Experimental Neuropsychology.*

163. Bates, E., D'Amico, S., Jacobsen, T., Szekely, A., Andonova, E., Devescovi, A., Herron, D., Lu, C.-C., Pechmann, T., Pleh, C., Wicha, N., Federmeier, K., Gerdjikova, I., Gutierrez, G., Hung, D., Hsu, J., Iyer, G., Kohnert, K., Mehotcheva, T., Orozco-Figueroa, A., Tzeng, A., & Tzeng, O. (in press). Timed picture naming in seven languages. *Psychonomic Bulletin & Review.*

164. Bates, E., Wilson, S. M., Saygin, A. P., Dick, F., Sereno, M., Knight, R. T., & Dronkers, N. F. (in press). Assessing brain-behavior relationships using voxel-based lesion-symptom mapping. *Nature Neuroscience.*

165. Bentrovato, S., Devescovi, A., D'Amico, S., Wicha, N., & Bates, E. (in press). Effects of grammatical gender and semantic context on word reading. *Journal of Psycholinguistic Research*.

166. Dick, F., Saygin, A. P., Moineau, S., Aydelott, J., & Bates, E. (in press). Language in an embodied brain: The role of animal models. *Cortex*.

167. Reilly, J., Weckerly, J., & Bates, E. (in press). La neuroplasticité et le développement: La morphologie et la syntaxe chez les enfants lésés [Plasticity and development: Morphology and syntax in children with lesions]. In J. Bernicot & J. Reilly (Eds.), Numéro Special: Le développement du langage chez les enfants atypiques [Special issue: Language development in atypical children]. *Enfance*.

168. Rubio, M. A., Basho, S., Haist, F., Wulfeck, B., Reilly, J. S., Buracas, G. T., Buxton, R. B., Bates, E., & Mller, R.-A. (in press). Hemodynamic effects of overt speech and paced production in semantic fluency tasks. *Neuroimage* (abstract).

169. Szekely, A., D'Amico, S., Devescovi, A., Federmeier, K., Herron, D., Iyer, G., Jacobsen, T., & Bates, E. (in press). Timed picture naming: Extended norms and validation against previous studies. *Behavior Research Methods, Instruments, & Computers*.

170. Thelen, E., & Bates, E. (in press). Connectionism and dynamic systems: Are they really different? Introduction to J. Spencer & E. Thelen (Eds.) Connectionism and dynamic systems. Special Section, *Developmental Science*.

171. Wicha, N. Y. Y., Bates, E., Moreno, E. M., & Kutas, M. (in press). Potatoes not Popes: Human brain potentials to gender expectation and agreement in Spanish spoken sentences. *Neuroscience Letters*.

172. Wulfeck, B., Bates, E., Krupa-Kwiatkowski, M, & Saltzman, D. (in press). On-line grammaticality sensitivity in children with early focal brain injury and specific language impairment. In B. Wulfeck & J. Reilly, J., (Eds.), Plasticity and development: Language in atypical children. Special issue, *Brain and Language*.

Chapters and Conference Proceedings

1. Bates, E. (1974). The acquisition of conditional verbs by Italian children. *Proceedings from the 10th Regional Meetings of the Chicago Linguistic Society*. Chicago: University of Chicago, 27–36.

2. Bates, E. (1975). Peer relations and the acquisition of language. In M. Lewis & L. Rosenblum (Eds.), *Friendship and peer relations: The origins of behavior*. New York: John Wiley & Sons, 259–292.

3. Bates, E. (1976). Pragmatics and sociolinguistics in child language. In D. Morehead & A. Morehead (Eds.), *Normal and deficient child language*. Baltimore: University Park Press, 247–307.

4. Bates, E., Benigni, L., Bretherton, I., Camaioni, L., & Volterra, V. (1977). From gesture to the first word: On the nature of cognitive and social prerequisites. In M. Lewis & L. Rosenblum (Eds.), *Interaction, conversation and the development of language*. New York: John Wiley & Sons, 247–307.

5. Benigni, L., & Bates, E. (1977). Interazione sociale e linguaggio: Analisi pragmatica dei pronomi allocutivi italiani. In R. Simone & G. Ruggiero (Eds.), *Atti del' VIII Congresso Internazionale di Studi, Societa di Linguistica Italiana.* Rome: Bulzoni, 141–165.

6. Bates, E. (1978). Functionalism and the biology of language. *Papers & Reports in Child Language.* Stanford University, Department of Linguistics.

7. Bates, E., & MacWhinney, B. (1979). A functionalist approach to the acquisition of grammar. In E. Ochs & B. Schieffelin (Eds.), *Developmental pragmatics.* New York: Academic Press, 167–209. (Reprinted in R. Dirven & V. Fried (Eds.), *Functionalism in linguistics.* Amsterdam: John Benjamins, 1987.)

8. Bates, E. (1979). On the emergence of symbols: Ontogeny and phylogeny. In A. Collins (Ed.), *Children's language and communication: The Minnesota Symposium on Child Psychology, Vol. 12.* Hillsdale, NJ: Erlbaum Associates, 121–157.

9. Bretherton, I., & Bates, E. (1979). The emergence of intentional language and action: Similarities and differences. *Papers & Reports in Child Language.* Stanford University, Department of Linguistics.

10. Bates, E., Kintsch, W., Fletcher, C., & Giuliani, V. (1980). Recognition memory for surface forms in dialogue: Explicit vs. anaphoric reference. *Proceedings of the 16th Regional Meeting of the Chicago Linguistic Society: Parasession on Pronouns and Anaphora.* Chicago: University of Chicago, Chicago Linguistic Society.

11. Bates, E., Bretherton, I., Shore, C., & McNew, S. (1983). Names, gestures, and objects: Symbolization in infancy and aphasia. In K. Nelson (Eds.), *Children's language: Volume IV.* Hillsdale, NJ: Erlbaum, 59–125.

12. Bates, E., Bretherton, I., Beeghly-Smith, M., & McNew, S. (1982). Social factors in language acquisition: A reassessment. In H. Reese & L. Lipsett (Eds.), *Advances in child development & behavior: Volume 16.* New York: Academic Press, 8–68.

13. Bates, E., & MacWhinney, B. (1982). Second language learning from a functionalist perspective: Pragmatic, semantic, and perceptual strategies. In H. Winitz (Ed.), *Foreign and native language acquisition: Annals of the New York Academy of Sciences.* New York: New York Academy of Sciences, 190–214.

14. Bates, E., & MacWhinney, B. (1982). Functionalist approaches to grammar. In E. Wanner & L. Gleitman (Eds.), *Child language: The state of the art.* New York: Cambridge University Press, 173–218.

15. Bates, E., MacWhinney, B., & Smith, S. (1983). Pragmatics and syntax in psycholinguistic research. In H. Wode & S. Felix (Eds.), *Language at the cross-roads: Interdisciplinary perspectives on language acquisition research.* Tuebingen, West Germany: Gunter Narr Publishing Company, 11–31.

16. Bretherton, I., & Bates, E. (1984). The development of representation from 10 to 28 months: Differential stability of language and symbolic play. In R. N. Emde & R. H. Harmon (Eds.), *Continuities and discontinuities in development.* New York: Plenum, 229–259.

17. Bretherton, I., O'Connell, B., Shore, C., & Bates, E. (1984). The effect of contextual variation on symbolic play: Development from 20 to 28 months. In I. Bretherton (Ed.), *Symbolic play: Representation of social understanding.* New York: Academic Press, 271–297.

18. Bates, E., Bellugi, U., & Levelt, W. J. M. (1985). Cross-linguistic studies of grammatical processing in aphasia. *Conference report to the Sloan Foundation and the Maison des Sciences de l'Homme.* University of California, San Diego: March.

19. Wulfeck, B., Juarez, L., Bates, E., & Kilborn, K. (1986). Sentence interpretation strategies in healthy and aphasic bilingual adults. In J. Vaid (Ed.), *Language processing in bilinguals: Psycholinguistic and neurological perspectives.* Hillsdale, NJ: Erlbaum, 199–220.

20. Bates, E., & MacWhinney, B. (1987). Competition, variation and language learning. In B. MacWhinney (Ed.), *Mechanisms of language acquisition.* Hillsdale, NJ: Erlbaum, 157–194.

21. Bates, E., & Marchman, V. (1987). What is and is not universal in language acquisition. In F. Plum (Ed.), *Language, communication and the brain.* New York: Raven Press, 19–38.

22. Bates, E., O'Connell, B., & Shore, C. (1987). Language and communication in infancy. In J. Osofsky (Ed.), *Handbook of infant development.* New York: Wiley, 149–203.

23. Bates, E., & Snyder, L. (1987). The cognitive hypothesis in language development. In I. Uzgiris & J. McV. Hunt (Eds.), *Research with scales of psychological development in infancy.* Champaign: University of Illinois Press, 168–206.

24. Bates, E., & MacWhinney, B. (1988). What is functionalism? *Papers & Reports in Child Language Development, Vol. 27.* Department of Linguistics, Stanford University.

25. Bates, E., & Devescovi, A. (1989). A cross-linguistic approach to sentence production. In B. MacWhinney & E. Bates (Eds.), *The crosslinguistic study of sentence processing.* New York: Cambridge University Press, 225–256.

26. Bates, E., & MacWhinney, B. (1989). Cross-linguistic research in language acquisition and language processing. *Proceedings of the World Conference on Basque Language and Culture.* San Sebastian: Basque Regional Government.

27. Bates, E., & MacWhinney, B. (1989). Functionalism and the Competition Model. In B. MacWhinney & E. Bates (Eds.), *The crosslinguistic study of sentence processing.* New York: Cambridge University Press, 3–76.

28. Bates, E., & Wulfeck, B. (1989). Cross-linguistic studies of aphasia. In B. MacWhinney & E. Bates (Eds.), *The crosslinguistic study of sentence processing.* New York: Cambridge University Press, 328–374.

29. Bates, E., & Thal, D. (1990). Associations and dissociations in language development. In J. Miller (Ed.), *Research on child language disorders: A decade of progress.* Austin, Texas: Pro-Ed, 147–168.

30. Chen, S., Tzeng, O., & Bates, E. (1990). Sentence interpretation in Chinese aphasia. In H. Burmeister & P. Rounds (Eds.), Variability in second language acquisition. *Proceedings of the Tenth Meeting of the Second Language Research Forum, Vol. I.* Eugene, Oregon: Department of Linguistics, University of Oregon.

31. Shore, C., Bates, E., Bretherton, I., Beeghly, M., & O'Connell, B. (1990). Vocal and gestural symbols: Similarities and differences from 13 to 28 months. In V. Volterra & C. J. Erting (Eds.), *From gesture to language in hearing and deaf children.* Amsterdam: Springer-Verlag, 79–92.

32. Thal, D., & Bates, E. (1990). Continuity and variation in early language development. In J. Fagen & J. Colombo (Eds.), *Individual differences in infancy: Reliability, stability, prediction*. Hillsdale, NJ: Erlbaum, 359–386.

33. Bates, E. (1990). Language about me and you: Pronominal reference and the emerging concept of self. In D. Cicchetti & M. Beeghly (Eds.), *The self in transition*. Chicago: University of Chicago Press, 165–182.

34. Bates, E., Thal, D., & MacWhinney, B. (1991). A functionalist approach to language and its implications for assessment and intervention. In T. Gallagher (Ed.), *Pragmatics of language: clinical practice issues*. San Diego: Singular Publishing Group, 133–162.

35. Bates, E., Thal, D., & Marchman, V. (1991). Symbols and syntax: A Darwinian approach to language development. In N. Krasnegor, D. Rumbaugh, R. Schiefelbush & M. Studdert-Kennedy (Eds.), *Biological and behavioral determinants of language development*. Hillsdale, NJ: Erlbaum, 29–65.

36. Bates, E. (1992). Sviluppo normale e anormale del linguaggio. In A. Benton, H. Levin, G. Moretti, & D. Riva, (Eds.), *Neuropsicologia dell'età evolutiva* [Developmental Neuro-psychology] (pp. 112–127). Milan: Franco Angeli.

37. Dixon, S., Feldman, H., & Bates, E. (1992). Two years: Learning the rules—language and cognition. In S. Dixon & M. Stein, *Encounters with children: Pediatric behavior and development, 2nd edition*. St. Louis, Missouri: Mosby Year Book Medical Publishers, 247–264.

38. Bates, E., Thal, D., & Janowsky, J. (1992). Early language development and its neural correlates. In S. Segalowitz & I. Rapin (Eds.), *Handbook of neuropsychology: Child neuropsychology (Vol. 7)*. Holland: Elsevier, 69–110.

39. Li, P., Bates, E., Liu, H., & MacWhinney, B. (1992). Cues as functional constraints on sentence processing in Chinese. In H. C. Chen & O. Tzeng (Eds.), *Language processing in Chinese*. Advances in Psychology Series. North Holland: Elsevier Science Publishers, 207–234.

40. Bates, E., & Elman, J. (1993). Connectionism and the study of change. In M. Johnson (Ed.), *Brain development and cognition: A reader*. Oxford: Blackwell Publishers, 623–642.

41. Bates, E., & Appelbaum, M. (1994). Methods of studying small samples. In S. Broman & J. Grafman (Eds.), *Atypical cognitive deficits in developmental disorders: Implications for brain function*. Hillsdale, NJ: Erlbaum, 245–280.

42. Bates, E., Elman, J., & Li, P. (1994). Language in, on and about time. In M. Haith, J. Benson, R. Roberts, & B. Pennington (Eds.), *The development of future-oriented processes*. Chicago: The University of Chicago Press, 293–321.

43. Bates, E. (1995). Conclusioni [Epilogue]. In M. C. Caselli & P. Casadio, *Il primo vocabolario del bambino: Guida all'uso del questionario MacArthur per la valutazione della comunicazione e del linguaggio nei primi anni di vita*. Milan: FrancoAngeli, 94–100.

44. Bates, E., Dale, P., & Thal, D. (1995). Individual differences and their implications for theories of language development. In P. Fletcher & B. MacWhinney (Eds.), *Handbook of child language*. Oxford: Basil Blackwell, 96–151.

45. Volterra, V., & Bates, E. (1995). L'acquisizione del linguaggio in condizioni normali e patologiche. In G. Sabbadini (Ed.), *Manuale di neuropsicologia dell'età evolutiva*. Bologna: Zanichelli, 183–202.

46. Bates, E., Wulfeck, B., Hernandez, A., & Andonova, E. (1996). The Competition Model: Implications for language processing, language development and language breakdown. In B. Kokinov (Ed.), *Perspectives on Cognitive Science, Volume 2.* Sofia: New Bulgarian University, 7–72.

47. Tzeng, O. J. L., Hung, D. L., & Bates, E. (1996). Cross-linguistic studies of aphasia: A Chinese perspective. In M. Bond (Ed.), *Handbook of Chinese psychology.* Oxford: Oxford University Press.

48. Bates, E. (1998). Presentazione [Prologue]. In C. Laicardi (Ed.), *Genitori competenti: scale di valutazione comportamentale (SVC) per genitori di bambini da due a sei mesi.* [Competent parents: Scales for the evaluation of behavioral development for parents of infants between two and six months]. Rome: Il Pensiero Scientifico Editore, XIII–XV.

49. Bates, E., Camaioni, L., & Volterra, V. (1998). The acquisition of performatives prior to speech. In A. Kasher (Ed.), *Pragmatics: Critical concepts.* London; New York: Routledge, Vol. 6, 274–295. (Originally printed in 1975, Merrill-Palmer Quarterly).

50. Devescovi, A., D'Amico, S., Smith, S., Mimica, I., & Bates, E. (1998). The development of sentence comprehension in Italian and Serbo-Croatian: Local versus distributed cues. In B. D. Joseph & C. Pollard (Series Eds.) & D. Hillert (Vol. Ed.), *Syntax & semantics: Vol. 31. Sentence processing: A cross-linguistic perspective.* San Diego, CA: Academic Press, 345–377.

51. Dick, F., & Bates, E. (1998). A continuum of language compression: Agrammatics, college students, and everyone in between. *Proceedings of the XIIth Meeting of the Cognitive Science Society.*

52. Stiles, J., Bates, E., Thal, D., Trauner, D., & Reilly, J. (1998). Linguistic, cognitive and affective development in children with pre- and perinatal focal brain injury: A ten-year overview from the San Diego longitudinal project. In C. Rovee-Collier, L. Lipsitt, & H. Hayne (Eds.), *Advances in Infancy Research.* Norwood, NJ: Ablex, 131–163.

53. Bates, E., Elman, J., Johnson, M., Karmiloff-Smith, A., Parisi, D., & Plunkett, K. Innateness and emergentism. (1998). In W. Bechtel & G. Graham (Eds.), *A companion to cognitive science.* Malden, MA & Oxford: Blackwell Publishers, 590–601.

54. Bates, E. (1999). Plasticity, localization and language development. In S. H. Broman & J. M. Fletcher (Eds.), *The changing nervous system: Neurobehavioral consequences of early brain disorders.* New York: Oxford University Press, 214–253.

55. Bates, E. (1999). On the nature and nurture of language. In R. Levi-Montalcini, D. Baltimore, R. Dulbecco, & F. Jacob (Series Eds.) & E. Bizzi, P. Calissano, & V. Volterra (Vol. Eds.), *Frontiere della biologia* [Frontiers of biology]. The brain of homo sapiens Rome: Giovanni Trecanni.

56. Bates, E., & Goodman, J. (1999). On the emergence of grammar from the lexicon. In B. MacWhinney (Ed.), *The emergence of language.* Mahwah, NJ: Lawrence Erlbaum, 29–79.

57. Bates, E., Vicari, S., & Trauner, D. (1999). Neural mediation of language development: Perspectives from lesion studies of infants and children. In H. Tager-Flusberg (Ed.), *Neurodevelopmental disorders.* Cambridge, MA: MIT Press, 533–581.

58. Hernandez, A. E., & Bates, E. (1999). Bilingualism and the brain. In *MIT Encyclopedia of Cognitive Sciences*. Cambridge, MA: MIT Press, 80–81.

59. Iyer, G., Saccuman, C., Bates, E., & Wulfeck, B. (2000). A study of Age-of-Acquisition ratings in Adults (Abstract). *Proceedings of the 22nd Annual Conference of the Cognitive Science Society*. New Jersey: Lawrence Erlbaum Associates, 1033.

60. Bates, E., & Elman, J. L. (2000). The ontogeny and phylogeny of language: A neural network perspective. In S. Parker, J. Langer, & M. McKinney (Eds.), *Biology, brains, and behavior: The evolution of human development*. Santa Fe: School of American Research Press, 89–130.

61. Devescovi, A., & Bates, E. (2000). Psicolinguistica. [Psycholinguistics]. In N. Dazzi & G. Vetrone (Eds.), *Psicologia: una introduzione alle scienze umane* [Psychology: An introduction to the human sciences]. Rome: Carocci, 239–276.

62. Bates, E., & Roe, K. (2001). Language development in children with unilateral brain injury. In C. A. Nelson & M. Luciana (Eds.), *Handbook of developmental cognitive neuroscience*. Cambridge, MA: MIT Press, 281–307.

63. Bates, E., & Elman, J. (2002). Connectionism and the study of change. In M. Johnson (Ed.), *Brain development and cognition: A reader* (2nd ed). Oxford: Blackwell Publishers. [revised/updated/extended version of Bates, E., & Elman, J. Connectionism and the study of change. In M. Johnson (Ed.), *Brain development and cognition: A reader*. Oxford: Blackwell Publishers, 1993, 623–642.]

64. Bates, E., Thal, D., Finlay, B. L., & Clancy, B. (2003). Early language development and its neural correlates. In F. Boller & J. Grafman (Series Eds.) & S. J. Segalowitz & I. Rapin (Vol. Eds.), *Handbook of neuropsychology, Vol. 8, Part II, Child neuropsychology*, (2nd ed., pp. 525–592). Amsterdam: Elsevier Science B.V. [extensively revised/updated version of Bates, E., Thal, D., & Janowsky, J. Early language development and its neural correlates. In S. J. Segalowitz & I. Rapin (Eds.), *Handbook of neuropsychology: Child neuropsychology* (Vol. 7). Holland: Elsevier, 1992, 69–110.]

Part I

GESTURES AND WORD LEARNING

Chapter 1

Gesture and the Emergence and Development of Language

Virginia Volterra
Maria Cristina Caselli
Olga Capirci
Elena Pizzuto
Institute of Cognitive Sciences and Technologies
Consiglio Nazionale delle Ricerche (CNR), Rome

> *Nature is a miser. She clothes her children in hand-me-downs, builds new machinery in makeshift fashion from sundry old parts . . .*
>
> (Bates, 1979, p. 1)

PREFACE (BY VIRGINIA VOLTERRA)

During the autumn of 2002, just a few weeks before we would discover about her disease, Liz and I were walking through Rome, talking about work and a dream we had. We wanted to write something together again, something about gesture—a topic in which we had been interested since we started our lifelong collaboration and profound friendship, about thirty years ago. We were aware that many of our old ideas about the role of gesture in children's linguistic development were suddenly becoming extremely "modern" and we were planning to articulate our current perspective (old and new at the same time) by doing a critical review of recent work carried on in different laboratories and countries.

As we had done many times in the past, we started to write the manuscript "a due mani" (two-handed) but despite the attempts we made during the first half of this awful 2003, we did not have enough energy to complete that work.

The present chapter is meant to be a modest, partial attempt to realize that dream: it has been written "a quattro mani" (four-handed) by four people of the "Nomentana Lab" who share a common debt: a debt of immense

3

gratitude to Liz who has forever marked their life with her unique, intense depth and generosity, as a scientist and as a human being.

INTRODUCTION

We would like to frame our observations within the context of current discussions of the origins of language, a topic that has been debated, from different perspectives, since antiquity. Early accounts of language origins often contained speculations about the relationship between language and gesture, including the idea that our hominid ancestors communicated through hand signs, which served as the "missing link" in language evolution. Adam Kendon (2002) recently provided a very elegant review of theories about a gestural origin of language showing the relationship between these theories and a deep interest in deaf people and their signed communication. For example the eighteenth-century Neapolitan philosopher, Giambattista Vico, in *La Scienza Nuova* (1744/1953) formulated his theory on the origin of language according to which in the beginning, humans were mute and communicated by gesture, not by speech. Similar ideas on the first forms of language being rooted in action or gesture were debated at about the same time in Paris by such thinkers as Condillac and Diderot. For Condillac, language began in the reciprocation of overt actions, making its first form a language of action. This led Condillac to write about the language of gesture, both as this was practiced in the pantomimes of antiquity and as it might be observed among deaf people (Kendon, 2002: 37).

In the nineteenth century comparative linguists like Bopp, Schleicher, Humboldt, and Muller, speculating on a universal language from which all modern languages were supposed to originate, formulated various hypotheses on the use of onomatopoeia and of so-called "acoustic gestures," which may have originally accompanied expressive gestures but then became more sophisticated, and were progressively detached from gestures (Leroy, 1969).

The issue was even too much debated and in 1866 the Société de Linguistique banned papers on language origins, stating that: "The Society will accept no communication concerning either the origin of language or the creation of a universal language." The London Philological Society did the same in 1872. The ban was so effective that the topic of language origins was almost ignored until the second half of the twentieth century when scientists from different disciplines like anthropology, paleontology, primatology, and linguistics came together for a symposium at the 1970 meeting of the American Anthropological Association. Many of the papers presented were collected and published a few years later in a volume entitled *Language Origins* (Wescott, Hewes & Stokoe, 1974). In order to get this book into print, Stokoe established a small publishing company, Linstok Press. This book put forward again the theory of a gestural origin of language showing that a great accumulation of ethological, neurological, and paleontological data relevant to the study of language made it possible to develop a scenario for the origins of language.

It is not accidental that around the same years a large body of research was developed in two areas strictly related to the above issue: sign language and language acquisition in deaf signing children. The study of the visual–gestural or signed languages used by deaf people has shown that gestures can, and indeed do develop into full-blown linguistic systems, with functions and properties that are largely comparable to those of vocal languages. This general result highlights the links and continuity that relate gestures to language systems. Due to the gestural substance of these languages, the comparative, crosslinguistic and crossmodal exploration of signed and spoken languages also provides unique insights with respect to the distinctive features of human language, the extent to which these can be influenced by the modality of production, and their evolutionary path (Armstrong, Stokoe & Wilcox, 1995).

The study of language acquisition by children exposed to sign language has highlighted interesting relationships between gestures and signs and between the acquisition of spoken and signed languages. Such comparisons have promoted remarkable advancements in the study of language development in human infants. Significant insights into the organization and evolution of language have been gained through studies aimed at clarifying the interplay between the vocal and the gestural modality in early development, and the more general cognitive roots and developmental precursors of language (Volterra & Erting, 1990).

The most recent formulation of a theory of a gestural origin of language has been provided by Corballis (2002) who, in his recent book *From Hand to Mouth*, has proposed that gesture has existed side by side with vocal communication for most of the last two million years, a hypothesis that has also been put forward by other scholars (Hewes, 1976; Armstrong, Stokoe & Wilcox, 1995; Deacon, 1997).

According to Corballis, something over 30 million years ago great apes differentiated from the Old World monkeys, and by around 16 million years ago larger brains probably heralded an increase in thinking, including enhanced representation of objects in the brain and the capacity of using a form of protolanguage. Around 5 or 6 million years ago, bipedalism was the main characteristic of early hominids that distinguished them from the other great apes and that had freed their hands and arms for more effective gesturing. But the advance from protolanguage to true grammatical language may not have begun until the genus *Homo* emerged, sometime around two million years ago. This branch of hominids was distinguished

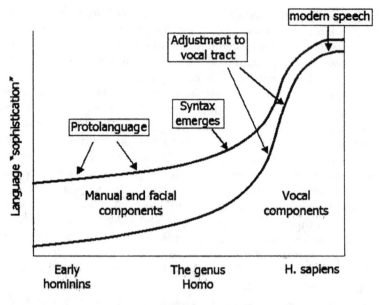

FIG. 1.1.

by an increase in brain size, the invention of stone tools, and the beginnings of multiple migrations out of Africa, and it is likely that language became increasingly sophisticated from then on. For most of this period, language would have been primarily gestural, although increasingly punctuated by vocalizations. An indirect evidence of the gestural origin of language is that articulate speech would have required extensive changes to the vocal tract along with the cortical control of vocalization and breathing. The evidence suggests that these were not completed until relatively late in the evolution of the genus *Homo* (see Fig. 1.1, from Corballis, 2002: 118).

The adaptations necessary for articulate vocalization may have been selected, not as a replacement for manual gestures, but rather to augment them. Since many species show a left-hemispheric dominance for vocalization (a bias that may go back to the very origins of the vocal cords), as vocalizations were increasingly incorporated into manual gesture, this may have created a left-hemispheric bias in gestural communication as well. *Homo sapiens* discovered that language could be conveyed more or less autonomously by speech alone, and this invention may have been as recent as 50,000 years ago (Corballis, 2002). Gesture was not simply replaced by speech. Rather, gesture and speech have co-evolved in complex interrelationships throughout their long and changing partnership. If this account is correct, then both modalities should still exhibit evidence of their prolonged co-evolution, reflected in certain universal (or near-universal) interdependencies, as well as predispositions that reflect the comparative recency or antiquity of these abilities (Deacon, 1997).

The tight relationship between language and gesture described above is compatible with recent discoveries regarding the shared neural substrates of language and meaningful actions that, in the work developed by Rizzolatti's laboratory (Gallese, Fadiga, Fogassi & Rizzolatti, 1996; Rizzolatti & Arbib, 1998) have been likened to gestures. Specifically, Rizzolatti and his colleagues have demonstrated that hand and mouth representations overlap in a broad frontal-parietal network called the "mirror neuron system," which is activated during both perception and production of meaningful manual action and mouth movements. The discovery of "mirror neurons" in the monkey brain provided a significant support to the notion of a gestural origin of language. These neurons respond both when the monkey makes a grasping movement and when it observes the same movement made by others. Since the mirror-neuron system is present in both monkeys and humans, it was most likely present in the common ancestor, providing a basis for a form of communication that was voluntary and flexible rather than fixed (Corballis, 2002).

In the present chapter we review a set of studies conducted in our laboratory that bear on the broader issues outlined above. These studies provide evidence on the continuity between prelinguistic and linguistic development, and on the interplay between the gestural and the vocal modalities in both typically developing children and in children with Down and Williams syndromes, whose development proceeds in atypical conditions. Corballis' (2002) evolutionary views on a slow transition from gesture to vocal language appear to be supported by our developmental data, as this transition, and the interdependency between gesture and speech, seem still evident in children's communicative and linguistic development. As observed by Deacon, it is of course unlikely that language development recapitulates "language evolution in most respects (because neither immature brains nor children's partial mapping of adult modern languages are comparable to mature brains and adult languages of any ancestor)" (Deacon, 1997 p. 354), but we can gain useful insights into the organization and evolution of both language and gesture by investigating the interplay between these modalities in the communication and language systems of children with typical and atypical development.

EARLIER WORK ON GESTURE AND THE EMERGENCE OF LANGUAGE

The first investigation on the role of gesture in the emergence of language conducted at our institution was a longitudinal (for that time pioneering) study by Bates, Camaioni, and Volterra (1975). That study involved three infant girls aged 2, 6, and 12 months, at the beginning of the study, observed (with home visits at two-week intervals) over a period of eight months. At the end of this period the three infants overlapped one another in development.

The study aimed to explore:

- the continuity from precommunicative schemes, to preverbal communication, to verbal interaction;
- cooccurring developments in other domains, such as nonverbal cognition and social relations;
- the kinds of performative intentions (e.g., declaring, ordering, asking) that emerged from the above developments.

The results indicated that the primary cognitive prerequisite for performative intentions was Piaget's sensorimotor stage 5, in particular the ability of tool use (see also Bates, Benigni, Bretherton, Camaioni, & Volterra, 1977). In the same period in which the children we observed used supports or sticks to pull objects (8/10 months of age) they also began:

- to use objects as "tools" to obtain adult attention, while producing communicative behaviors like showing, giving, communicative pointing called *protodeclarative*;
- to invoke adult help in obtaining objects by means of ritualized request or communicative pointing called *protoimperative*.

The first one-word labeling appeared within the same kinds of communicative sequences in a later period, corresponding to Piaget's sensorimotor stage 6, when other abilities like deferred imitation, memory for absent objects or people, and initial form of "pretend" play began to emerge.

The first stage involving intentional communication, but not necessarily speech, was termed the *illocutionary phase* (after Austin, 1962), while the following stage, involving the use of words in the same performative sequences, was termed the *locutionary phase*. The use of terms like phase and stage did not imply sudden and qualitative shift but rather a gradual transition from:

- wordlike sounds in the service of performative functions (e.g., the sound "Mmmm!" used to accompany all requests);
- semi-referential words, in which a relation between sound and referent can be determined only within a ritualized, function-based range (e.g., the word "da!" as an accompaniment to the act of exchanging objects);
- referential words which appear to "stand for" their referents in a range of contexts (e.g., "bau bau" to designate dogs).

In related work (e.g., Bates, 1976; Camaioni, Volterra, & Bates, 1976) the nature of performatives was explored and described in greater detail (for example another behavior noted was "showing off" through the repetition of an arm movement or a facial expression for eliciting adult attention), but the main conclusions reached by the study were confirmed. Of particular relevance for the present review was the finding that the onset of intentional communication between the ages of 9 and 13 months was marked in part by the emergence of a series of gestures—GIVING, SHOWING, POINTING, and RITUALIZED REQUEST—that preceded the appearance of first words.

A subsequent, crosscultural and crosslinguistic study compared the gestural and vocal repertoires of 25 Italian and American infants observed between 9 and 13 months of age (Bates, Benigni, Bretherton, Camaioni, & Volterra, 1979; Volterra, Bates, Benigni, Bretherton, & Camaioni, 1979). Striking parallels between early vocal production and gestural schemes of symbolic play were found. The findings can be summarized as follows (Bates, Bretherton, Snyder, Shore, & Volterra, 1980: 408–409):

- V-symbols (vocal) and G-symbols (gestural) emerge around the same time, and are correlated across the sample in frequency of use, rate of acquisition, and number of different schemes observed by the experimenters and reported by the mothers.
- Patterns of correlation with other measures are quite similar for V- and G-symbols. Both correlate with aspects of tool use and imitation, while neither correlates with spatial relations or object permanence.
- Both kinds of symbols are initially acquired with prototypical objects, in highly stereotyped routines or scripts. At roughly parallel rates, they gradually "decontextualize" or extend out to a wider and more flexible range of objects and events.
- There is tremendous overlap in content for both V- and G-symbols, when "vocabularies" are compiled across the whole sample. There are words for such concerns as eating, dressing, play with vehicles, telephones, games of exchange and peekaboo, sleeping, bathing, and doll play. The repertoires of conventional[1] gestures involve precisely the

---

[1]It may be useful to clarify that in the studies reviewed here, as in the work of other researchers, the terminology used for different types of gestures observed in children's development is not homogeneous, and it has often considerably changed over the years, even in the work of the same author(s), reflecting parallel changes in methodology and/or perspectives. In this review we have generally chosen not to alter the terminology used in the original studies we refer to. However, it must be noted that gestures that in early work were called "performatives" were subsequently reanalyzed and reclassified as "deictic." More content-loaded gestures that were initially classified as "conventional" or "referential," or also "symbolic play schemes," were subsequently reclassified as "representational" (see the subsequent sections of this chapter and Capirci, Iverson, Pizzuto & Volterra, 1996).

same set of concerns: eating, dressing, telephones, exchange games, etc. In short, the two types of symbols refer to, name, or in some sense "mean" the same things.

Already at that time, important differences between vocal and gestural "names" were noted. First, it was clear that children were encouraged by parents to rely much more on vocal symbols for communication. Second, some important differences between the vocal and gestural modalities were to be considered, including differences in short-term memory and a relative propensity for sequential vs. simultaneous presentation of information. Third, unlike the vocal symbols of speech, the symbolic gestures used by 1-year-olds typically involve actions directly on the associated object. Young children are much more likely to name objects vocally while they are manipulating them. However, as observed by Bates et al. (1980: 409) "gestural symbols provide a more unique, defining kind of kinesthetic feedback from their objects. Simply put, you can do more things to a cup while saying 'cup' that you can while drinking from it. For this reason, we might expect the gestural symbols of 1-year-olds to be more 'closely tied' to their objects than equivalent vocal symbols. By this we mean that gestures may require more perceptual input, and/or that physical contact with the object may more likely to trigger a gestural scheme than a word."

Taken together, these findings highlighted the remarkable similarities between production in the gestural and the vocal modalities during the first stages of language acquisition. They also raised interesting issues with regard to the communicative and linguistic value of early words and gestures. Symbolic actions produced in the gestural modality were often considered to be non-communicative or non-referential despite reports that these gestural schemes can be used productively to communicate about a specific referent in a decontextualized, symbolic manner (Volterra et al., 1979). Consequently, they were often referred to and analyzed separately from verbal production as "symbolic play" regardless of their level of decontextualization. In contrast, words were in general considered to be communicative or referential irrespective of the context or contexts in which they were used. This distinction is highly problematic, however, because it implies that only signals produced in the vocal modality can potentially become referential and be used to name new objects or events in a variety of different contexts.

These issues were addressed by Caselli (1983a) in a longitudinal diary study of one Italian infant from the age of 10 to 20 months. Caselli showed that many of the gestures usually set aside as "schemes of symbolic play" (e.g., holding an empty fist to the ear for TELEPHONE, waving the hand for BYE_BYE, or raising the arms, palms up, for ALL_GONE) were in fact frequently used by the child to communicate in a variety of situations and contexts similar to those in which first words were produced. These gestures, characterized as "referential gestures," differed from deictic gestures (such as prototypical POINTING or SHOWING) in that they denoted a precise referent and their basic semantic content remained relatively stable across different situations. The form and meaning of these gestures seemed to be the result of a particular agreement established in the context of child–adult interaction, while their communicative function appeared to develop within routines similar to those which Bruner (1983) has considered fundamental for the emergence of spoken language.

Caselli's (1983a) findings were confirmed by further observations. Caselli, Volterra, and Pizzuto (1984) conducted qualitative analyses of longitudinal diary data on the spontaneous vocal and gestural productions of four typically-developing Italian children (age range: 10–30 months). These authors reported that, at the one-word stage, the children's gestural utterances were comparable to their vocal productions. As children moved to the two-word stage, numerous gesture–word combinations were observed (e.g., "POINT (to chair)–mommy," requesting that mommy sit on the chair), and two-gesture combinations (e.g., "EAT–POINT (to food)," requesting to be fed). These types of combinations seemed to precede the first two-word utterances. When two-word utterances appeared, however, a marked difference between the vocal and the gestural modalities was found: combinations of two symbolic, referential words (e.g., "mommy open") were common, but combinations of two referential gestures were never observed.

Since the end of the 70s, research in our laboratory has developed in new directions as we began to explore language development in deaf children and, shortly thereafter, the visual–gestural language used within the Italian (adult) Deaf community, a language that had never been described until we began our investigations, and that is now widely known as Italian Sign language or LIS. The knowledge we began to gain by studying a visual–gestural language like LIS undoubtedly stimulated us not only to compare the acquisition of signed vs. spoken language, but also to refine our methodology in the analysis of the gestures, signs, and words observable in children exposed to a signed or a spoken language.

As noted earlier, comparative research on signed vs. spoken language acquisition can shed new light on the study of language acquisition, most notably in determining which aspects of the acquisition process are dependent on the modality of production and reception, and which ones are unaffected by modality. This is particularly true for studying the role of gesture in the emergence of language. When hearing children acquiring a spoken language make the transition from prelinguistic gestural communication to language, a modality change occurs. In contrast, deaf children acquiring a signed language communicate prelinguistically and linguistically in the same visual–gestural modality. Thus, comparisons between hearing children acquiring a spoken language and deaf children acquiring a signed language may be particularly valuable for clarifying the relationship between prelinguistic communication and language. However, in order to pursue appropriate comparisons it is necessary to use the same criteria, and a uniform terminology, for identifying and distinguishing gestures, signs and words in the communicative productions of both deaf and hearing children.

These methodological concerns were taken into account by Caselli and Volterra, who compared the emergence and development of language in two deaf children of deaf parents and two hearing children of hearing parents (Caselli, 1983b, 1990; Caselli & Volterra, 1990; Volterra, 1981). The children were observed at different ages (one pair during their first year, the other pair during their second year of age), using the same criteria for classifying their gestural and/or linguistic productions (signs or words). This comparison showed that the same stages and timing characterized the development of communication and language across children, independently of the modality of language reception and expression.

In a first, initial period both deaf and hearing children used only deictic gestures, while referential gestures, signs, and words appeared in a subsequent period. Referential gestures, signs, and words were initially used imitating more or less correctly the model offered by the adult, in response to adult elicitations, in ritualized exchanges that often referred to complex schemes of action not yet analyzed. In a subsequent period, gestures, signs, and words were separated from the action scheme or ritualized exchange, appeared to represent only part of the scheme (for example an object or an action), and were used spontaneously to communicate needs or states, or to name objects, actions and events. Importantly, several referential gestures produced by both the hearing and the deaf children appeared to undergo a similar process of gradual decontextualization, eventually assuming symbolic-like properties.

Both deaf and hearing children began to combine two signs or two words in a single utterance at the same age (around 17–18 months), when their observed vocabularies of signs or words comprised about 20–40 distinct items. The combinations the children produced were comparable under one important aspect: hearing–speaking children combined two referential words at the same stage of symbolic development that deaf–signing children combined two referential signs. Interestingly, the hearing children never combined two referential gestures. Caselli and Volterra thus concluded that in hearing children acquiring spoken languages the capacity to produce symbols can be displayed in both the gestural and the vocal modality, but the specifically linguistic capacity to *produce* and *combine* symbol in the same modality is manifested only in the modality of the linguistic input to which children are exposed. Caselli and Volterra also underscored that, when the vocal and gestural communicative productions of both deaf and hearing children are analyzed according to the same criteria and a uniform terminology, the linguistic advantage reported by some authors (e.g., Bonvillian, Orlansky, & Novack, 1983) in the acquisition of signed languages disappears (see also Volterra & Iverson, 1995).

In the same years in which we were developing our own research, several colleagues around the world had been exploring, from different perspectives, the use of communicative gestures in the first two years of life, and/or early communication in children acquiring signed languages. A collection of papers edited by Volterra and Erting (1990) brought together several studies on these topics, arranged in different sections based on the hearing status of the children examined (hearing and deaf) and the linguistic input they received (spoken or signed). In their concluding remarks, Erting and Volterra (1990) underscored the many points of agreement among the different studies, most notably with respect to the evidence that both hearing and deaf children use gestures to communicate, and that there is a progression in the use of gestures over time. Erting and Volterra also noted relevant discrepancies, especially as concerned the terminology and classificatory criteria used, and the methodological issues these raised. For example, if a child production is labeled as a "sign," the implication is that it is part of a linguistic system and therefore a symbolic act. But, if the same production is labeled as a "gesture," its symbolic status is unclear. Often an author's choice of terms depends upon whether the child is hearing or deaf, or upon the linguistic input to which the child is exposed. Erting and Volterra stressed the need of using a uniform terminology and of defining explicit criteria for deciding upon the status of a gestural production in early infancy: the same criteria should be applied to examine children's vocal, gestural and signed productions in order to determine their communicative, symbolic, and linguistic status.

Further evidence on the relevance of gestures in the emergence of language in typically developing children was provided by the first results of two new research lines we began pursuing at the end of the 80s. One stemmed from work finalized to develop and validate the Italian version of the MacArthur Communicative Development Inventory (MCDI), the now well known parental report instrument designed to explore and assess children's early communicative and linguistic development (Dale, Bates, Reznik, & Morisset, 1989; Fenson, Dale, Reznick, Thal, Bates, Hartung, Pethick, & Reilly, 1993).[2] Casadio and Caselli (1989) explored children's

---

[2]This work, which eventually resulted in the creation of the PVB, the Italian version of the MacArthur CDI (see next section), is another research line inspired by Liz, and it would have never been started nor developed without her constant encouragement, support, and most stimulating collaboration.

early word repertoire (receptive and expressive) and production of communicative action-gestures using both a preliminary elaboration of the Italian MCDI (see next section) and a structured interview designed to obtain detailed information from parents on the contexts and the degree of conventionalization/symbolization of children's early word and gesture use. The repertoire of words and action-gestures explored with these parental report tools included:

- a list of 294 words distinguished in different categories related to people, animals, objects, actions, and relations that are commonly encoded in early language (e.g. mommy, dog, water, telephone, feeding-bottle, go, sleep, above),
- a list of 62 action-gestures also distinguished in different categories which, in addition to deictic and referential gestures as defined thus far, comprised real actions (e.g., eating with a spoon), pretend or symbolic play schemes (e.g., pretending to eat with a spoon in the absence of food), and routines (e.g., peekaboo) that are commonly observed in children.

Data were provided on a sample of twenty 14-month-old children. The qualitative analyses of the parental reports showed that at this age the number of words children comprehended was markedly larger than the number produced. There were interesting "meaning correspondences" (in a broad sense of the term "meaning") between *words comprehended* and *action-gestures produced* by the children (i.e., in many cases the meaning of words comprehended referred to actions the children produced or which were also encoded by referential gestures noted in children's production). The number of distinct action-gestures produced was larger than that of words produced. The productive action-gestural and vocal systems of the individual children were also found to be highly distinct: in most cases action-gestures and words were related to different types of objects or actions (e.g., if children used a word for 'food' it was unlikely that they had a referential gesture for 'food' or 'eat'). Only a few children had words and action-gestures that somehow conveyed comparable meanings. Information on the contexts of early word and gesture use also indicated that many words were used while performing an action or holding an object related to the word produced. In addition, the parental interview data showed that although parents tended to attribute a communicative value more often to words than gestures, both the words and the referential gestures identified in the children's productive repertoires appeared to undergo a similar process of decontextualization: they were initially produced only in specific and ritualized contexts (nonreferential use), and only later were they used in a symbolic/referential way to anticipate or evoke absent referents.

A second and related investigation aimed at providing new data on children's use of gestures and words during the first two years of life (Caselli, Volterra, Camaioni, & Longobardi, 1993). That study employed a different parental questionnaire, which was originally devised for collecting information from parents of deaf children (Luchenti, Ossella, Tieri, & Volterra, 1988) and subsequently adapted to investigate the communicative and linguistic development of hearing children (Camaioni, Caselli, Longobardi, & Volterra, 1991). In addition to detailed questions on children's vocal and gestural behaviors in different contexts, this questionnaire included:

- a restricted list of early words (N = 15) and deictic and referential gestures (N = 15), designed to be used with 12- and 16-month-old children (and excluding real as well as symbolic action schemes);
- a much larger vocal vocabulary list comprising 680 items subdivided into 18 different semantic and grammatical categories (e.g., nouns for people, animals, objects; verbs for different actions and states; function words such as articles, prepositions, pronouns).

The items included in these lists were selected from those identified as relevant on the basis of previous studies. The questionnaire was given to the parents of 23 children, with instructions to compile when their children reached the ages of 12, 16, and 20 months. The major results of this study showed that at 12 months the children made extensive use of gestures, at 16 months both gestures and words were used in similar fashion, and only at 20 months did the vocal modality become the predominant mode of communication.

MORE RECENT STUDIES

Compared to earlier work, in the more recent studies reviewed below we have extended the investigation of the interplay between gestures and language by examining, with different methodologies:

- larger samples of typically developing children;
- the patterns observable at more advanced stages of communicative–linguistic development;
- input–output relationship in the acquisition of both spoken and signed language;
- the role of gestures in the communicative–linguistic system of children with atypical learning conditions.

The Growth of Expressive and Receptive Vocabulary
and Its Relationship With Action and Gesture

Evidence on this topic was provided by research conducted using the final version of the "Italian MCDI" or "Primo Vocabolario del Bambino" (hereafter: PVB), the parental questionnaire elaborated by Caselli and Casadio (1995) who have collected normative data on a large sample of about 700 children in the age range from 8 to 30 months. The PVB comprises two forms, labeled "Gestures and Words" and "Words and Sentences," designed to collect information on children's early word comprehension and production and action-gesture repertoire, and children's more advanced lexical-grammatical repertoire and sentence structure. In the form that is relevant for the present discussion, Gestures and Words, the repertoire of words potentially comprehended or produced includes 408 items (distinguished in 19 different broad semantic and grammatical categories that range from words for natural sounds, nouns for people, animals, familiar objects, body parts, verbs and adjectives for a variety of actions and states that are commonly encoded in child language, adverbials, pronouns and a subset of function words). The repertoire of action-gestures, listed in a separate subsection, comprises 63 items, distinguished in 7 categories. As in the Casadio and Caselli (1989) study, these categories include not only deictic and referential gestures as defined in several studies, but also real actions and pretend or symbolic play schemes, as well as routines that the children use spontaneously and/or in imitating actions or routines proposed by the adult.

On the basis of data on 315 children (age range: 8–17 months) whose parents compiled the Gestures and Words form of the PVB, Caselli and Casadio (1995) have shown that there is a complex interrelationship between early lexical development in comprehension and production and action-gestures. First, in this age range there are interesting asynchronies between the receptive and the expressive vocabulary, with the first being significantly larger than the second one. Second, in early development the productive repertoire of action-gestures appears to be larger than the vocal repertoire. For example, at 11–13 months the mean number of action-gestures produced is 29, compared to a mean number of 8 words. Third, and what is more interesting, at this early age there is a significant correlation, and also a meaning correspondence, between words comprehended and action-gestures produced. In addition, action-gestures and words appear to develop in parallel through the age of 17 months: at 16–17 months children are reported to produce a mean number of about 40 action-gestures and 32 words. The range of meanings covered by action-gestures and words also appear to be comparable.

These results on a large sample of children support and significantly expand those provided by Casadio and Caselli (1989) and Caselli et al. (1993) on much smaller samples of children. In addition—and although certainly more research is needed to ascertain with more precision the developmental relations between actions, gestures and word—these findings (especially those concerning word comprehension and action-gestures production) suggest that the link between real actions, actions represented via gestures, and children's vocal representational skills may be deeper than it has been ascertained thus far.

Gestures in the Transition From the One-Word to the Two-Word Stage

As noted above, in our own work preliminary evidence from diary and longitudinal observations (e.g., Caselli et al., 1984; Caselli & Volterra, 1990) suggested that, in typically developing children, gestures are used productively not only in the earliest stages of language development but also when two-word utterance appear. It is well known that the ability to combine two linguistic symbols marks a milestone in the language learning process. From that point on, several major changes in the child's linguistic abilities occur: vocabulary grows at a very fast rate, two- and multi-word utterances become progressively more frequent and articulated in their meaning and structure, and the acquisition of grammar begins.

Crosslinguistic investigations of a wide variety of languages have shown that the developmental progression from one- to two-symbol utterances takes place in a similar fashion regardless of the particular language and culture to which children are exposed, and can thus be characterized as a universal feature of language learning, in the spoken as in the signed modality (see the studies collected in Slobin, 1985, 1992, 1997). But what is the role of gestures, and how are different types of gestures, as compared to different types of words, distributed in *both* children's repertoire *and* expressive utterances during the transition from the one-word to the two-word stage? Data on these questions were provided by two related studies focused on children's vocal and gestural repertoires (Iverson, Capirci, & Caselli, 1994) and the structure of their vocal, gestural and gestural-vocal or crossmodal utterances (Capirci, Iverson, Pizzuto, & Volterra, 1996). The major results of both studies are summarized and reconsidered here from a unitary perspective that relates the changes in the composition of children's gestural and vocal repertoires to the functions and structure of their vocal and/or gestural utterances (Pizzuto et al., 2000; Capirci, Caselli, Iverson, Pizzuto & Volterra, 2002).

The data used for these studies were videotaped, 45-minute recordings of 12 children observed at home, in different contexts of spontaneous interaction with their mothers (e.g., play with familiar objects, meals or snack time), at two age points: at 16 months, when their vocal utterances consisted for the most of one element, and at 20 months, when two-word utterances appeared in an appreciable number.

All communicative gestures and words identified in the children's production were distinguished in two major categories: deictic and representational. Deictic gestures included the REQUEST, SHOW, and POINT gestures that have been extensively described in the literature (e.g., Bates et al., 1979). Deictic words included demonstrative and locative expressions, personal and possessive pronouns. Representational gestures included both gestures iconically related to actions performed by or with the referent (e.g., wiggling the nose for RABBIT, flapping the arms for BIRD or FLY), and conventional gestures (e.g., shaking the head for NO, turning and raising the palms up for ALL_GONE, culturally-specific gestures proper to the Italian repertoire, such as bringing the index finger to the cheek and rotating it for GOOD or opening-closing four fingers, thumb extended, for CIAO = 'bye-bye'). Representational words included for the most content words that in the adult language are classified as common and proper nouns, verbs, adjectives (e.g., 'mommy', 'flowers', 'Giacomo', 'open', 'good'), affirmative and negative expressions (e.g., 'yes', 'no', 'allgone'), but also conventional interjections and greetings such as 'bravo!', or 'bye bye'.

The notion of utterance was extended to cover not only vocal productions but also gestural and crossmodal (gestural and vocal) productions. In addition, the information conveyed by different combinations of vocal and/or gestural elements was analyzed and three major types of two-element utterances were distinguished: *equivalent, complementary,* and *supplementary.*[3] *Equivalent* combinations included only crossmodal productions of two representational units that typically referred to the same referent and conveyed the same meaning (e.g., BIG = *grande* 'big'; BYE_BYE = *ciao* 'bye-bye', where the notation "=" denotes the comparable meaning). *Complementary* combinations, like the equivalent ones, typically referred to a single referent, but had one distinctive feature, denoted by an ampersand (&) between the two combined elements: they always included one deictic element (gestural or vocal) which provided non-redundant information, singling out or disambiguating the referent indicated by the accompanying representational element or by another, cooccurring deictic element (e.g., POINT (to flowers) & *fiori* 'flowers'; POINT (to drawing of fish) & FISH; *questa*

---

[3]Our distinction between complementary and supplementary utterances differs from that proposed by Goldin-Meadow and Morford (1985, 1990). We extended the use of these terms to the classification of both vocal and crossmodal or gestural utterances, and we attribute to them a different meaning as defined above.

& *pappa* 'this & food'; POINT (to toy) & *etto* 'this'). *Supplementary* combinations differed from the other two types in that they referred either to the same or to two distinct referents, but in all cases each of the combined elements added information to the other one, a feature we notated with a plus sign (+) between the two combined elements. Vocal combinations of two representational words provided the clearest example of this class of utterances (e.g., *piccolo* + *miao miao* 'little + kitty'), but eight other different subtypes were identified (e.g., the crossmodal utterances POINT (to pigeon) + *nanna* 'sleep'; POINT (to game) + *te* 'you', ALL_GONE + *acqua* 'water').

Details on our classificatory/coding procedure and its rationale can be found in Iverson et al. (1994) and Capirci et al. (1996). Two points should be noted, however. First, the label "representational" was applied in these studies (as in subsequent studied discussed below) to those gestures that in much previous work were defined as "referential" (and with a variety of other terms). Second, and even though we are aware of several important problems that still need to be solved, our classification explicitly attempts to provide more accurate information on the relationship between gestures and words by using comparable classificatory criteria (and terminology) in their analysis. This issue has often been neglected in much, even recent research on the topic, where for example deictic words are not distinguished from content-loaded words (our "representational" words), or deictic gestures are attributed more or less complex "representational-like" meanings that to some extent obscure their basic deictic functions (e.g., Butcher & Goldin-Meadow, 2000; Goldin-Meadow & Morford, 1985, 1990; see also relevant discussions in Capirci et al., 1996).

The results concerning the children's gestural and vocal repertoires showed that at both 16 and 20 months gestures constituted a noticeable portion of all children's repertoires (Mean N of types: 9.58 and 10, respectively). At 16 months, six of the twelve children we observed had more or as many gestures as words types. At 20 months, a clear and significant shift toward the vocal modality was observed: ten out of twelve children had more words than gestures.

We also found differences, and developmental changes, in the distribution of deictic and representational elements in the gestural as compared to the vocal repertoire. In fact, while all children had deictic gestures in their repertoire at both age points (with POINT being by far more frequently used compared to REQUEST and SHOW), the same was not true of deictic words: gestural deixis preceded vocal deixis in the repertoire of half the children in our sample, and deictic gestures did not appeared to be supplanted by deictic words, because they continued to be present in the repertoires of all children at 20 months.

Representational gestures were also found, along with representational words, in the repertoires of all children at both ages, and in many children representational gesture types moderately increased from 16 to 20 months. However, and not surprisingly for children exposed to a spoken language, at both ages the repertoire of most children was composed more of representational words (Mean N = 22 and 58, respectively, at the two age points) than representational gestures (Mean N = 6.58 and 7), and a marked increase in the number of representational elements took place in the vocal but not in the gestural modality.

These data demonstrate that, for representational as well as for deictic elements, the clear shift toward the vocal modality observed at 20 months cannot be attributed simply to a contraction of the children's gestural repertoire, but was due to a parallel, and comparatively much greater expansion of the vocal repertoire.

The data on the *different utterance types* produced by the children at 16 and 20 months evidenced distinct developmental patterns for one- as compared to two-element utterances. Within *one-element utterances*, significant developmental changes were noted from 16 to 20 months. At 16 months, most children produced more one-gesture than one-word utterances, and thus showed a clear preference for the gestural modality in the production of one-element utterances. At 20 months, most children shifted to the vocal modality: they produced more one-word than one-gesture utterances, and this increase in the production of one-word utterances was highly significant, while at the same time the number of one-gesture utterances remained essentially the same. It was also found that most one-word utterances consisted of a representational (not a deictic) word. The opposite was found in one-gesture utterances, composed for the most by deictic gestures.

The data on the composition and the information conveyed by the children's *two-element utterances* provided a more complex and articulate picture of the role that gestures played at both 16 and 20 months of age.

First, we found that at both 16 and 20 months the most frequent type of two-element utterances were crossmodal combinations of a gestural and a vocal element, which also increased significantly from 16 to 20 months (Mean N at the two age points: 15 and 33). These utterances were in fact significantly more frequent not only of two-gesture utterances (almost absent from the children's production), but also of two-word utterances, which began to be consistently produced only at 20 months. Thus, while in one-element utterances the use of gestures declined from 16 to 20 months, in two-element utterances gestures continued to be a constituent structural element. No clear shift towards the exclusive use of the vocal modality was observed, even though—as expected—two-word utterances increased sharply and significantly from 16 to 20 months.

It is of interest to relate this finding to the data on the development of the children's gestural as compared to the vocal repertoire. The significant expansion of the children's vocal repertoire observed at 20 months appeared to have a rather direct effect on the production of one-element utterances (where a shift to the vocal modality was noted at the same age), and was clearly related to the significant increase of two-word utterances. In principle, the growth of the vocal repertoire could have led also to a decrease in the production of crossmodal gesture-word utterances. The fact that these utterances increased instead of decreasing is an additional strong indication of the important role that gestures continue to play even when the children's vocal repertoire and combinatorial abilities had considerably expanded.

Quite differently from crossmodal and two-word utterances, utterances consisting only of gestures remained in a very small number at both 16 and 20 months (Mean N = 1 and 2, respectively), and never included combinations of two representational elements. Taken together with the limited use of one-representational gestural utterances we noted in our children, this result indicates that the exclusive use of representational gestural elements (either alone or in combinatorial structures) is a marginal phenomenon in hearing children who are exposed to a vocal language input. The developmental patterns we noted for the different types of two-element utterances further clarified the role that deictic as compared to representational gestures and words play in children's growing linguistic system. Our results highlighted the special role that deictic gestures (notably POINT) play in development. This role was most evident in two-element utterances, where combinations of a POINT with a representational word were the most productive type of utterance the children used.

The results on the distribution of equivalent, complementary, and supplementary combinations of gestures and/or words provided new information on the structure of crossmodal and vocal communication in the transition from one- to two-word speech. We found that at both age points the most frequent type of two-element utterances produced were crossmodal complementary combinations of a deictic gesture (by far most commonly a POINT) and a representational word (e.g., POINT (to food) & *pappa* 'food'). This type of utterance, which we proposed could be interpreted as a kind of crossmodal "nomination" (somewhat comparable to its vocal-only counterpart made of a deictic word and a name as in *questa* & *pappa* 'this & food'), also increased significantly from 16 to 20 months.

At 16 months, when supplementary utterances of two words had just barely appeared, the second most frequent type of two-element utterances were supplementary crossmodal utterances composed of a deictic gesture and a representational word (e.g., POINT (to balloon) + *grande* 'big'). This type of utterance, which we proposed can be likened to a kind of crossmodal "predication," also increased from 16 to 20 months (Mean N = 5.58 and 12 respectively), but this increase was not significant. In contrast, and quite predictably, the increase of supplementary vocal-only utterances

(Mean N = 0.41 and 9.66 at 16 and 20 months respectively) was highly significant.

Finally, equivalent crossmodal combinations of two representational elements (e.g., BIG = *grande* 'big') were present in an appreciable number at both age points (Mean N = 3.75 and 5.5), but were always in smaller proportions compared to the other crossmodal utterances types, and their small increase at 20 months was not significant. In fact, these utterances appeared to be characterizable more as "bimodal one element utterances," where each of the two representational elements somehow "reinforces" or emphasizes the other, than true combinations of distinct elements.

We also performed correlation and two-step regression analyses to evaluate whether single gesture and gesture-word utterances predicted total vocal production. Total vocal production was defined as the total number of all tokens of single- or two- and multiword utterances produced, with or without an accompanying gesture. The correlational and variance patterns we found indicated that both single-gesture and, more significantly, gesture-representational word utterances produced at 16 months were good predictors of total language output at 20 months.

In sum, as noted elsewhere (Capirci et al., 1996), our results suggested that gesture-word utterances serve three different functions for young children as they attempt to communicate. First, the redundancy provided by representational gestures in equivalent combinations may function to reinforce the child's intended message and seems to help the child who is both vocally uncertain and still moderately unintelligible to ensure that her message is understood. Second, the gestural indication contained in complementary utterances provides disambiguating information that helps to locate and identify the single referent in the child's utterances. Third, in supplementary utterances, the gesture and the word refer to two distinct elements and, as a result, the child's intended message is extended.

From a more general perspective, the sheer presence of a consistent number of two-element crossmodal utterances at 16 months, when children's vocal communication is mostly limited to one-word utterances, and the persisting use of such utterances at 20 months, when children begin to produce two- and multiword utterances, suggest that a reappraisal of this developmental period is necessary. The definition of one-word stage appears to be reductive: at this stage, children's utterances are not limited to one-element, but already include two-element crossmodal combinations which appear to convey both nomination and predication structures. On the same grounds, at the two-word stage, a redefinition of the transitional phenomena that lead children to the acquisition of syntax and grammar may be warranted. At this stage a large portion of children's prototypical nomination and predication structures are still expressed via two-element crossmodal utterances. This suggests that in the transition to language proper gestures, most notably POINT gestures, may play an even more crucial role than has been recognized thus far (see also Greenfield & Smith, 1976).

The Role of Gestural Input in Hearing Mother–Child Interaction

The results summarized above stimulated us quite naturally to extend the investigation to the role and functions of gestures in maternal input. Toward this end, Iverson, Capirci, Longobardi, and Caselli (1999) reexamined the data used for the Iverson et al.'s (1994) and Capirci et al.'s (1996) studies focusing on the gestures produced by the mothers of the 12 children who participated in these earlier studies. Iverson et al.'s study aimed also to assess whether maternal use of gestures changed as children's speech became more complex from the first observation point at which the children were examined (16 months) to the second one (20 months). The mothers' gestures were identified and classified in three major categories: deictic and representational (as defined in the previous section), and emphatic. This last category included gestures that do not have a well identifiable meaning but are often executed during speech in a rhythmic fashion to stress or highlight aspects of discourse structure and/or the content of accompanying speech, essentially comparable to "beats" as described by McNeill (1992) or Magno Caldognetto and Poggi (1995). All maternal utterances containing both speech and gesture were categorized in three major classes according to the informational role played by gesture with respect to speech: *reinforce* (e.g., nodding YES while saying "Yes, I know that mommy is ugly"), *disambiguate* (e.g., POINT to floor while saying "Put it over there"), and *add* (e.g., POINT to toy telephone while saying "pretty").

Iverson et al. (1999) found that the majority of gestures produced by mothers at both observation points were deictic or representational, while emphatic gestures were rarely observed. Among deictic gestures, POINT was most common. Comparison of maternal gesture patterns at 16 months with those at 20 months revealed no significant differences in the production of any of the gesture types over time. The finding that emphatic gestures were produced so infrequently in this sample is especially interesting given the extensive use of such gestures in Italian culture (Kendon, 1995; Magno Caldognetto & Poggi, 1995).

At both observation points the majority of maternal gestures served to reinforce the message conveyed in speech. Utterances in which gesture disambiguated the verbal message were somewhat less frequent, while utterances in which gesture added information to that conveyed in speech were relatively uncommon. No significant differences were found in the number of utterances in each of the three categories at the two observation points.

Mothers' gestures, in other words, rarely provided information that was not already present in the spoken message. In marked contrast to what is typically reported for adult–adult interactions, in which gesture generally complements or supplements information conveyed in speech (McNeill, 1992), this suggests that Italian mothers are also gesturing less with their children than they would with another adult. This is particularly striking in the light of the fact that, at both observations, the proportion of maternal utterances containing gesture was much lower than that found in the children.

In summary, analyses of maternal production revealed that when mothers gestured, their gestures tended to cooccur with speech, and consisted primarily of deictic gestures that served to indicate referents in the immediate context. In effect, mothers appeared to be using a kind of "gestural motherese" characterized by fewer and more concrete gestures redundant with and reinforcing the message conveyed in speech. Not only were mothers' gestures tightly linked to the immediate linguistic and extralinguistic context, but they appeared to be used with the goal of underscoring, highlighting, and attracting attention to particular words and/or objects. Gestures that that would not fulfill this function, such as the emphatic gestures widely used by Italian adults when speaking to other adults, appeared to be almost completely absent from the communicative repertoire of the mothers examined in this study.

Signed and Spoken Language Input: Data From the Study of a Bilingual Child

More detailed evidence on the relationship between maternal input, language modality and gestural-linguistic development was provided by a study on the spontaneous communication of a bilingual hearing child of deaf parents, exposed to sign and spoken language from birth (Capirci, Iverson, Montanari, & Volterra, 2002).

The hearing child of deaf parents who participated in this study (Marco), was observed at monthly intervals between the ages of 10 and 30 months. Both of Marco's parents used Italian Sign Language (LIS) as their primary means of expression, but they frequently used Italian words (voiced or only mouthed) to accompany their signing when interacting with their child. Marco was also exposed to spoken Italian in the nursery he began to attend during the period in which he was observed. Marco was thus exposed from the beginning of his life to LIS and simultaneous signed/spoken communication at home, and to spoken Italian at the nursery.

The analysis of Marco's production focused on his manual gestures, signs and words, and utterance production patterns. To avoid overestimating Marco's sign production, specific, and quite conservative criteria were used to distinguish signs from gestures. Communicative gestural signals were defined as signs only when: a) they resembled adult LIS forms, and b) their form differed from those that have been identified in the production of typically developing monolingual children. All of Marco's manual signals that failed to meet these criteria were classified as gestures, and further distinguished in the two major classes of deictic and representational gestures according to the criteria proposed in Iverson et al. (1994), and Capirci et al. (1996).

The results of the study showed that Marco's earliest communications consisted primarily of gestures, a finding consistent with all the evidence we have reviewed in the present chapter, indicating that even in a bilingual signing/speaking child the earliest communicative signals are produced in the gestural modality. Acquisition of new words and signs was initially rather slow, and was subsequently followed by a period of rapid growth that occurred first in the word (between the ages of 19 and 22 months) and then in the sign vocabulary (beginning at 25 months). Marco's initial preference for gestural communication was eventually replaced by a preference for verbal and signed communication. By the end of the observation period, Marco's word and sign vocabularies were approximately the same size (82 signs and 93 words), and he used sign and speech to communicate with roughly equal frequency. Two-word utterance first emerged in Marco's production at 16 months, and began to increase markedly in number from 25 months on. Two-sign utterances first emerged at 25 months, outnumbering two-word utterances by 29 months. Interestingly, two-word combinations increased before two-sign combinations, with each increase occurring after rapid growth in word and sign vocabulary size respectively.

In order to examine any effect of simultaneous exposure to signed and spoken languages on early communicative development, Marco's gestural and verbal production at 16 and 20 months was compared to that of the group of 12 monolingual children observed at 16 and 20 months in the Iverson et al. (1994) and Capirci et al. (1996) studies previously described. The results of this comparison showed that, aside from an enhanced communicative use of the manual modality, Marco's communication patterns generally followed those observed among children exposed only to speech. Marco's overall vocabulary size and overall verbal/manual productivity fell well within the respective ranges observed in the monolingual children. All of these results are consistent with those of earlier studies on (deaf) signing children (e.g., Caselli, 1983b; Caselli & Volterra, 1990), and further support the view that there is no "sign advantage" in children exposed to a signed language input.

However, an interesting difference was observed when the proportions of deictic and representational gestures produced by Marco were compared to those of the monolingual children. While Marco used proportionately more representational than deictic gestures at both ages—a finding consistent with data also reported by van den Bogaerde and Mills (1995)—monolingual children produced deictic gestures much more frequently than representational gestures. Although it is possible that this difference may have been influenced by the conservative criteria used for distinguishing signs from gestures, it seems likely that Marco's relatively extensive use of representational gestures was a result of increased facility in the manual modality. Specifically, exposure to sign language may have enhanced the child's appreciation of the representational potential of the manual modality, and this may have been in turn generalized to gesture use.

The study aimed also to clarify whether the signed/spoken input to which Marco was exposed had any significant effect on his production of different utterance patterns, especially with respect to combinations of representational gestures, and of crossmodal combinations of gestural and vocal elements (obviously leaving aside two-sign combinations that are peculiar to language development in the signed modality). Since bilingual signers/speakers have access to linguistic symbols in two modalities, they may in principle be able to produce crossmodal combinatorial structures that are simply not available to monolingual children (e.g., gesture-sign, word-sign). Crossmodal combinations can be used to convey two different pieces of information in a single, integrated utterance, thereby eliminating the problem of coordinating articulatory movements necessary for the production of two words. Crossmodal combinations, in other words, appear to reflect a compromise between "readiness" to produce word combinations and constraints on the ability to produce two words in succession. These constraints may differ in a bilingual signing/speaking child.

In order to ascertain to what extent Marco's two-element utterances were comparable to those noted in monolingual children, Marco's production at 16 and 20 months was again compared to that of the monolingual children of the study previously described. This comparison revealed that at 16 months Marco's relative distribution of combinations across structure types was quite similar to that for monolingual children. However, at 20 months Marco's overall production of crossmodal combinations was well above the group mean for monolingual children. In fact, Marco produced more crossmodal combinations than any of the monolingual children. Interestingly, though not surprisingly, these combination included not only gesture-word but also sign-word combinations. In addition, at both ages, Marco combined two representational gestures (albeit in a small number of cases), producing structures that were never used by his monolingual peers, and thus appeared to be influenced by his exposure to a signed input.

The large number of crossmodal combinations produced by Marco raised the question of whether these enhanced his communicative potential relative to his monolingual peers. In other words, did Marco make use of sign-word (in addition to gesture-word) combinations to convey two different pieces of information, something that his monolingual non-signing peers can only do using gesture-word?

To address this issue, all of Marco's two-element utterances were classified according to the informational content they conveyed, distinguishing them into the equivalent, complementary, and supplementary type. It was found that at 16 months of age, the overall pattern of production of equivalent, complementary, and supplementary combinations for Marco was roughly similar to that of the monolingual children taken as a group. At 20 months, however, a striking difference emerged. While Marco's production of complementary and supplementary combinations remained similar to that of the monolingual children, he produced many more equivalent combinations than did the monolingual children taken as a group (Marco = 60 vs. group mean = 5.5). One additional relevant differences between Marco and the hearing monolinguals was that Marco's equivalent combinations included not only gesture=word combinations, but also an almost equal number of sign=word combinations (e.g., producing the LIS sign WORK together with the word *lavoro* 'work').

Why was Marco making such great use of equivalent sign=word combinations? It is reasonable to hypothesize that this reflected the nature of the bimodal sign/speech input to which he was exposed: informationally redundant sign=word combinations may be the product of extensive experience with simultaneous communication in everyday interactions (see also van den Bogaerde, 2000). It is of particular interest to note that Marco did not appear to fully exploit the potential of the input to which he was exposed. In principle, considering the large number of representational gestural elements in Marco's repertoire (both gestures and signs), one could have expected that he produced supplementary gesture+word or sign+word combinations. But this was not found, and the types of complementary and supplementary combinations produced by Marco were on the whole comparable to those noted in his monolingual peers. These data provide an additional indication that exposure to a signed input does not affect the informational content of early two-element utterances, regardless of whether they are gestural, vocal, or crossmodal.

Gestures and Words in Children With Atypical Development: Down and Williams Syndromes

While we have devoted many years to the study of the relationship between language and gesture in typically-developing children, in deaf children and in children exposed to a signed input, we are only beginning to study the nature and development of gesture in children with atypical patterns of language and cognitive development. Our recent investigations on this topic have been focused on the role of gesture in language development and use in children with two different genetic syndromes: one, Down Syndrome (hereafter: DS), is fairly well known, the other, Williams Syndrome (hereafter: WS), is a rare genetic condition associated with a microdeletion on chromosome 7q11.23 (Bellugi & St. George, 2001). Children with WS usually present a number of severe medical anomalies, including mental retardation with a specific cognitive profile.

The behavioral phenotypes of these two genetically determined syndromes appear to mirror each other. Children with DS usually exhibit impairments in language acquisition. Problems in morphology and syntax are frequently reported (Chapman, 1995; Vicari, Caselli, & Tonucci, 2000; Fabbretti, Pizzuto, Vicari, & Volterra, 1997). Fowler (1995) has pointed out that the linguistic difficulties of persons with DS may be a consequence of specific difficulties at the phonological level, both in speech perception and in the re-elaboration of acoustic information into a representational form that can be retrieved to serve memory, production, and comprehension. In contrast, children with WS appear to have an unusual command of language: although their comprehension is usually far more limited than their expressive language, this latter tends to be grammatically correct, complex and fluent at least at a superficial level, while under closer inspection it appears verbose and pseudo-mature (Volterra, Capirci, Pezzini, Sabbadini, & Vicari, 1996).

Relatively few studies have examined the relationship between gesture and developing language in children with DS or WS, and such studies have often focused on a limited set of gestures (Franco & Wishart, 1995; Bertrand, Mervis, & Neustat, 1998; Laing et al., 2002). Our own work on the topic is summarized below.

A first study conducted by Caselli et al. (1998) explored the relationship between action-gestures and words in children with DS compared to typically developing (hereafter: TD) children. Caselli et al. (1998) administered the Words and Gestures form of the PVB parental questionnaire (Caselli & Casadio, 1995) to the parents of 40 Italian children with DS (Mean chronological age, hereafter CA: 28.3 months). The scores obtained by the children with DS in the production of action-gestures and words were compared with those of a group of 40 TD children taken from Caselli and Casadio's (1995) normative sample, matched on the basis of receptive vocabulary size. Caselli et al. (1998) found that the children with DS had significantly larger action-gestures repertoires than their TD comparison group. However, this difference only emerged at higher word comprehension levels, i.e., among children with comprehension vocabularies above 100 words. These findings are in agreement with results reported by Singer Harris, Bellugi, Bates, Jones, and Rossen (1997) in a similar (MCDI based) study on American children with DS, and suggest that there may be some sort of "gestural advantage" in children with DS. These children may compensate for poor productive language abilities through greater production of gestures. However, it must be noted that inventories such as the PVB or the MCDI only provide information about whether or not a particular behavior is in a child's repertoire. The data do not provide any information on the frequency with which children produce gestures when communicating. Furthermore, in the PVB and MCDI actions and gestures are grouped in a single category, and it is thus difficult to assess what is the role of gestures proper in children's developing communicative and language system.

These issues were addressed in a more recent study on the spontaneous production of gestures and words in children with DS conducted by Iverson, Longobardi, and Caselli (2003). In this study five children with DS (three boys and two girls) were examined. The DS children had an average CA of 47.6 months, an average mental age (hereafter: MA) of 22.4 months, and an average language age of 18 months. Language age was assessed on the basis of the PVB expressive vocabulary scores. Each child with DS was matched with a TD child on the basis of gender, language age, and observed expressive vocabulary size. It must be noted that although the children in the two groups were of comparable language age, all the children with DS were still at the one-word stage, whereas all the TD children had already reached the two-word stage. The ten children participating in the study were videotaped for 30 minutes as they interacted spontaneously with their mothers. Their vocal and gestural productions were analyzed according to the coding scheme proposed by Iverson et al. (1994) and Capirci et al. (1996) described earlier in this chapter.

The results of the study provided evidence for a tight link between gesture and language in children with DS, and revealed interesting similarities as well as differences between the two groups of children examined. Relative to their language-matched TD peers, children with DS produced similar amounts of gesture and words, and combined gestures and words with comparable frequencies. However, relevant difference in the types and distribution of gesture-word combinations were found. When children with DS combined gestures and words, they did so primarily in an informationally redundant fashion. The vast majority of combinations produced by these children were in fact equivalent combinations in which the two representational elements referred to the same referent and conveyed the same meaning (e.g., headshake for NO = 'no'; BYE-BYE = 'bye'). Complementary combinations, in which a gesture is typically used to single out a referent that is being simultaneously labeled in speech were uncommon, and supplementary combinations, in which combined elements add information to one another were virtually non-existent in the production of the children with DS. TD children, on the other hand, made wide use of both complementary and supplementary combinations. Since complementary and especially supplementary combinations can be considered to be cognitively more sophisticated (i.e., convey greater amounts of information) than equivalent combinations, this suggests that children with DS may be somewhat delayed in the production of more advanced types of gesture-word combinations.

In contrast with children with DS, children with WS have been generally described as appearing to prefer the vocal modality. It has been reported that children with WS display a delay in starting to produce gestures (Bertrand et al., 1998), and that they show a limited use of gestures either with a declarative or an instrumental function (Laing et al., 2002).

A study conducted by Capirci, Iverson, Pirchio, Spampinato, and Volterra (2001) aimed to clarify similarities and differences in the use of gestures and words by children with WS, children with DS and TD children. Three preschool children with WS (CA range: 39–51 months; MA range: 26–36 months) were individually matched with three children with DS (CA range: 36–50 months; MA range 26–39 months) and with three TD children matched for mental age (CA range 24–34 months; MA range: 25–37 months). All the nine children examined had already reached the two-word stage. The children were observed at home, in 40-minute free play interactions with their mothers (20 minutes), and with an unfamiliar adult (20 minutes). All interactions were videotaped and all of the children's verbal and gestural communicative productions were fully transcribed and analyzed as described below. The children's utterances were categorized in three major classes: (1) vocal only (utterances consisting only of spoken words), (2) gestural only (utterances consisting only of gestures), (3) mixed, or vocal-gestural utterances (consisting of speech accompanied with gestures). The children's gestures were classified in the following categories: (1) pointing gestures, (2) conventional gestures (i.e., hands and/or body movements that are known to be used within the Italian culture and are associated with stable meaning, e.g., rotating the index finger on the cheek for GOOD), (3) iconic gestures (i.e., hands and body movement referring to objects, people, places, or events by some idiosyncratic representation of their form or function, e.g., flapping the hands for BIRDIE, or raising the arms high for TALL), (4) beats (gestures without a clear and stable meaning, that serve to highlight or emphasize aspects of discourse structure and/or the content of accompanying speech, comparable to those that in Iverson & al.'s (1999) study were classified as "emphatic" gestures). Mixed utterances were further coded according to the information conveyed by the gestural elements, and were distinguished into three major types: (1) reinforce (e.g., waving the hand in the gesture meaning 'hello' while saying "hello"), (2) disambiguate (e.g., pointing to a ball while saying "this one is mine"), (3) add (e.g., waving the hand in the gesture meaning 'hello' while saying "mommy").

The results showed that all the children observed produced a greater amount of vocal than gestured utterances. However, the children with DS produced more utterances containing gestures than did the children of the other two groups. With respect to the type of gestures produced, it was found that almost all the children produced pointing more than other gestures. Children with DS again differed: they produced more iconic gestures than did children with WS and TD children. The information conveyed by gestures in the utterances produced by the two groups of children with genetic syndromes was on the whole comparable to that observed in TD children: gestures were used mainly to reinforce the meaning of verbal utterances, even though gestures with "disambiguate" and "add" functions were also observed.

Children with WS thus appeared to be similar to TD children with respect to the frequency, type, and function of gestures produced, and this result does not support the indications provided by previous studies on a more limited use of gestures by children with WS. In contrast, children with DS produced more and different types of gestures compared to both children with WS and TD children. This result is in agreement with earlier indications on a possible enhancement of gestural communication in children with DS, as provided by Caselli et al.'s (1998) and Singer-Harris's (1997) studies, and as often reported by clinicians. However, this result also differs from the one reported by Iverson et al. (2003), who did not find any "gestural enhancement" in the DS children they studied.

The studies under discussion are all based on relatively small samples of children, and thus their results must be interpreted with caution. While more research is certainly needed, it is also useful to consider the methodological and developmental differences that may explain the discrepancies observed, especially with respect to the role of gestures in children with DS.

From a methodological standpoint, it must be noted that the broader set of action-gestures examined in the Caselli et al.'s (1998) study is not comparable to the much more restricted set of communicative gestures analyzed by both Iverson et al. (2003) and Capirci et al. (2001). The nature of the data used (parental reports vs. observations of children's spontaneous production in different contexts), the different measures used to match children with DS and TD children, the partially different methodologies used for analyzing and coding the children's gestural and vocal productions, all of these factors render very difficult to draw precise comparisons between these studies, and to reach more definite conclusions. In addition, the important role that individual differences may play needs to be further investigated.

Furthermore, it is of interest to recall that the children with DS in the Iverson et al. (2003) study were all at the one-word stage, whereas those of the Capirci et al. (2001) study were at the two-word stage. This developmental difference in language production abilities may be one of the factors involved in determining the somewhat contrasting results of these two observational studies. In other words, one cannot exclude the possibility that children with DS may use less gestures at the one-word as compared to the two-word stage. From this perspective, the results of the studies in question may be less contradictory than it appears at first sight: rather, they may have explored different facets of the developmental process at different developmental stages (Karmiloff-Smith, 1997).

There is ample evidence that the gap between cognition and language skills (especially language production) becomes progressively wider with development among children with DS (Chapman 1995; Fabbretti, et al., 1997). However, with increasing cognitive skills and social experience, and progressively greater difficulty with productive language, children with DS may be able to make use of actions produced in the context of object-related activities and social routines as communicative gestures. Once this happens, they may begin to develop relatively large repertoires of gestures and make enhanced use of gesture to compensate for poor productive language, particularly if they are encouraged to do so through the provision of signed language input (for a review see Abrahamsen, 2000). Thus, while gesture and language may develop in tandem during the early stages of communicative development in children with DS, the nature of the gesture-language link may begin to change as children's cognitive abilities begin to outstrip their productive language skills. A very recent study conducted in our laboratory has focused on the role of gestures in older children with WS (Bello, Capirci, & Volterra, 2004). This study investigated lexical organization and lexical retrieval in children with WS by examining both naming accuracy and the use of accompanying gestures in a picture-naming task such as the Boston Naming Test. This test consists of 60 line drawings representing different objects that children are requested to name. Ten children with WS (Mean CA = 10 yrs;11 months; Mean MA = 5 yrs;11 months) were administered the test. These children's performance, and their use of gestures during the task, were compared to those of two distinct groups of TD children: ten TD matched by chronological age (Mean CA = 10 yrs; 8 months) and ten TD matched by mental age (Mean MA = 6 yrs).

It was found that the overall naming accuracy of children with WS was in accord with their mental age. However, compared to both their MA- and CA-matched TD children, the children with WS showed a higher overall rate of gesture production, displayed a richer gestural repertoire than typically developing children, and used a significantly larger number of iconic gestures. The majority of iconic gestures noted in all children (WS and TD alike) appeared to represent the function, rather than the form, of the object depicted (e.g., a child produced a gesture meaning 'brush' moving the extended index finger in the air, as though mimicking the movement of a painting brush). There were few cases of iconic gestures reproducing the form of the represented object (i.e., for 'globe' a child traced a circle in the air with the index finger). In all three groups of children, iconic gestures tended to cooccur with circumlocutions. The analysis of these circumlocutions and of the gestures cooccurring with them indicated that, when the children could not provide the name for an object, they sought the word in the appropriate semantic space, and this appeared to be at least partially expressed and/or codified in the gesture produced. These findings seem to support recent theories on the key role of coverbal gesturing in speech production (e.g., McNeill, 1992), and indicate that the production of iconic gestures, more than other gesture categories, may be triggered by problems in accessing the word for a given object.

CONCLUSIONS

In the present chapter we have reviewed studies conducted within our laboratory on the role of gesture in the emergence and development of language. If we consider these studies from a unitary perspective, remarkable changes can be noted over the years. In earlier work, gestures were explored primarily as relevant features of the "prelinguistic" stage, as behaviors that preceded and prepared the emergence of language, which was more or less explicitly identified with speech. At the time, even among scientists, there were very few people who would think of language apart from speech, and it was very difficult to focus on gestures as behaviors that deserved to be fully investigated on their own right, and that continued to be of considerable interest even beyond the stage at which children begin to produce their first recognizable spoken words.

Subsequent studies on deaf signing children who acquire language through their intact visual–gestural modality led us to reconsider the use of gestures also in hearing children. Going back to our "traditional" studies on the acquisition of language under typical conditions, we were able to see that the use of gestures did not stop with the emergence of words but, rather, increased and played an important role in the transition from the one-word to the two-word stage. We would like to try to summarize our present view referring to the developmental scheme in Fig. 1.2, a scheme which was inspired by, and indeed mirrors the evolutionary scheme by Corballis presented in the introduction of this chapter.

Before one year of age, children begin to communicate intentionally mainly through gestures, and these gestures are often accompanied by vocalizations. Vocalizations become progressively more sophisticated and sim-

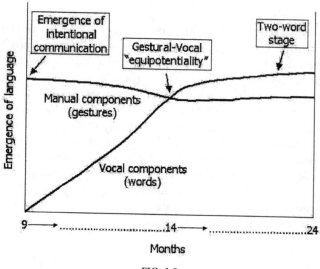

FIG. 1.2.

ilar to the words used in the adult language to which the children are exposed. Around 14 months there is a basic "equipotentiality" between the gestural and vocal channels. In this bimodal period, as aptly summarized by Abrahamsen (2000), "words are not as distinct from gestures and gestures are not as distinct from words as they first appear." As our earlier studies have shown, words and gestures appear to encode similar meanings, and go through a similar decontextualization process. In the following months, the repertoire of spoken words increases dramatically, but gestures are not simply replaced by speech. Rather both the vocal and the gestural modalities are used together, and crossmodal combinations mark the transition to the two-word stage.

The main hypotheses underlying much current work on the interplay between gesture and speech is that there is a continuity between an earlier "preverbal" and a subsequent, somehow functionally "equivalent" linguistic form, and that the use of gesture is a robust developmental phenomenon, exhibiting similar features across different children and cultures. The output systems of speech and gesture may draw on underlying brain mechanisms common to both language and motor functions (Iverson & Thelen, 1999). Within this broad framework, evidence on children with atypical patterns of language and cognitive development may be particularly relevant to assess the resilience of gesture as a developmental phenomenon.

In the studies we have conducted thus far on children with atypical development such as children with Down and Williams Syndromes, we have found that during the early stages of language learning the developmental patterns followed by gesture and speech are on the whole similar to those observed in typically developing children with similar language production abilities. Relevant differences are also observable (e.g., the greater use of redundant, equivalent combinations of gestures and words noted in children with DS, or the different use of iconic gestures found in children with WS compared to typically developing children). Further research is clearly needed to explore the ways in which the role of gesture in relation to speech changes developmentally, and the extent to which this role may vary among individuals with language difficulties.

The studies reviewed in the present chapter, based on children who varied in cultural experience (Italian vs. North American), input language (spoken vs. signed, English vs. Italian) and cognitive profiles (typical development, Down Syndrome, Williams Syndrome), strongly support the view that there is a remarkable continuity between prelinguistic and linguistic development, and that symbolic skills that are most evident in vocal linguistic productions are inextricably linked to, and co-evolve with more general cognitive and representational abilities, as is most apparent in the tight relationship between gestures and words, which continues through adulthood (McNeill, 1992, 2000).

This view appears to be particularly plausible in the light of the neurophysiological studies on "mirror neurons" we mentioned earlier (Gallese et al., 1996; Rizzolatti & Arbib, 1998) that have discovered powerful links between motoric and representational abilities in both monkey and human brains, with strong implications for a clearer understanding of the relationship between structured action, gestures and vocal language in humans. A central question that has always been hotly debated since ancient times, and which is still much discussed at present, is whether language development in human infants is driven primarily by specialized (and species-specific) innate structures that are for the most unrelated to those underlying more general cognitive and symbolic abilities, a sort of "language instinct" as characterized by one of the proponents of this view (Pinker, 1994), or whether on the contrary it is intricately but solidly linked to more general cognitive and neuro-sensory-motor structures that language shares with other domains (e.g., memory, sensory-motor coordination), and that are put in the service of language in a unique way, as proposed by other leading scholars (Deacon, 1997; Elman et al., 1996; Tomasello, 1999). Proponents of the first view underscore the dissociation of language from other cognitive domains, and the discontinuity between prelinguistic and linguistic development. Proponents of the second view highlight the interrelation between language and other cognitive domains, and the continuity between prelinguistic and linguistic development. As observed by Tomasello (1999), language did not come out of nowhere nor did it arise as some bizarre genetic mutation unrelated to other aspects of human cognition and social life. Natural language is a symbolically embodied social institution that arose historically from previously existing social-communicative activities. Long before children learn to speak, they are able to communicate, meaningfully and intentionally, with their caretakers. In learning a language, children are acquiring a more effective and elaborate means of doing something that they can already do in a more primitive fashion. As suggested by Bates' earlier and more recent work: ". . . *Language is a new machine built out of old parts*" (Bates & Goodman, 1997), "*emerging from a nexus of skills in attention, perception, imitation, and symbolic processing that transcend the boundaries of 'language proper'*" (Bates & Dick, 2002).

Liz Bates has been for a long time a strong advocate of this second view, a view which we fully share not on "a priori" bases, but on the grounds of our research. Much of this research has been inspired by Liz's work, and often developed together during Liz's frequent visits at "her" Nomentana Lab in Rome. Liz focused from the start on key questions that only later were to be "rediscovered" and recognized as being of central relevance for an appropriate understanding of human symbolic skills. Many of Liz's "old ideas" appear today surprisingly "new" and are supported by the most recent findings in both behavioral and neurophysiological studies.

ACKNOWLEDGMENTS

The research reported in the present chapter was supported in the framework of the European Science Foundation EUROCORES programme "The Origin of Man, Language and Languages" (OMLL).

REFERENCES

Abrahamsen, A. (2000). Explorations of enhanced gestural input to children in the bimodal period. In K. Emmorey & H. Lane (Eds.), *The Signs of Language Revisited: An antology to honor Ursula Bellugi and Edward Klima.* Mahwah: Erlbaum, pp. 357–399.

Armstrong, D. F., Stokoe, W. C., & Wilcox, S. E. (1995). *Gesture and the Nature of Language.* Cambridge University Press.

Austin, J. L. (1962). *How to do things with words.* New York: Oxford University Press.

Bates, E. (1976). *Language and Context. The acquisition of pragmatics.* New York: Academic Press.

Bates, E. & Benigni, L., Bretherton, I., Camaioni, L., Volterra, V. (1979). *The emergence of symbols: cognition and communication in infancy.* New York: Academic Press.

Bates, E., Benigni, L., Bretherton, I., Camaioni, L., & Volterra, V. (1977). From gesture to the first word: on cognitive and social prerequisites. In L. Lewis and L. Rosenblum (Eds.), *Interaction, conversation and communication in infancy.* New York: John Wiley, pp. 247–307.

Bates, E., Bretherton, I., Snyder, L., Shore, C., & Volterra, V. (1980). Vocal and gestural symbols at 13 months. *Merrill Palmer Quarterly, 26,* (4), 407–423.

Bates, E., Camaioni, L., & Volterra, V. (1975). The acquisition of performatives prior to speech. *Merrill Palmer Quarterly, 21,* (3), 205–226.

Bates, E., & Dick, F. (2002). Language, gesture, and the developing brain. *Developmental Psychobiology, 40*(3), 293–310.

Bates, E. & Goodman, J. C. (1997). On the inseparability of grammar and the lexicon: Evidence from acquisition, aphasia and real-time processing. *Language and Cognitive Processes,* 12(5–6), 507–584.

Bello, A., Capirci, O. & Volterra, V. (2004). Lexical production in children with Williams syndrome: spontaneous use of gesture in a naming task. *Neuropsychologia, 42,* 201–213.

Bellugi, U. & St. George, M. (Eds.). (2001). *Journey from cognition to brain to gene. Perspectives from Williams syndrome.* Cambridge MA: MIT Press.

Bertrand, J., Mervis, C. B., & Neustat, I. (1998). Communicative gesture use by preschoolers with Williams syndrome: a longitudinal study. Paper presented at the *International Conference of Infant Studies.* Atlanta, GA.

Bonvillian, J. D., Orlansky, M. D., & Novack, L. L. (1983). Developmental milestones: Sign language acquisition and motor development. *Child Development, 54,* 1435–1445.

Bruner, J. (1983). Child's talk: learning to use language. New York: Norton.

Butcher, C. & Goldin-Meadow, S. (2000). Gesture and the transition from one- to two-word speech: when hand and mouth come together. In D. McNeill (Ed.), *Language and gesture.* Cambridge: Cambridge University Press: 235–257.

Camaioni, L., Caselli, M. C., Longobardi, E., & Volterra, V. (1991). A parent report instrument for early language assessment. *First Language, 11,* 345–359.

Camaioni, L., Volterra, V., & Bates, E. (1976). *La comunicazione nel primo anno di vita.* Torino: Boringheri.

Capirci, O., Iverson, J., Montanari, S. & Volterra, V. (2002). Gestural, signed and spoken modalities in early language development: The role of linguistic input. *Bilingualism Language and Cognition,* 5 (1), 25–37.

Capirci, O., Iverson, J. M., Pirchio, S., Spampinato, K. & Volterra, V. (2001). Speech and gesture in discourse produced by children with Williams syndrome and with Down syndrome. Paper presented at the *Xth European Conference on Developmental Psychology,* August 22–26, Uppsala: Sweden.

Capirci, O., Iverson, J. M., Pizzuto, E., & Volterra, V. (1996). Gestures and words during the transition to two-word speech. *Journal of Child Language, 23,* 645–673.

Capirci, O., Caselli, M. C., Iverson, J. M., Pizzuto, E., & Volterra, V. (2002). Gesture and the Nature of Language in infancy: the role of gesture as transitional device enroute to two-word speech. In D. Armstrong, M. Karchmer, & J. Van Cleeve (Eds.). *The Study of Sign Languages—Essays in Honor of William C. Stokoe.* Washington, D.C.: Gallaudet University Press, pp. 213–246.

Casadio, P., & Caselli, M. C. (1989). Il primo vocabolario del bambino. Gesti e parole a 14 mesi. *Età Evolutiva, 33,* 32–42.

Caselli, M. C. (1983a). Gesti comunicativi e prime parole. *Età Evolutiva, 16,* 36–51.

Caselli, M. C. (1983b). Communication to language: deaf children's and hearing children's development compared. *Sign Language Studies, 39,* 113–144.

Caselli, M. C. (1990). Communicative gestures and first words. In V. Volterra & C. J. Erting (Eds.), *From gesture to language in hearing and deaf children.* New York: Springer-Verlag, pp. 56–67.

Caselli, M. C., & Casadio, P. (1995). *Il primo vocabolario del bambino. Guida all'uso del questionario MacArthur per la valutazione della comunicazione e del linguaggio nei primi anni di vita.* Milano: Franco Angeli.

Caselli, M. C., Vicari, S., Longobardi, E., Lami, L., Pizzoli, C. & Stella, G. (1998). Gestures and words in early development of children with Down syndrome. *Journal of Speech, Language and Hearing Research, 41,* 1125–1135.

Caselli, M. C., & Volterra, V. (1990). From Communication to language in hearing and deaf children. In V. Volterra & C. Erting (Eds.) *From gesture to language in hearing and deaf children.* Berlino: Springer Verlag, pp. 263–277 (1994—2nd Edition Washington, D.C.: Gallaudet University Press).

Caselli, M. C., Volterra, V., Camaioni, L., & Longobardi, E. (1993). Sviluppo gestuale e vocale nei primi due anni di vita. *Psicologia Italiana,* IV, 62–67.

Caselli, M. C., Volterra, V., & Pizzuto, E. (1984, April). The relationship between vocal and gestural communication from the one-word to the two-word stage. Paper presented at the *International Conference on Infant Studies,* New York, NY.

Chapman, R. S. (1995). Language Development in Children and Adolescents with Down Syndrome. In P. Fletcher & B. MacWhinney (Eds.), *The Handbook of Child Language.* Oxford: Blackwell, pp. 641–663.

Corballis, M. C. (2002). *From hand to mouth—The origins of language.* Princeton, NJ: Princeton University Press.

Dale, P. S., Bates, E., Reznick, J. S., & Morisset, C. (1989). The validity of a parental report instrument of child language at twenty months. *Journal of Child Language, 16,* 239–429.

Deacon, T. (1997). *The symbolic species. The coevolution of language and the human brain.* The Penguin Press.

Elman, J. L., Bates, E., Johnson, M. H., Karmiloff-Smith, A., Parisi, D. & Plunkett, K. (1996). *Rethinking Innateness.* Cambridge, Mass: MIT Press.

Erting, C., Volterra, V. (1990). Conclusion. In V. Volterra, C. Erting (eds), *From gesture to language in hearing and deaf children.* Berlino: Springer Verlag, pp. 299–303. (1994—2nd Edition Washington, D.C.: Gallaudet University Press).

Fabbretti, D., Pizzuto, E., Vicari, S., & Volterra, V. (1997). A story description task with Down's syndrome: lexical and morphosyntactic abilities. *Journal of Intellectual Disability Research, 41,* 165–179.

Fenson, L., Dale, P. S., Reznick, J. S., Thal, D., Bates, E., Hartung, J. P., Pethick, S., & Reilly, J. S. (1993). *Communicative Development Inventories.* San Diego, CA: MacArthur.

Fowler, A. E. (1995). Language variability in persons with Down syndrome. In L. Nadel & D. Rosenthal (Eds.), *Down syndrome: Living and learning in the community.* New York: Wiley-Liss.

Franco, F., Wishart, J. G. (1995). The use of pointing and other gestures by young children with Down syndrome. *American Journal of Mental Retardation, 2,* 160–182.

Gallese, V., Fadiga, L., Fogassi L. & Rizzolatti, G. (1996). Action recognition in the premotor cortex. *Brain, 119,* 593–609.

Goldin-Meadow, S. & Morford, M. (1985). Gesture in early child language: Studies of hearing and deaf children. *Merrill-Palmer Quarterly, 31,* 145–176.

Goldin-Meadow, S. & Morford, M. (1990). Gesture in early child language. In V. Volterra & C. J. Erting (Eds.), *From gesture to language in hearing and deaf children.* New York: Springer-Verlag, pp. 249–262.

Greenfield, P. M. & Smith, J. H. (1976). *The structure of communication in early language development.* New York: Academic Press.

Hewes, G. W. (1976). The current status of the gestural theory of language origin. *Annals of the New York Academy of Sciences,* vol. 280, 482–604.

Iverson, J. M., Capirci, O., & Caselli, M. C. (1994). From communication to language in two modalities. *Cognitive Development, 9,* 23–43.

Iverson, J. M., Capirci, O., Longobardi, E., Caselli, M. C. (1999). Gesturing in Mother-child Interaction. *Cognitive Development, 14,* 57–75.

Iverson, J., Longobardi E., & Caselli, M. C. (2003). The Relationship between Gestures and Words in Children with Down Syndrome and Typically-Developing Children in the Early

Stages of Communicative Development. *International Journal of Language and Communication Disorders, 38,* 179–197.

Iverson, J. M., Thelen, E. (1999). Hand, mouth, and brain: The dynamic emergence of speech and gesture. *Journal of Consciousness Studies, 6,* 19–40.

Karmiloff-Smith, A. (1997). Crucial differences between developmental cognitive neuroscience and adult neuropsychology. *Developmental Neuropsychology, 13(4),* 513–524.

Kendon, A. (1995). Gestures as illocutionary and discourse structure markers in Southern Italian conversation. *Journal of Pragmatics, 23,* 1–33.

Kendon, A. (2002). Historical observations on the relationship between research on sign languages and language origins theory. In D. Armstrong, M. Karchmer, J. Van Cleeve (Eds.), *The Study of Sign Languages—Essays in Honor of William C. Stokoe.* Washington, D.C.: Gallaudet University Press, pp. 35–52.

Laing, E., Butterworth, G., Ansari, D., Gsodl, M., Longhi, E., Paterson, S. & Karmiloff-Smith, A. (2002). Atypical development of language and social communication in toddlers with Williams syndrome. *Developmental Science 5 (2),* 233–246.

Leroy, M. (1969). *Profilo storico della linguistica moderna.* Bari: Laterza.

Luchenti, S., Ossella, T., Tieri, L., & Volterra, V. (1988). Una scheda di osservazione per il bambino sordo alla prima diagnosi audiologica. *Giornale di Neuropsichiatria dell'Età Evolutiva, 8,* 4, 313–328.

Magno Caldognetto, E., & Poggi, I. (1995). Conoscenza e uso di gesti simbolici: Differenze di sesso e di età. *Atti del Convegno Internazionale di Studi "Dialettologia al Femminile".* Padova, Italy: CLEUP, pp. 399–412.

McNeill, D. (1992). *Hand and Mind—What gestures reveal about thought.* Chicago: University of Chicago Press.

McNeill, D. (Ed.). (2000). *Language and Gesture.* Cambridge: Cambridge University Press.

Pinker, S. (1994). *The language instinct: How the mind creates language.* New York: William Morrow.

Pizzuto, E., Capirci, O., Caselli, M. C., Iverson, J. M., & Volterra, V. (2000). Children's transition to two-word speech: Content, structure and functions of gestural and vocal productions. Paper presented at the *7th International Pragmatics Conference,* Budapest, July 9–14 2000.

Rizzolatti, G., & Arbib, M. A. (1998). Language within our grasp. *TINS, 21,* 188–194.

Singer Harris, N., Bellugi, U., Bates, E., Jones, W., & Rossen, M. (1997). Contrasting profiles of language development in children with Williams and Down Syndromes. *Developmental Neuropsychology, 13(3),* 345–370.

Slobin, D. I. (Ed.). (1985). *The crosslinguistic study of language acquisition. Vol. 1: The data, Vol. 2: Theoretical issues.* Mahwah, NJ: Lawrence Erlbaum Associates.

Slobin, D. I. (Ed.). (1992). *The crosslinguistic study of language acquisition. Vol. 3.* Hillsdale, NJ: Lawrence Erlbaum Associates.

Slobin, D. I. (Ed.). (1997). *The crosslinguistic study of language acquisition. Vol. 4.* Mahwah, NJ: Lawrence Erlbaum Associates.

Tomasello, M. (1999). *The cultural origins of human cognition.* Cambridge, MA: Harvard University Press.

van den Bogaerde, B. (2000). *Input and Interaction in Deaf Families* (Doctoral dissertation). Utrecht, NL: LOT.

van den Bogaerde, B., & Mills, A. (1995). *Propositional content in different modes: An analysis of the language production of deaf and hearing children of deaf parents.* Paper presented at the Child Language Seminar, Bristol, April 7–9.

Vicari, S., Caselli, M. C., & Tonucci, F. (2000). Asynchrony of lexical and morphosyntactic development in children with Down Syndrome. *Neuropsychologia, 38,* 634–644.

Vico, G. (1744). *La Scienza Nuova.* Naples: Stamperia Muziana [1954 edition by F. Nicolini, *Giambattista Vico—Opere.* Verona: Stamperia Valdonega., pp. 531–550]

Volterra, V. (1981). Gestures signs and words at two years: When does communication become language? *Sign Language Studies, 33,* 351–362.

Volterra, V., Bates, E., Benigni, L., Bretherton, I., Camaioni, L. (1979). First words in language and action: A qualitative look. In E. Bates, *The emergence of symbols: cognition and communication in infancy.* New York: Academic Press, pp. 141–222.

Volterra, V., Capirci, O., Pezzini, G., Sabbadini, L., & Vicari, S. (1996). Linguistic Abilities in Italian Children with Williams Syndrome. *Cortex, 32,* 663–677.

Volterra, V., Erting, C. (Eds.). (1990). *From gesture to language in hearing and deaf children.* Berlino: Springer Verlag. (1994—2nd Edition Washington, D.C.: Gallaudet University Press).

Volterra, V., Iverson, J. M. (1995). When do modality factors affect the course of language acquisition? In K. Emmorey, J. Reilly (Eds.), *Language, Gesture, and Space.* Hillsdale, NJ: Erlbaum, pp. 371–390.

Wescott, R., Hewes, G., & Stokoe, W. C. (Eds.). (1974). *Language origins.* Silver Spring, MD: Linstok Press.

Chapter 2

Commonality and Individual Differences in Vocabulary Growth

Philip S. Dale
Judith C. Goodman
University of Missouri–Columbia

A CRUCIAL METHODOLOGICAL INNOVATION[1]

We live in an era of high-tech everyday life. Computer chips can be found in automobiles, toys, washing machines and toasters. The study of language use and acquisition is no exception. Among the techniques currently in fashion are computerized analysis of language samples (MacWhinney, 2000), split video monitors with a soundtrack that matches one image for the study of language comprehension (Hirsh-Pasek & Golinkoff, 1996), evoked-potential recording to trace the division of labor between the two hemispheres in language processing (Mills, Coffey-Corina & Neville, 1997), magnetic resonance imaging (MRI) to identify the brain locus of specific aspects of language processing (Raichle, 1994), and molecular genetic techniques to identify and characterize the influence of specific genes on language (Plomin & Dale, 2000; Meaburn, Dale, Craig & Plomin, 2002).

In contrast to these technologically complex methods, this chapter is based largely on the revival and improvement of a very old and low-tech approach to studying language; one that is not only practical and cost effective, but is also, for certain purposes, simply *better* than the alternatives. It is *parent report*: the systematic utilization of the extensive and representative experience of parents (and potentially other caregivers) with their children. Parent report, in the form of diary studies, is in fact the oldest form of

---

[1] Portions of this section have been adapted from Dale (1996) and Fenson et al. (1994).

child language research. A long series of "baby biographies," often examining language, began with Tiedemann's 1787 diary of infant behavior and includes such distinguished examples as Darwin's 1877 study (both excerpted in Bar-Adon & Leopold, 1971). The tradition continues fruitfully, as in Dromi (1987) and Tomasello (1992).

Despite the scientific significance of these studies, there has been an understandable reluctance to use parent report more generally for purposes of language assessment or substantive investigation. Unlike Dromi and Tomasello, most parents do not have specialized training in language development and may not be sensitive to subtle aspects of structure and use. Furthermore, a natural pride in their own child and a failure to critically test their impressions may cause a parent to overestimate developmental level; conversely, frustration in the case of delayed language may lead to underestimates.

One of the most striking developments in the study of child language, and indeed developmental psychology more generally, over the past 20 years is the revival of parent report as a trustworthy, and trusted, research technique. The work of Elizabeth Bates and her colleagues in Italy and the United States has been central to this revival.[2] Indeed, the single most widely used language assessment instrument for young children included in published research today is a product of Bates's research program: The MacArthur Communicative Development Inventories (MCDI; Fenson, Dale, Reznick, Bates, Thal, & Pethick, 1994).

The MacArthur Communicative Development Inventories had their genesis in free-form interviews with parents (Bates et al., 1975). They continued to evolve through structured interviews using a standard set of open-ended probes (Bates, Benigni, Bretherton, Camaioni & Volterra, 1979), to a highly structured checklist administered orally, to a self-administered checklist format, the Early Language Inventory (never published, but widely used in research). Gradually a range of aspects of early language and communication was incorporated in the research program, including preverbal communication and symbolic skills, morphology, and syntax. A more complete account of this development, including the emergence of an impressive body of validation evidence for these measures, may be found in Fenson et al. (1994) and Dale (1996). By 1988, there was clear evidence for the research and clinical utility of this type of measure, together with a body of detailed, item-by-item information necessary to develop scales with adequate psychometric properties. With funding from the MacArthur Foundation Network on Early Childhood Transitions, a final, substantial revision

---

[2]Rescorla's development and research on the Language Development Inventory (Rescorla, 1989) has also played an important role, especially in demonstrating the clinical usefulness of this approach.

was undertaken, along with a very large (N = 1,803) norming project, and several validation studies.

Following the principle that parents can best evaluate *emerging* aspects of language, two forms of the Inventory were developed, one for children between 8–16 months (*MacArthur Communicative Development Inventory: Words and Gestures*, or MCDI:WG) and one for children between 16 and 30 months (*MacArthur Communicative Development Inventory: Words and Sentences*, or MCDI:WS). Both instruments are often used with somewhat older children whose communicative development is delayed. The MCDI:WG includes two major components. The first is a 396-item vocabulary checklist organized into 19 semantic categories. Parents indicate for each word if the child *understands* the word, or if the child *understands and says* the word. The second component is a list of 63 communicative, social, and symbolic gestures. The MCDI:WS also has two major components. The first is a vocabulary checklist of 680 words organized in 22 semantic categories. Parents are asked only to indicate if they have heard their child *say* the word. The second major component utilizes an innovative sentence pair format to assess grammar, e.g., to judge whether "kitty sleep" or "kitty sleeping" sounds most like the way their child is talking. (See Marchman & Thal, this volume, for more discussion of the grammar component.)

The central place of vocabulary in the MCDI is itself notable. Vocabulary development was relatively neglected in research on early language development during the 1960s and 1970s. One source of this neglect was the difficulty of studying vocabulary in young children, for whom structured testing is often unfeasible. Probably more important, however, was the intense focus on syntax that stemmed from Chomsky's (1957) emphasis on the complexity, creativity, and abstractness of syntactic structure, and the exciting discovery of some of this complexity and creativity in the language of quite young children (Brown, 1973). The linguistics and psycholinguistics of the era emphasized the distinction between lexicon and grammar. On first consideration, lexical development appeared to be less creative, less combinatorial, and less pattern-governed than syntax. Nevertheless, by the late 1970s interest in vocabulary development also revived. Several sources contributed to this revival. One was interest in the cognitive foundations of lexical development (Bloom, 1973; Gopnik & Meltzoff, 1986). Another was interest in individual differences (Nelson, 1973). But we suggest that the main reason was a renewed appreciation of the fundamental challenge of learning a word. Consider what would appear to be the simplest condition of word learning. A fluent speaker of the language, such as a parent, undertakes to teach a learner a word by uttering the word, say, "gavagai" and pointing in the direction of a small furry white object, recognizably a rabbit (borrowing from Quine, 1960). What does "gavagai" mean? Does it mean 'rabbit'? Perhaps, but it might also plausibly mean 'white' or 'animal' or 'food' or 'tail' or 'my pet rabbit'. Each type of reference is a plausible use of the word. And even if we were correct in believing that "gavagai" meant 'rabbit', how would we know the range of animals to which this label might be correctly applied? That is, every word other than proper names is a label for a *category*, not a single object, action or quality. Learning the category boundaries for each word is a specific "problem of induction." Children are placed in exactly this situation, and must solve the problem for tens of thousands of words; the fact that they do so successfully means that some general principles of acquisition must be involved (Clark, 1995; Markman, 1994). While the MCDI provides measures of gesture and grammatical development, it is largely devoted to measuring vocabulary, and that will be the focus of the present chapter.

Advances in observational and measurement techniques have often directly stimulated theoretical advances, because they do not simply lead to more precise measurement of what is already studied, but to the observation and/or measurement of new entities or quantities. The development of the microscope and of the telescope are good examples of this, leading to the discovery of new forms of life and new objects in the sky, respectively. The same process occurs in the study of language development. As Bates and Carnevale (1993) wrote, "the field of child language has reached a new level of precision and sophistication in the way that we code and quantify linguistic data. Single-case studies, qualitative descriptions and compelling anecdotes will continue to play an important role. But they cannot and will not be forced to bear the full weight of theory-building in our field." The development of the MCDI made possible a measure of overall vocabulary size which was both comprehensive and cost-effective. Unlike structured tests of vocabulary, it was not biased toward nouns and other words which are easily pictured; unlike language samples, it was not biased toward high-frequency words. Furthermore, it was cost-effective enough to be used longitudinally with a substantial sample. Thus it provides a perspective on early language development, especially vocabulary development, that was not previously possible. In particular, it made possible the establishment of a database on vocabulary development which was could be used to characterize both commonality and individual differences in vocabulary development. The ability to draw on both commonality and individual differences provides a foundation for theorizing at the level of specific acquisition processes which is far better grounded than relying on either alone.

The authors of this chapter have been the beneficiaries, both personally and professionally, of the collaborative program of research which led to the MCDI. Liz Bates's collegiality, collaborative enthusiasm, and passionate commitment to addressing the "big questions" of child language development with multiple innovative techniques including parent report are responsible for the major themes of our own research. Her generous friendship and copious humor have made it a delight. In the remainder of this chapter we discuss some of the fruits of our own and related research, much of it done in collaboration with Bates. Three projects receive special emphasis in this far-from-comprehensive review. The first is the norming study for the MCDI (Fenson et al., 1994). At the time of its publication, it was a uniquely large-sample study of child language development, and both the design of the study and the consistency of the results did much to gain acceptance for parent report. It was a cross-sectional study, however, and two other studies have added important longitudinal perspectives. The first is the San Diego Longitudinal Study, conducted by Goodman in collaboration with Bates, which followed a group of 28 children longitudinally from 8 to 30 months with monthly assessment utilizing both the MCDI and laboratory measures of comprehension, production, and word learning. The second is the Twins' Early Development Study (TEDS), directed in the U.K. by Robert Plomin, in which Dale is a collaborator. Measures of language development at ages 2, 3, and 4 years were adapted from the MCDI. In addition to a very large sample size for a longitudinal study—more than 8,000 for most analyses—the twin design made possible the evaluation of genetic and environmental factors in early language development.

WHAT WE HAVE LEARNED ABOUT VOCABULARY GROWTH FROM THE MCDI

Vocabulary Size as Antecedent and Consequent

Does size matter? Does the number of words learned by a young child reflect important aspects of the present or past environment, or of significant organismic factors? Does it have any continuing, i.e., predictive, significance?

Which "Size?" Before addressing the question of vocabulary size directly, we must consider an issue which is begged by the use of the singular noun "size." Almost all parents and other observers of young children have an impression that they understand more words than they produce. Every pediatrician has had worried inquiries about children who have barely started to talk, even though they appear to understand much of the speech addressed to them. That impression is confirmed by more systematic research, which was greatly stimulated by Nelson's (1973) careful comparison of very early receptive and expressive vocabularies (see Bates, Dale & Thal, 1995 for a more complete review). Nevertheless, it is possible that even though receptive vocabulary exceeds expressive, the two might be sufficiently well correlated that a single number would characterize both developments. Here is a first payoff from the increased sample size that is made possible by the use of parent report. As Fenson et al. (1994) document, there is enormous variability in the development of both receptive and expressive vocabulary. But more surprising is the developmental asynchrony between the two. Figure 2.1 illustrates the magnitude of the dissociation. A substantial number of children appear to understand far more words than they produce, including some children who produce no words at all despite receptive vocabularies of 200 words or more. Thus no single number can represent children's early vocabulary accomplishment. A related and intriguing finding is that a measure of expressive gestural development is more highly correlated with vocabulary comprehension that it is with expressive vocabulary, despite the shared modality of gesture with the latter. Bates et al. suggest that this finding is consistent with much other research that suggests "most cognitive variables correlate with what the child *knows* about language (indexed by comprehension), as opposed to what the child *does* (indexed by production)" (p. 113). Lexical comprehension is thus the "leading edge" of early language development. However, because there is much more research on expressive vocabulary as well as information across the wider age range of 8 to 30 months, the remainder of this chapter will focus primarily on measures of expressive vocabulary.

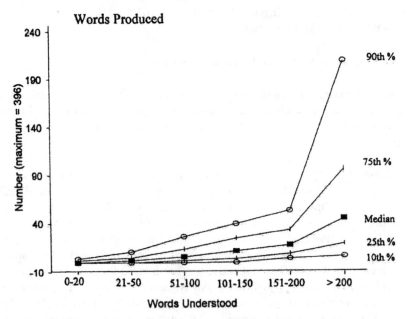

FIG. 2.1.   The relation between infants' word production and the size of their receptive vocabularies, plotted for children at selected percentile levels for word production. Reprinted, by permission, from Fenson et al., 1994.

Vocabulary Size as Consequence of Environmental Factors. A key question about the significance of early vocabulary size is the extent to which it reflects major aspects of the child's environment. Much previous research demonstrates the emergence of social class differences in language during the third year, e.g., Hart and Risley (1995). In the norming study for the MCDI, correlations between SES, as indexed by maternal education, and language measures became significant in the expected direction only for vocabulary production for the MCDI:WS. Even then the correlation was very small, accounting for less than 1% of the variance. However, the norming sample was underrepresentative of low-education parents. A later study by Arriaga, Fenson, Cronan & Pethick (1998) found a more significant effect of SES at the lower extreme. The effect of SES appears to be highly nonlinear, perhaps reflecting a "threshold" effect for language input.

SES is a highly global environmental measure, and one goal of research on language development is the identification of specific aspects of the environment that affect development. Two recent and intriguing findings will be mentioned here. The first is the role of childcare and childcare quality in early development. The National Institute of Child Health and Human Development Study of Early Childcare is a longitudinal prospective study, beginning at birth, of a group of socioeconomically and geographically diverse children. The MCDI:WG and the MCDI:WS were used as outcome measures for language at 15 and 24 months, respectively (NICHD Early Child Care Research Network, 2000). Childcare quality was evaluated on the basis of direct observation of children and caregivers in the facility. Childcare quality, especially frequency of language stimulation, was positively and significantly related to all three MCDI vocabulary measures: comprehension and production at 15 months and production at 24 months. This relation held even when numerous other factors were significantly controlled, including income level, maternal receptive vocabulary, and maternal stimulation of infant. The sensitivity of parent-reported vocabulary to childcare quality was very similar in pattern and magnitude to that found for a tester-administered measure, the Bayley Scales of Infant Development.

The second finding is related to the continuing and lively controversy over whether there is an enduring effect of recurring ear infections, i.e., otitis media. Ear infections may be viewed as an environmental variable, because they affect the amount and quality of input in a fluctuating and intermittent fashion. In a large, population-based study, Feldman, Dollaghan, Campbell, Colborn, Janosky, Kurs-Lasky, Rockette, Dale, and Paradise (2003) compared the cumulative duration of days of otitis media with middle-ear effusion (OME) during the first 3 years of life with reported development on the MCDI:WG at one year, on the MCDI:WS at two years, and on a newly developed upward extension, the CDI–III, at three years. At age one, the correlations were nonsignificant; at two years, either nonsignificant or of questionable clinical significance; and at three years, consistently moderately significant. Interestingly, maternal education and OME contributed independently to scores at three years, presumably by independently affecting input.

Vocabulary Size as Consequence of Genetic Factors.   The role of genetic factors has only recently begun to be considered seriously in the study of language despite the strong trend of much linguistic theorizing to invoke an innate basis for language. Behavioral genetic research can provide an increased understanding of genetic and environmental contributions to individual differences, and of the developmental interplay between nature and nurture. This understanding is likely to improve description, prediction, intervention, and prevention of language disorders (Gilger, 1995; Plomin & Dale, 2000). New analysis techniques make it possible to address even more relevant questions than the overall extent of genetic influence. In particular, they can explore the extent to which disorders are etiologically distinct from normal variation rather than simply being the low end of the continuum responsible for the normal range of variation. In addition, multivariate analyses can investigate the extent to which the same or different genetic (or environmental) factors influence two or more areas of development.

Although a body of evidence for a genetic influence on variability in language development is growing (see Stromswold, 2001, for a comprehensive review), relatively little of it has focused on early development, i.e., before age 3. Furthermore, the new analysis techniques require much larger samples than the classic univariate analysis of estimating heritability. Thus the Twins' Early Development Study (TEDS; Plomin & Dale, 2000), which has examined language and nonverbal development at 2, 3, and 4 years in a very large sample of twins in the UK, has broken fresh ground. As noted several times previously, only parent report—in this case a UK adaptation of the MCDI measures—can provide very large samples of data, although many of the TEDS analyses have been supplemented by smaller-scale studies with in-person assessment. Here we summarize only selected analyses of vocabulary measures; see Marchman and Thal (this volume) for more information on the relation between vocabulary and grammatical development.

How influential are genetic factors for early vocabulary development? Dionne, Dale, Boivin and Plomin (2003) estimated genetic factors to account for approximately 20% of the variance at age 2, and 12% at age 3, both highly significant statistically. In comparison, shared environmental influence, that is, aspects of the environment that are shared by the twins, accounted for 78% and 83% of the variance at the two ages, respectively. (Non-shared environmental factors, including measurement error, are responsible for the remainder of the variance.) Thus genetic factors play a significant role, but are considerably outweighed at this early age by environmental factors.

We can further ask if the same balance of genetic and environmental factors that accounts for variation across the entire distribution is responsible for the lowest extreme of the distribution, that is, children who are learning vocabulary very slowly. Specifically, we asked if genetic factors play a greater role at the lower tail of the distribution. A statistical technique called DF extremes analysis based on comparing the vocabulary scores of co-twins of low-vocabulary twins in identical vs. fraternal pairs (see Bishop, Price, Dale & Plomin, 2003, for further explanation) makes it possible to estimate the relative contribution of genetic and environmental factors to a condition defined in terms of a score below a cutoff on a continuum. Bishop et al. (2003) estimated this "group heritability" to be .24 for placement in the lowest 10% of the distribution of age 2 vocabulary. With a more extreme cutoff of lowest 5%, the group heritability was estimated at .32. Although neither of these figures is significantly different from the 20% heritability estimated at age 2 for the entire distribution, the pattern of results—higher figures for the extremes, and higher for the more extreme cutoff—suggests that it is at least possible that genetic factors play a greater role at the lower extreme. More recently, Spinath, Price, Dale & Plomin (in press), using a composite language measure based on MCDI vocabulary and grammar score, found significantly stronger genetic effects at the extremes (lowest 5% and lowest 10%) than for individual differences heritability across the full distribution; the same pattern was seen at all three ages.

We also note that many conditions that include childhood language impairment are known to have genetic involvement, and that studies of early vocabulary development as indexed by the MCDI in those clinical populations have confirmed both the validity of parent report and a dramatically slower rate of development. The clinical populations studied include children with Down Syndrome (Miller, Sedey, & Miolo, 1995), specific language delay (Thal, O'Hanlon, Clemmons & Fralin, 1999), and autism (Charman, Drew, Baird & Baird, 2003). And as will be seen in the next two sections, a very low vocabulary during the second year of life is a considerable risk factor for later difficulties.

The Predictive Significance of Early Vocabulary Size. We turn now from vocabulary size as consequent to size as antecedent. For early childhood measures especially, the most persuasive argument for their value is evidence for their ability to predict later ability. Human beings differ not only in their level of development at single points in time; they differ in their *trajectory*, their pattern of growth through time. There is a clinical as well as a basic science facet to the study of growth. For example, there is a dilemma familiar to almost every speech-language pathologist and pediatrician: how much concern and/or intervention is warranted in response to a young child whose early development is notably slow? The dilemma is sharpened by the development of well-normed and valid parent report measures such as the MCDI, which document the extensive variability characteristic of early development. We can determine with relative confidence whether a child's development falls, for example, in the lowest 10th percentile at 24 months. But longitudinal studies confirm anecdotal impressions that many late talkers do appear to catch up and score within the normal range by the time they begin school, though they are often still below norms for typically developing children or a matched control group (Thal, 1996; Bishop & Leonard, 2000; Dale et al., 2003). Thus we would not expect to find perfect prediction to the future, even if the measures were perfect. From the point of view of a basic science understanding of development, the pervasive presence of substantial differences in trajectory in such traits as IQ, personality, and psychopathology provides a window on developmental processes. It is the "failures" of early prediction which are likely to be the most illuminating, because simple linear predictions patterns are overdetermined, and hence ambiguous in their interpretation. In the next section, we address analyses of growth directly. Here we simply document the predictive ability of early vocabulary measures.

Bates, Bretherton and Snyder (1988) present the results of a groundbreaking study—in its methods, sample size, and analytical methods—of individual differences in early language development. Twenty-seven children were followed from 10 to 28 months, using a combination of observational, interview, and experimental methods. Of particular interest here is the pattern of predictions from 20 month vocabulary, based on an interview-administered vocabulary checklist. There was a significant and substantial prediction to 28 month vocabulary, whether based on a language sample (r = .64) or on a receptive vocabulary measure, the Peabody Picture Vocabulary Test–Revised (r = .51). Even more striking was the prediction of r = .83 from 20 month vocabulary to 28 month MLU. Indeed, "the single best estimate of grammatical status at 28 months (right in the heart of the 'grammar burst') is total vocabulary size at 20 months (measured right in the middle of the 'vocabulary burst')" (Bates & Goodman, 1997).

These correlations, reinforced by some quite specific correlations involving component subcategories of vocabulary, served as the basis for a complex theory of variation in language development, summarized in Figure 3 of Bates et al. (1988). The theory posited three distinct "strands" of development—comprehension, analyzed production, and rote output—which were realized in different measures at different ages. The strands did not represent polar opposites, but aspects of language learning that could each be strong or weak in a particular child.

Another intriguing finding of this study is the prediction from 20 month vocabulary to a novel label learning task, also administered at 20 months.

Children were exposed to a novel object label, "fiffin," and a novel action label, "gloop." Parent-reported vocabulary was correlated at $r = .51$ with correct responses to requests such as "Make the kitty gloop the fiffin." This *in vitro* demonstration of the relation of current vocabulary to learning was confirmed *in vivo* in the San Diego Longitudinal Study described later. In that study, the number of words children add to their vocabulary each month was determined not so much by age or even overall word-learning ability (i.e., their percentile level), but by the size of their vocabulary the previous month. There is a strong suggestion in these findings of "learning to learn," a phenomenon whereby a single learning mechanism can produce nonlinearities in development.

Utilizing a sample of 8,386 twins in TEDS, Dale et al. (2003) compared parent-report vocabulary at 2 years with similar measures at 3 and 4 years. (These measures were considerably shorter than the full CDI, undoubtedly reducing their reliability and validity to some extent.) The predictive correlations from age 2 to 3 and 4 were .62 and .50, respectively, quite comparable to the results of Bates et al. Of equally great interest as prediction across the full distribution is prediction from very low early scores. Dale et al. (2003) went on to classify 2-year-old children with vocabulary scores below the 10th percentile for that sample as showing early language delay (ELD), and contrasted them with the remainder of the sample. Two years later, at age 4, the vocabulary scores of the ELD group were *on average* one standard deviation below the mean, that is, at about the 16th percentile, though there was very great variability. A more comprehensive definition of language difficulty at 4 was adopted for further analysis, namely, scores below the 15th percentile on at least two of the three parent-provided measures (vocabulary, grammar, use of abstract language). Using this classification scheme, 40.2% of the ELD group was classified as having a continuing difficulty at 4, compared to just 8.5% of the remainder of the group. Thus the ELD group is 4.7 times more likely to have persisting difficulty as the typically developing group. These results are quite consistent with smaller-scale, but more fine-grained longitudinal analyses of late talkers (see Bates, Dale & Thal, 1995, for a review).

Far less is known about variation at the other extreme of the distribution, about the developmental course of children who get off to an usually rapid start to language, even though they too can offer a valuable window on processes of development. It might even be argued that precocity in development is more illuminating than delay. A complex system can be disrupted by a very wide range of factors, whereas it is likely that optimal performance can occur only under a highly constrained set of circumstances. Although there have been several studies of the language of precocious talkers at early stages (Bates, Dale & Thal, 1995), there is little information on the predictive significance of an unusually large early vocabulary. One such study is that of Robinson, Dale & Landesman (1990), who identified children at 20 months on the basis of vocabulary, MLU or verbal reasoning (language items on the Bayley Scales of Infant Development) at a level two standard deviations above the mean. Robinson et al. utilized the Early Language Inventory, a precursor of the MCDI:WS. Only limited norms were available at the time for the ELI; Robinson et al. adopted a criterion of 424 words on the ELI, which corresponds to the 90–95th percentile range on the MCDI:WS. Of the 30 children who met their overall criterion for precocity, 22 met the vocabulary criterion (most of the children satisfied at least two of the criteria). The precocity of the 20-month-olds was maintained over the five years of the project. For example, at 24 months the mean MLU was 3.14, equivalent to that of average children at 36 months; at 30 months the mean PPVT–R vocabulary age equivalent was 42.6 months; and at 6½ years, their Stanford–Binet IV Vocabulary age equivalent was 9 years, 10 months. Each of these scores is approximately two standard deviations above the mean, suggesting that early talkers maintain a significant advantage throughout early childhood. Interestingly, this language advantage did not translate into an equivalent advantage in early reading (Crain-Thoreson & Dale, 1992).

In sum, the MCDI has been the basis of a wealth of research on the social and genetic factors contributing to vocabulary development as well as on the predictability of growth across time. Predictability provides a window on how stable an individual's growth rate is over time. Another way of looking at change and continuity is through growth curve modeling, and we turn now to data from the San Diego Longitudinal Study.

GROWTH CURVE MODELING

Two flavors of research have dominated studies of child language acquisition. One involves collecting longitudinal language samples from a small number of children and examining those corpora for the development of some behavior, such as the use of negative markers. These results are then generalized to all children learning that language. The other is to run controlled studies on a larger number of children, for example, assessing whether children can fast-map a word meaning. These results are then generalized to naturalistic settings. Of course, to generalize most persuasively, it would be desirable to apply the longitudinal approach to large samples. By "systematizing" parent report, the MCDI provides a tool for collecting vocabulary data from a large number of children longitudinally. Parents hear their children in many settings, and these settings are far richer than the relatively impoverished and unfamiliar laboratories of controlled studies. Consequently, the results generalize to the real world where children learn language. Liz Bates has long realized the potential of applying the MCDI to fine-grained longitudinal research. Such research is critical for determining not only universals that generalized across children, but for characterizing and understanding the individual differences between them. Bates et al. (1995) have referred to this dual approach of searching for both the universals and the individual differences in the service of theory building as an attempt "to locate the seams and joints of the language processor, i.e. components that can develop at different rates because they depend on different cognitive and/or neural mechanisms." (p. 97).

A large longitudinal database makes it possible to describe both commonalities and individual differences in the rate and shape of vocabulary acquisition. But one can go a step further and use the data to test theoretical claims by modeling the data formally. A mathematical model of acquisition makes certain assumptions which can be viewed as hypotheses about the mechanisms underlying growth. Comparing the consequences of those assumptions with real growth data is a powerful form of hypothesis testing. One issue that can be addressed with growth curve modeling is the nature—and number—of the mechanism(s) underlying the vocabulary spurt. Children initially establish their lexicons slowly, adding a few words each month for about 6 months. After they produce about 50 to 100 words (typically, around 18–20 months of age), learning appears to speed up dramatically, a period known as the vocabulary spurt (Bloom, 1973; Nelson, 1973). This pattern of development generally has been interpreted as indicating that two different mechanisms are involved in early vocabulary development—first, one that allows children to slowly map words to their meanings and second, one that apparently comes on-line at about 18 months and underlies the period of rapid growth. Candidate new mechanisms include a realization that things have names (Baldwin, 1989) or that they are members of categories (Gopnik & Meltzoff (1987); an improved ability to segment word-sized chunks from fluent speech (Plunkett, 1993); and a shift from an associationistic to a referential lexical acquisition mechanism (Nazzi & Bertoncini, 2003). This sort of account is not surprising. Behavior changes dramatically and begs for an explanation. However, the changing-mechanism explanation is not the only possibility. Non-linear growth patterns can also result from a single nonlinear learning mechanism that operates according to the same rules throughout early vocabulary development, from the very first word. If one can formally model this nonlinear growth spurt using a single set of parameters that start the ball rolling before the period of slow, prespurt acquisition and remain constant through the spurt, it would lend support to this second model, based on a single, nonlinear learning mechanism.

Goodman, Bates, John-Samilo, Appelbaum, Carnevale and Elman (1999) have used this approach to model vocabulary development. The observed data to be modeled were collected from 28 children ranging in age from 8 to 30 months participating in the San Diego Longitudinal Study (Jahn-Samilo, Goodman, Bates, Appelbaum & Sweets, 2003). The children's parents filled out the MCDI monthly. The MCDI:WG form was used until the child was 16 months old or understood 50 words, whichever came later. The MCDI:WS form was used from that point on until children were 30 months old. The group data closely mirror the cross-sectional data collected by Fenson et al., (1994). Figure 2.2 presents the number of words children produced at each month of the study, with children grouped by percentile. The groups show a typical pattern of development, that is, slow initial growth followed by a spurt in the rate of word learning (only the bottom 10th percentile might be an exception). The different levels of ability do differ, however, in how early they begin to "take off" and in how steep their slopes are (determined by the number of words learned each month after the onset of the spurt). Essentially, one sees a "rich-get-richer-and-the-poor-stay-poor" pattern, suggesting that individual differences exist in the nature of the vocabulary spurt. The range of individual differences can be seen more clearly if we look at the 22 months of development for some individual children.

Figure 2.3 presents the growth curves for 6 children individually. While some children look like the average child of the grouped data, others vary in rate of development, the shape of development, or both. Individual differences in rate do not necessarily challenge the standard two-mechanism story of the vocabulary spurt. Rather, they may simply mean that whatever that second mechanism is, some children get it sooner than others. But suppose that the new mechanism responsible for the vocabulary spurt is the realization that things have names. While it is clear what it means to say that a precocious child realizes that all things have names or are members of categories, or can be segmented from the stream of speech BEFORE a more slowly-developing child realizes the same thing, differences in the shape of growth are harder to explain. Does the fast developing child with a very steep slope have, for example, MORE of a realization that all things have names? Does the child who is developing with only a gradual slope have only half an "Aha experience" that world's things have names or think that only some things names? The same question could be asked about other mechanisms that have been proposed to explain the vocabulary spurt. At least for now, it is not clear how to reconcile claims of a new mechanism coming on-line with individual variation in the shape of change.

An alternative approach is to assume that the same mechanisms that started the ball rolling and are responsible for the slower learning observed in the early phase of development are responsible for nonlinear growth spurts as well. Some preliminary curve-fitting that we have done lend support to this view (Goodman et al., 1999). The observed growth data from

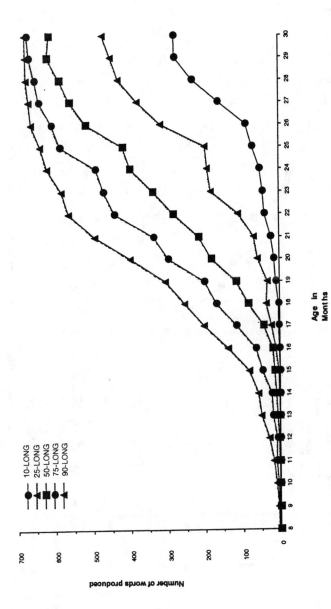

FIG. 2.2. Number of words produced by age for the 10th, 25th, 50th, 75th, and 90th percentiles.

55

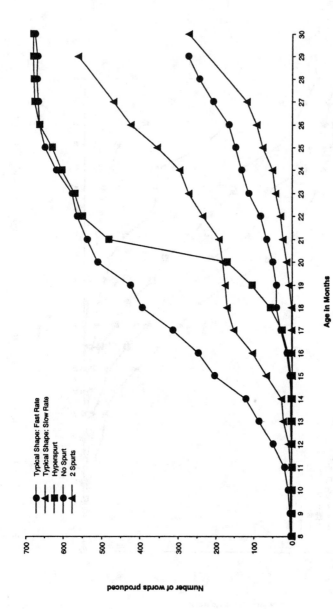

FIG. 2.3.   Vocabulary growth trajectories for five individual children.

the MCDI was compared to models generated by a class of dynamical, non-linear mathematical equations. Dynamical, non-linear equations allow the rate of change to vary across time. The rate of change at any given time also depends on the state of the system as a whole at that moment. The equation was of the form $dy/dt = ay^2 + by + c$. dy/dt represents a derivative, not division, and can be read as *the rate of change in y per unit of change in t.* The variable y represents the number of words, t represents time, and a, b, and c are parameters that are estimated to fit the growth observed for each child. The formula posits that the rate of change in y is a function of the current value of y. For each child, a was set to the largest number of words a child might know, 680 words on the MCDI:WS. The b and c parameters were allowed to vary, using a parametric search to find the values of b and c that fit each child best. This was done by using a deviation score (the average number of words separating the predicted vs. observed curve at each time point) as a measure of error. In the end, when we had converged on the best fit for every child, these deviation scores averaged 8.85, ranging from a low of 1.71 to a high of 19.94. In other words, our best theoretical estimates tended to deviate from the observed vocabulary totals by an average of only 9 words at any given month. Figure 2.4 shows the observed data and the fitted curves for several children. What one can see with these examples is that the shape of change predicted through curve fitting two parameters (b and c) matches the shape of change observed in children remarkably well. Despite large individual variations in the timing and size of the vocabulary spurt, a single class of equations can predict the rate and shape of developmental change.

The point here is *not* that this specific equation can most elegantly model children's behavior, but that it is possible to construct a single growth equation that, when applied continuously over time, may explain nonlinearities and apparent discontinuities in vocabulary acquisition. One does not need to posit one causal mechanism to help children to slowly learn those first words and a second causal mechanism to explain the rapid growth seen after they know 50 to 100 words. "The important insight here is that we need no external cause to change the course of development halfway through life. The rise and fall of this developmental system are prefigured in the same dynamic equation, set into motion at the beginning of its life." (Elman, Bates, Johnson, Karmiloff-Smith, Parisi & Plunkett, 1996, p. 199.)

VARIATION VIEWED LONGITUDINALLY

Common Patterns. Although the norming study of the MCDI (Fenson, et al, 1994) provided a wealth of data regarding the patterns of vocabulary growth across children, it presented still photographs of many children of different ages. A moving picture of the course of development—a fine-

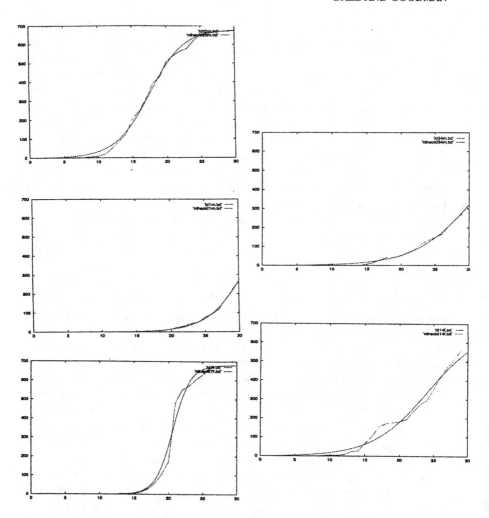

FIG. 2.4.   Observed vocabulary growth trajectories for the five children in
Fig. 2.3 plotted with the predicted growth trajectories based on a nonlinear
dynamic model. Each graph represents one child with age on the x-axis and
number of words produced on the y-axis.

grained look at individual growth patterns—can complement this enormous data set by confirming both the common patterns of development reported in the literature and the enormous variation in those patterns
shown by the norming study, and by identifying individual idiosyncrasies in
development.

Looking first at aggregate data, the major patterns of the norming study
are confirmed. For example, Fig. 2.5 shows the median number of words

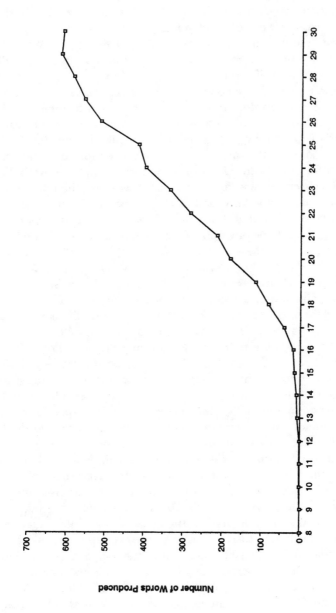

FIG. 2.5. Median number of words produced by children's age from the MCDI data collected in the San Diego Longitudinal Study.

comprehended and produced by children in this study for each month of age. In both measures we see the characteristic patterns of development that have been described in the literature. Initial word acquisition is slow but, particularly for production, the rate of acquisition speeds up considerably after a few months of acquisition.

Another commonality between the 2 datasets concerns variation. A core finding of the MCDI norming study is that enormous individual variation exists with respect to the acquisition of language skills. Language researchers and clinicians have long acknowledged variability in rate (cf. Shore, 1995), but the extent of the variation among children found in the cross-sectional study for both comprehension and production, as shown in Figs. 2.6a and 2.7a respectively, was far greater than expected. The longitudinal study found the same fan-like variation (Figs. 2.6b and 2.7b). It may be counterintuitive to call variation a "common pattern," but the enormous variations in rate and shape of vocabulary growth by now seem as well-nigh universal phenomena as the vocabulary spurt.

Of course, one wants to know what factors influence the rate of growth. The norming study (Fenson et al., 1994) noted that the no single factor such as gender, birth order or maternal education, accounts for a substantial amount of the variation across children. One possibility is that some children are simply faster learners, so that at any given level of vocabulary knowledge they are adding more words each month. Do children in the 90th percentile learn more words than children in the 10th percentile for a given month even at the same vocabulary size, such as when each group knows 100 words? The first group would be much younger, of course. Examining the data longitudinally allows us to look at this aspect of growth rate. A new common pattern emerges, namely, the number of words children add to their vocabulary each month is not determined by their age or by their overall word-learning ability (i.e., what percentile they fall in), but by the size of their vocabulary the previous month. Figure 2.8 plots the number of words added to receptive vocabulary each month as a function of vocabulary size the previous month. Further, children are grouped by rate of growth (percentile rankings). Although all of the children range in age from 8 to about 16 months, there is very little overlap in the number of words that children in the 10th, 50th, and 90th percentiles learn in a month. Rather as the number of words the children know increases, the number of words they add each month increases as well. This implies that the rich get richer because they can use words that they know to learn more words. For example, a child knows the word *eat* and hears someone say, "Mmm, Mommy's eating a kumquat!" she can infer a good bit about the word *kumquat* (see also Goodman, McDonough, and Brown, 1998). A similar picture emerges for production at least up to a productive vocabulary of 200 words (Fig. 2.9). Once children know 200 words, however, some addi-

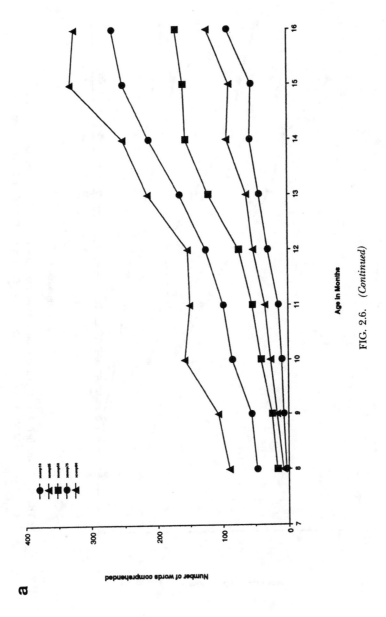

Age in Months

FIG. 2.6. *(Continued)*

a

Number of words comprehended

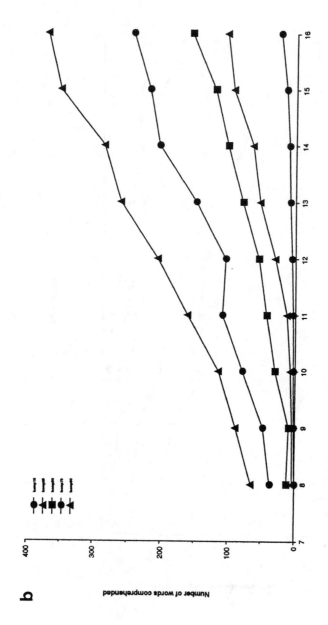

FIG. 2.6. Number of words comprehended by age in months at five percentile levels, from the cross-sectional MCDI norming study (2.6a, p. 61) and the San Diego Longitudinal Study (2.6b, p. 62).

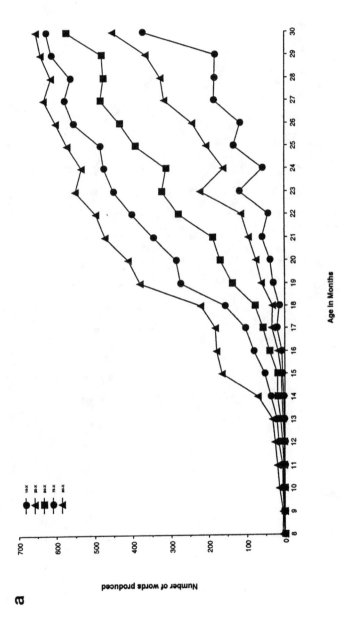

FIG. 2.7. (Continued)

63

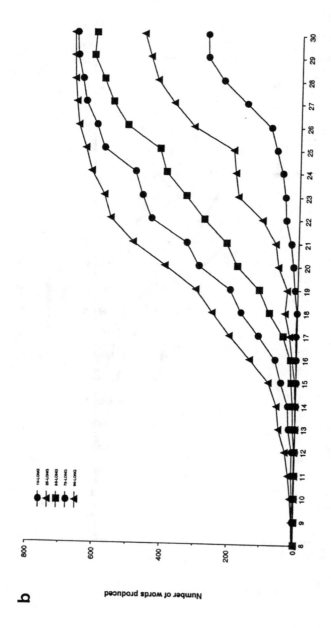

FIG. 2.7. Number of words produced by age in months at five percentile levels, from the cross-sectional MCDI norming study (2.7a, p. 63) and the San Diego Longitudinal Study (2.7b, p. 64).

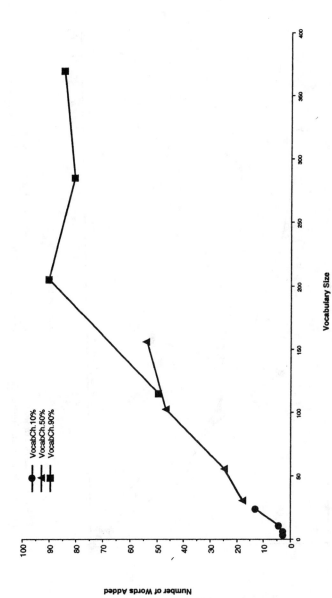

FIG. 2.8. Number of words added to the children's receptive vocabulary each month as a function of vocabulary size for the 10th, 50th, and 90th percentiles in the San Diego Longitudinal Study.

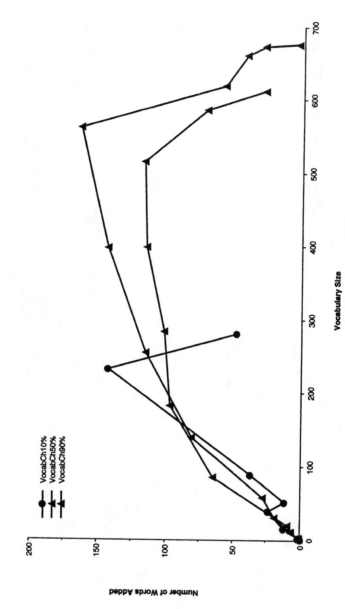

FIG. 2.9.   Number of words to the children's productive vocabulary each month as a function of vocabulary size for the 10th 50th, and 90th percentiles in the San Diego Longitudinal Study.

tional factor also influences the number of words added each month such that children in the 90th percentile who produce between 200 and 600 words add more new words to their vocabulary each month than children in the 50th who know between 200 and 600 words. Perhaps they are more willing to take risks and say the word or perhaps they are more able to retrieve words. This is a topic requiring further study.

Individual Differences.   The San Diego Longitudinal Study allows us to examine not only group differences in vocabulary growth, but differences at the individual level as well. Thus one can begin to assess how universal the prototypic growth pattern truly is. For example, do all children start out adding a few words to their vocabulary each month and then show a vocabulary spurt when they produce between 50 and 100 words? As noted in the growth curve section above, children vary not only in the rate at which they learn new words, but also in the shape of their growth trajectories. Figure 2.3 shows a variety of different patterns from individual children. (1) and (2) show the standard slow-early-development-followed-by-a-vocabulary-spurt that the literature has taught us to expect, but one child began learning words earlier and continues to add them at a faster rate than the other child. Children (3), (4), and (5), however, deviate in the shape of growth. (3) shows a hyperspurt; that is she got a slow start, but when s/he spurted, that spurt was far more dramatic than for most children. (4), on the other hand, shows slow, steady development with no evidence of a spurt by 30 months of age. (5) shows a vocabulary spurt that levels off and then resumes again later. Any theory of language development must account not only for children who vary in rate, but also for children who show a different pattern. As discussed earlier, the common explanations that rely on changes in mechanism (e.g., children realize that all things have names, are members of categories, etc.) are not particularly satisfying here. Understanding the range of variation in patterns of acquisition will be critical in figuring out the underlying mechanisms responsible for vocabulary learning.

CROSSLINGUISTIC COMPARISONS AND STUDIES OF BILINGUALISM

Crosslinguistic comparisons of child language have been among the most powerful sources of theory development. The response of the human child's ability to learn language to the distinctive patterns of each language, both the variations that occur and the limitations ("constraints") to that variation, provides some of the clearest evidence for specific theoretical processes (cf. the remarkable series of crosslinguistic acquisition surveys edited by Slobin beginning with Slobin, 1985). For the most part, however, only modest numbers of children have been examined in each language until recently, sometimes as small as n = 1. Small samples may give a plausible estimate of the central tendency of a distribution, but little information on the variability. The success of the MCDI has stimulated the development of similar instruments for other languages, and thus provides the potential for larger samples for comparison across languages.

It is important to note that each of these versions is an *adaptation* of the MCDI, not just a simple translation. Languages and cultures differ substantially in both the form and content of their communication systems. Even in the earliest phases, differences in gestural communication, vocabulary, and grammar will be noticeable. For example, Ogura, Yamashita, Murase & Dale (1993) included bowing as an early emerging gesture in Japanese, while Jackson-Maldonado, Thal, Marchman, Newton, Fenson and Conboy (2003) included *tortillitas* ('little tortillas'), a variant of the pat-a-cake game that is played in Mexico. A current listing of adaptations and their status is available on the MCDI website, at http://www.sci.sdsu.edu/cdi/.

Limitations of space preclude a review of the results of this fruitful line of research. But it is notable that nearly all of the main results from English-speaking children are replicated in studies of Italian, Spanish, Hebrew, Japanese, Chinese, and other languages. In particular, there is enormous variability in rate of lexical acquisition, a positive acceleration is noted in the second year of life, comprehension and production are substantially dissociated with a "fan effect" relating them, gestural communication is more strongly related to receptive vocabulary than productive vocabulary, and vocabulary production is strongly related to grammatical development (see Marchman & Thal, this volume). The single area of possible variation concerns the noun predominance in early vocabulary. Even in languages such as Italian and Japanese, whose structure might be expected to make verbs more salient by e.g., allowing subject and other NPs to be deleted, or by favoring verbs in final position, nouns are generally predominant. However, serious methodological debates continue on this issue, and it is possible that in some languages—Mandarin provides the strongest evidence so far—nouns do not show a dominance. If this is the case, the reasons for it are likely to be highly illuminating. It may be that the pragmatics of sentence use are more important than more obvious structural features. For further discussion, see Gentner (1982), Caselli, Bates, Casadio, Fenson, Fenson, Sanders, and Weir (1995), Jackson-Maldonado, Thal, Marchman, Bates et al. (1993), and Tardif, Shatz & Naigles (1997).

In addition to comparisons of monolingual children across languages, the availability of MCDI adaptations in other languages provides a powerful tool for the study of bilingual development. One such study is described in Marchman & Thal (this volume).

SOME FUTURE DIRECTIONS

The research reviewed above provides considerable evidence for the utility of comprehensive parent report to ground developmental theorizing about vocabulary development. In this concluding section, we sketch two research programs in progress to assess aspects of vocabulary development. They might be contrasted as the "wide-angle lens" approach and the "microscopic lens" approach. The first is an extension of the growth curve modeling approach described earlier in this chapter. In this approach, the basic unit of analysis is the widest possible: not an examination of vocabulary size or even composition at a single moment in time, but the shape of change over time. The second zooms in on the acquisition of individual words, seeking to identify and evaluate the causal influence of structural and environmental factors.

Growth Curve Modeling and Psychological Theories

A nonlinear dynamic model with two free parameters does a good job of modeling individual growth trajectories in vocabulary despite variation in the shapes of the curves. This result lends plausibility to the idea that we do not need to posit changing psychological mechanisms to explain nonlinear development. Nonetheless, without knowing what b and c represent, we do not know what is responsible for change. We don't know whether these variables represent the amount of input, or some general intelligence, or some language-specific intelligence, or something entirely different. Translating these parameters to psychological mechanisms will not be a simple exercise. However, one can proceed in several directions to try to identify the mechanisms that are driving nonlinear change in vocabulary and nonmonotonic changes in the rate of growth—that is, an initial revving up followed by a slowing down.

One approach would be to examine how the parameters correspond to observed measures collected for the children. For example, preliminary correlations between b and c and various CDI and laboratory measures indicate that b and c do not seem to bear a strong and consistent relationship to absolute scores for vocabulary size at any given month, nor do they correlate with other aspects of communication like word comprehension and gesture. In other words, b and c are not some fancy equivalent of Spearman's g which be interpreted as simple estimates of "good learning rate" that correlate in a linear fashion with just about anything else that we measure in these children. But perhaps that should not surprise us: the parameters in this model are nonlinear in nature, integrated at every point across this period of growth. Hence, we shouldn't expect them to work as linear predictors of any and all aspects of language and communicative development.

However, if these variables index some aspect of absolute learning efficiency, then they might map onto performance in a novel word-learning task. The lab component of the San Diego Longitudinal Study included a novel word learning task. One could add the number of exposures a child needed to learn a novel word as a separate parameter indicating general mapping ability, and assess the effect on b and c. Similarly, the laboratory sessions included free play between these children and their parents. This could provide an estimate of the amount of input each child receives and could be added as an additional variable in the model to see how b and c then change. If b and c depend in part on the amount of input, then they should change when this variable is added independently.

The b and c parameters conflate many factors that influence word learning. We need to better specify how several factors interact in determining the dynamics of vocabulary acquisition over time. Nonetheless, the results to date suggest that the dominant two-mechanism view of the vocabulary shift is not necessary. That is, a dramatic shift in mechanism is not logically needed to explain a dramatic shift in observable behavior. A more parsimonious view is that one mechanism underlies the slow, initial development of the lexicon as well as the more rapid increase known as the vocabulary spurt.

Building an Integrated Model of Vocabulary Development

The vocabulary of English, like that of other languages, is enormous; even the vocabulary likely to be heard by children is of the order of magnitude of tens of thousands of words. And yet there are remarkable commonalities of order of acquisition. Indeed, it is precisely those commonalities which make possible the construction of a valid vocabulary checklist for young children. Why are some words learned before others? Roger Brown (1958) suggested one important factor, at least for nouns. Most objects can receive a multiplicity of names, e.g., *plant, flower, jonquil*, which refer to narrower or broader categories. Some developmental theories might predict a progression from larger to smaller categories, whereas other might predict a progression from smaller to larger categories. In fact, Brown noted, children are most likely to begin an intermediate level of generality, with *flower* before the superordinate term *plant* and before the subordinate term *jonquil*. He concluded that it is the functional equivalence of items in the intermediate categories that makes the category labels easier to learn. Brown also related this feature of early naming to parental language: mothers are more likely to use these terms just because they do correspond to functionally equivalent categories. Later this notion of intermediate, functionally equivalent category labeling would be elaborated into the concept of basic level categories by Rosch (Rosch, Mervis, Gray, Johnson, & Boyes-Braem, 1976).

Other factors have been nominated as potentially influential. For example, early vocabularies have high proportions of nouns, concrete words appear to be learned before abstract words, "simple words" are learned before "complex" words, and time and emotion words appear to be particularly challenging. However, more precise empirical research on this question has been difficult, primarily because of a lack of relevant data. Structured tests are inappropriate for very young children, and in any case, cannot assess more than a small proportion of vocabulary. Language samples are heavily biased by differences in word frequency, and thus substantially underestimate vocabulary. Furthermore, it is essential to have an adequate sample of children to estimate mean ages of acquisition.

The high reliability and validity of parent report measures such as the MCDI, together with the remarkable consistency found between developmental trends in the parent report data and reports in the developmental psycholinguistics research literature (Fenson et al. 1994), suggests that the inventories may be taken to provide "high-resolution" data on vocabulary growth. Goodman, Dale and Li (2003) therefore took the age of acquisition of each word (defined as the age at which 50% of the children in the norming sample were reported to produce it) included in one or both of the MCDI instruments as the "dependent variable" for prediction by hypothesized causal factors. We excluded words which were not acquired by 30 months using this definition, items which were multiword forms (e.g., *on top of*), and proper names (e.g., a pet's or babysitter's name).

There are at least two qualifications to be made to this research approach. First, the present data can be used only to examine factors influencing *early* vocabulary growth, up through 30 months. Additional factors may become important later, and the relative importance of predictors found in the present study may change later. For example, there are virtually no superordinate words on the MCDI (at most, *animal, food,* and *toy* might qualify), so it is not possible to investigate the impact of basic vs. superordinate category labels. Second, the MCDI vocabulary checklists, while lengthy, cannot provide an exhaustive "atlas" of any child's vocabulary. It is very likely that any particular child will know other words as well. But the checklists have been developed on the basis of multiple revisions, with input from observational studies and open-ended parent report. They capture the majority of young children's vocabulary, and are likely to be highly representative of the overall composition with respect to major subcategories.

In contrast to previous research using norms based on written or adult-directed spoken language, we estimated parental frequency directly by searching all parental speech transcripts in the Childes database for every use of the items on the MCDI (Li, Burgess, and Lund, 2000). Some words did not appear in any parental transcript, and they too were excluded. This resulted in a final list of 562 words, which were grouped into six categories: 256 common nouns, e.g., *ball, frog, juice*; 21 people words, e.g., *doctor, girl, mommy*; 90 verbs, e.g., *bite, hug, take*; 55 adjectives, e.g., *big, happy, tired*; 68 closed class words, e.g., *that, in, some*; and 72 other words, e.g., *please, lunch, park*.

Input frequency plays a special role in developmental theorizing. In virtually any theory of lexical acquisition, words that are experienced more often can be expected to be acquired earlier. A first comparison of input frequency and age of acquisition across these categories yields a counterexample to the hypothesized negative correlation of frequency and age of acquisition; see Fig. 2.10. On examination, this counter-intuitive result is not so surprising: closed class words are produced most frequency in parental input (mean frequency = 14,727) but learned the latest, while nouns are produced least frequently in input (mean frequency = 540) but learned the earliest. However, when the relation is examined *within* categories, it is, as hypothesized, consistently negative: the more frequent a word, the earlier it is acquired. The correlations vary in size, but are substantial: for nouns, $r = -.55$ (p < .01); for people words, $r = -.52$ (p < .02); for verbs, $r = -.22$ (p < .04); adjectives, $r = -.28$ (p < .04); for closed class words, $r = -.24$ (p < .05); and for other words $r = -.34$ (p < .01). When similar analyses were performed using adult-based word frequency norms, such as Kucera–Francis (Francis & Kucera, 1982), the relations were substantially smaller and often non-significant. These results provide persuasive evidence for two conclusions: first, that parental frequency makes a difference, and second, that the role of additional predictors is more appropriately explored within each of these categories, as rather different processes may be involved. For example, frequency may be more important for nouns, which form a very large set of items of roughly similar semantic complexity, than for closed-class items, which constitute a smaller set, are nearly all high frequency, and are characterized by great syntactic and semantic heterogeneity.

A second set of potentially influential factors are phonological in nature. We examined length of words, difficulty of the initial consonant, and complexity of the first stressed syllable (on the grounds that initial unstressed syllables are often deleted by young children).[3] All three were related to age of acquisition for the category of common nouns and the category of other words. Interestingly, the majority of words in the "other words" category are also nouns, e.g., *home, snack, day*. The relation generally remained significant even when input frequency was partialled out, though it accounted for

---

[3]The phonological measures were developed in collaboration with Carol Stoel-Gammon, whose help is gratefully acknowledged.

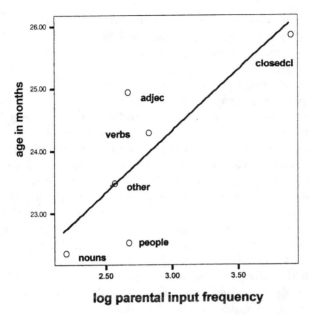

FIG. 2.10.   Mean parental input frequency and age of reported acquisition for words in six categories.

less of the variability in age of acquisition. An additional, intriguing phonological result concerns stress pattern. Even young infants discriminate stress patterns and learn the characteristic trochaic (strong–weak) pattern of English (Jusczyk, Cutler, & Redanz, 1993). The trochaic bias is so strong that it is difficult to find comparisons across stress patterns with sufficient sample size in our set of words. However, combining all two-syllable words with unequal stress results in 165 trochaic and 13 iambic items. Iambic words have a higher input frequency than trochaic words, (on average, 1029 vs. 583) but are learned significantly later (26.7 vs. 23.6 months).

Even though we are limited to acquisition prior to 30 months, the nonlinear growth trends discussed earlier in this chapter suggest that there are likely to be developmental shifts during this period, e.g., nonlinear growth trends. We divided the words into those acquired before and after the average child is reported to produce 100 words (19.2 months, on average). We then assessed whether parental frequency and age of acquisition were related, separately for the slow, early period of acquisition and during the time of a rapid spurt in acquisition. For the early-learned words, there were no significant correlations for any of the categories, whereas for the later-learned words, the correlations were significant for the common noun, people, adjective, and closed-class categories. With respect to phonological factors, there was one quite striking developmental shift. Words beginning with /b/ make up 10% of the entire MCDI word list, in contrast to only 5%

of the words in Webster's Pocket Dictionary (1997; see Stoel-Gammon, 1998). But they make up 24% of the first 100 words.

The results thus far obtained support several conclusions. First, input frequency does play a role, but primarily with respect to other words within the same lexical category. Furthermore, measures that are based on actual parental input are more appropriate than measures derived from a different modality (writing) or for a different audience (adult-directed speech). Comparative analysis of early- and late-appearing words suggest that frequency effects begin only after a critical mass of words or a particular age has been reached. Other factors must influence the acquisition of children's first words. Phonological factors, particularly the difficulty of the first consonant, may be important here. Later, phonological factors play only a weak role. More generally, there is a great deal of variability in age of acquisition which is yet to be explained. We are currently examining the role of semantic factors, such as animacy and concreteness, and syntactic factors, such as verb argument structure. Taken together, the findings will demonstrate the effects of a variety of variables on the age of acquisition of individual words. We expect most of these variables to interact with lexical category, age, and vocabulary size.

CONCLUDING THOUGHTS

The assessment of vocabulary size made possible by the MCDI has made at least two major contributions to the study of language development. The first is primarily empirical. A wide range of cross-sectional, longitudinal, modeling, crosslinguistic and bilingual approaches reviewed in this chapter have converged on a set of growth patterns for comprehension and production vocabulary, and the relationship between them. These patterns include both prototypic trends and enormous individual variability, along with idiosyncratic patterns. Furthermore, vocabulary size is clearly a developmentally significant index, sensitive to both genetic and environmental factors, and predictive of multiple aspects of later development.

Equally important, if perhaps less expected, is the contribution of this "low-tech" measure to the enterprise of theory-building. The availability of vocabulary growth information over time from longitudinal studies, and from studies of large numbers of children, has given us a characterization of central tendencies and variation in vocabulary growth. And that information has made it possible to address some deep questions of acquisition mechanism, most notably in this chapter, the number and nature of basic learning processes.

Liz Bates stepped out of the nature vs. nurture debate long ago. She preferred to ask how nature and nurture interact, and in particular, what sort of innate mechanisms would be required to take the linguistic input to which humans are exposed and generate both universal and unique patterns of language development. A remarkable, sizable and varied body of data has emerged based on her methodological and theoretical insights. These data are beginning to illuminate the ways in which nature constrains vocabulary acquisition, and the way that environmental factors influence the composition, rate, and shape of vocabulary growth. We believe that the methodological and theoretical work of the coming decades will build on this foundation she has given us, and enable us to be much clearer on just how children infer the meaning of a word, and of so many words. We leave the last word to Liz:

> ... we have argued in favor of continuity in the mechanisms, motives, and representations that underlie the evolution and development of language. None of these arguments should be taken as a denial of the undeniable fact that language is special. It is our prized possession, something that no other species really shares. Our children burst into language learning with talent and enthusiasm, and they seem to be ideally suited for it. But the beauty of language will not be compromised if we rob it of some mystery; continuity can give birth to discontinuity, and exquisite products can be constructed with humble tools. (Bates, Thal & Marchman, 1991, p. 59)

REFERENCES

Arriaga, R. I., Fenson, L., Cronan, T., & Pethick, S. J. (1998). Scores on the MacArthur Communicative Development Inventory of children from low- and middle-income families. *Applied Psycholinguistics, 19,* 209–223.

Baldwin, D. (1989). Establishing word-object relations: A first step. *Child Development, 60,* 381–398.

Bar-Adon, A., & Leopold, W. F. (Eds.). (1971). *Child language: A book of readings.* Englewood Cliffs, NJ: Prentice-Hall.

Bates, E., Benigni, L., Bretherton, I., Camaioni, I., & Volterra, V. (1979). *The emergence of symbols.* New York: Academic Press.

Bates, E., Bretherton, I., & Snyder, L. (1988). *From first words to grammar: Individual differences and dissociable mechanisms.* New York: Cambridge University Press.

Bates, E., & Carnevale, G. (1993). New directions in research on language development. *Developmental Review, 18,* 436–470.

Bates, E., Dale, P. S., & Thal, D. (1995). Individual differences and their implications for theories of language development. In P. Fletcher & B. MacWhinney (Eds.), *Handbook of child language,* 96–151. Oxford: Basil Blackwell.

Bates, E., & Goodman, J. C. (1997). On the inseparability of grammar and the lexicon: Evidence from acquisition, aphasia and real-time processing. *Language and Cognitive Processes, 12,* 507–586.

Bates, E., Thal, D., & Marchman, V. (1991). Symbols and syntax: A Darwinian approach to language development. In N. A. Krasnegor, D. M. Rumbaugh, R. L. Schiefelbusch, & M. Studdert-Kennedy (Eds.), *Biological and behavioral determinants of language development.* Hillsdale, NJ: Erlbaum.

Bishop, D. V. M., & Leonard, L. B. (Eds.). (2000). *Speech and language impairments in children: Causes, characteristics, intervention, and outcome*. Philadelphia: Taylor & Francis.

Bishop, D. V. M., Price, T. S., Dale, P. S., & Plomin, R. (2003). Outcomes of early language delay: II. Etiology of transient and persistent language difficulties. *Journal of Speech-Language-Hearing Research, 46*, 561–575.

Bloom, L. (1973). *One word at a time*. The Hague: Mouton.

Brown, R. (1958). How shall a thing be called? *Psychological Review, 65*, 14–21.

Brown, R. (1973). *A first language*. Cambridge, MA: Harvard University Press.

Caselli, M. C., Bates, E., Casadio, P., Fenson, J., Fenson, L., Sanders, L., & Weir, J. (1995). A crosslinguistic study of early lexical development. *Cognitive Development, 10*, 159–199.

Charman, T., Drew, A., Baird, C., & Baird, G. (2003). Measuring early language development in preschool children with autism spectrum disorder using the MacArthur Communicative Development Inventory (Infant Form). *Journal of Child Language, 30*, 213–236.

Clark, E. V. (1995). Later lexical development and word formation. In P. Fletcher & B. MacWhinney (Eds.), *Handbook of child language*, 393–412. Oxford: Blackwell.

Crain-Thoreson, Catherine., & Dale, Philip S. (1992). Do early talkers become early readers? Linguistic precocity, preschool language and emergent literacy. *Developmental Psychology, 28*, 421–429.

Dale, P. S. (1996). Parent report assessment of language and communication. In K. N. Cole, P. S. Dale, D. J. Thal (Eds.), *Assessment of language and communication*, 161–182. Baltimore: Paul H. Brookes.

Dale, P. S., Price, T. S., Bishop, D. V. M., & Plomin, R. (2003). Outcomes of early language delay: I. Predicting persistent and transient difficulties at 3 and 4 years. *Journal of Speech-Language-Hearing Research, 46*, 544–560.

Dionne, G., Dale, P. S., Boivin, M., & Plomin, R. (2003). Genetic evidence for bidirectional effects of early lexical and grammatical development. *Child Development, 74*, 394–412.

Elman, J. L., Bates, E. A., Johnson, M. H., Karmiloff-Smith, A., Parisi, D., & Plunkett, K. (1996). *Rethinking innateness: A connectionist perspective on development*. Cambridge, MA: MIT Press.

Feldman, H. M., Dollaghan, C. A., Campbell, T. F., Colborn, D. K., Janosky, J., Kurs-Lasky, M., Rockette, H. E., Dale, P. S., & Paradise, J. L. (2003). Parent-reported language skills in relation to otitis media during the first three years of life. *Journal of Speech-Language-Hearing Research, 46*, 273–287.

Fenson, L., Dale, P. S., Reznick, J. S., Bates, E., Thal, D. J., & Pethick, S. J. (1994). Variability in early communicative development. *Monographs of the Society for Research in Child Development, 59* (5, Serial No. 242).

Francis, W. N., & Kucera, H. (1982). *Frequency analysis of English usage: Lexicon and grammar*. Boston: Houghton Mifflin.

Gentner, D. (1982). Why nouns are learned before verbs: Linguistic relativity versus natural partitioning. In S. Kuczaj (Ed.), *Language development, vol 2*. Hillsdale, NJ: Erlbaum.

Gilger, J. W. (1995). Behavioral genetics: Concepts for research and practice in language development and disorders. *Journal of Speech & Hearing Research, 38*, 1126–1142.

Goodman, J. C., Bates, E., Jahn-Samilo, J., Appelbaum, M., Carnevale, G., & Elman, J. (1999, July). Early lexical development and the dynamics of change. VIIIth Congress of the International Association for the Study of Child Language, San Sebastian, Spain.

Goodman, J. C., Dale, P. S., & Li, Ping. (2003, April). Determinants of the age of acquisition of children's early vocabulary. Society for Research in Child Development, Tampa, Florida.

Goodman, J. C., McDonough, L., & Brown, N. (1998). The role of semantic context and memory in the acquisition of novel nouns. *Child Development, 69*, 1330–1344.

Gopnik, A., & Meltzoff, A. N. (1986). Relations between semantic and cognitive development in the one-word stage: The specificity hypothesis. *Child Development, 57*, 1040–1053.

Gopnik, A., & Meltzoff, A. N. (1987). The development of categorization in the second year and its relation to other cognitive and linguistic developments. *Child Development, 58,* 1523–1531.

Hart, B., & Risley, T. (1995). *Meaningful differences in the everyday experience of young American children.* Baltimore: Paul H. Brookes.

Hirsh-Pasek, K., & Golinkoff, R. M. (1996). *The origins of grammar: Evidence from early language comprehension.* Cambridge, MA: MIT Press.

Jackson-Maldonado, D., Thal, D. J., Marchman, V., Bates, E., et al. (1993). Early lexical development in Spanish-speaking infants and toddlers. *Journal of Child Language, 20,* 523–549.

Jackson-Maldonado, D., Thal, D. J., Marchman, V., Newton, T., Fenson, L., & Conboy, B. (2003). *El Inventario del Desarollo de Habilidades Comunicativas: User's guide and technical manual.* Baltimore: Paul H. Brookes.

Jahn-Samilo, J., Goodman, J. C., Bates, E., Appelbaum, M., & Sweets, M. (2003). Vocabulary learning in children from 8 to 30 months of age. Manuscript in preparation.

Jusczyk, P. W., Cutler, A., & Redanz, N. J. (1993). Infants' preference for the predominant stress patterns of English words. *Child Development, 64,* 675–687.

Li, P., Burgess, C., & Lund, K. (2000). The acquisition of word meaning through global lexical co-occurrences. In E. V. Clark (ed.), *Proceedings of the Thirtieth Stanford Child Language Research Forum.* Stanford, CA: Center for the Study of Language and Information, 167–178.

MacWhinney, B. (2000). *The CHILDES Project: Tools for Analyzing Talk, Third Edition.* Mahwah, NJ: Erlbaum.

Markman, E. M. (1994). Constraints on word meaning in early language acquisition. In L. Gleitman & B. Landau (Eds.), *The acquisition of the lexicon,* 199–229. Cambridge, MA: MIT Press/Elsevier.

Meaburn, E., Dale, P. S., Craig, I. W., & Plomin, R. (2002). Genotyping of 270 language-impaired children for the FOX2P gene guanine-to-adenine nucleotide mutation in the forkhead DNA-binding domain. *NeuroReport, 13,* 103.

Miller, J. F., Sedey, A. L., & Miolo, G. (1995). Validity of parent report measures of vocabulary development for children with Down Syndrome. *Journal of Speech and Hearing Research, 38,* 1037–1044.

Mills, D., Coffey-Corina, S., & Neville, H. (1997). Language comprehension and cerebral specialization from 13 to 20 months. *Developmental Neuropsychology, 13,* 395–445.

Nazzi, T., & Bertoncini, J. (2003). Before and after the vocabulary spurt: Two modes of word acquisition? *Developmental Science, 6,* 136–142.

Nelson, K. (1973). Structure and strategy in learning to talk. *Monographs of the Society for Research in Child Development, 38* (1–2, Serial No. 149).

NICHD Early Child Care Research Network. (2000). The relation of child care to cognitive and language development. *Child Development, 71,* 960–980.

Ogura, T., Yamashita, Y., Murase, T., & Dale, P. S. (1993, July). Some preliminary findings from the Japanese Early Communicative Development Inventory. Paper presented at the Sixth International Congress for the Study of Child Language, Trieste, Italy.

Plomin, R., & Dale, P. S. (2000). Genetics and early language development: A UK study of twins. In D. V. M. Bishop & L. B. Leonard (Eds.), *Speech and language impairments in children: Causes, characteristics, intervention, and outcome,* 35–51. Philadelphia: Taylor & Francis.

Plunkett, K. (1993). Lexical segmentation and vocabulary growth in early language acquisition. *Journal of Child Language, 20,* 43–60.

Raichle, M. E. (1994). Images of the mind: Studies with modern imaging techniques. *Annual Review of Psychology, 45,* 333–356.

Rescorla, L. (1989). The Language Development Survey: A screening tool for delayed language in toddlers. *Journal of Speech and Hearing Disorders, 54,* 587–599.

Quine, W. V. O. (1960). *Word and object.* Cambridge, England: Cambridge University Press.

Robinson, N. M., Dale, P. S., & Landesman, S. (1990). Validity of Stanford-Binet IV with linguistically precocious toddlers. *Intelligence, 14*, 173–186.

Rosch, E., Mervis, C. B., Gray, W. D., Johnson, D. M., & Boyes-Braem, P. (1976). Basic objects in natural categories. *Cognitive Psychology, 8*, 382–439.

Shore, C. (1995). *Individual differences in language development.* Thousand Oaks, CA: Safe Publications.

Slobin, D. I. (Ed.). (1985). *The crosslinguistic study of language acquisition, vol. I.* Hillsdale, NJ: Erlbaum.

Spinath, F. M., Price, T. S., Dale, P. S., & Plomin, R. (in press). The genetic and environmental origins of language disability and ability: A study of language at 2, 3, and 4 years of age in a large community sample of twins. *Child Development.*

Stoel-Gammon, C. (1998). Sounds and words in early language acquisition: The relationship between lexical and phonological development. In R. Paul (Ed.), *Exploring the speech-language connection*, 25–52. Baltimore: Paul H. Brookes.

Stromswold, K. (2001). The heritability of language: A review of twin and adoption studies. *Language, 77*, 647–723.

Tardif, T., Shatz, M., & Naigles, L. (1997). Caregiver speech and children's use of nouns versus verbs: A comparison of English, Italian, and Mandarin. *Journal of Child Language, 24*, 535–565.

Thal, D. J., O'Hanlon, L., Clemmons, M., & Fralin, L. (1999). Validity of a parent report measure of vocabulary and syntax for preschool children with language impairment. *Journal of Speech, Language and Hearing Research, 42*, 482–496.

Webster's Pocket Dictionary. (1997). Springfield, MA: Merriam-Webster.

Part II

THE COMPETITION MODEL
AND CONNECTIONISM

Chapter 3

New Directions in the Competition Model

Brian MacWhinney
Carnegie Mellon University

The Competition Model stands as one Elizabeth Bates's major theoretical contributions to psycholinguistics. It was my honor to work with her for over twenty years in the development of this model from our first co-authored paper in 1978 up through our applications of the model to second language and aphasia in the late 1980s and early 1990s. The classic version of the model can be found in the volume that we co-edited in 1989 (MacWhinney & Bates, 1989). Recently Bates, Devescovi, & Wulfeck (2001) have summarized a wide range of newly accumulated data, particularly on the application of the model to crosslinguistic studies of aphasia. In addition, a recent article by Dick et al. (2001) shows how the comparison of normals and aphasics in a Competition Model framework can illuminate the issue of the distributed nature of language localization in the brain.

The current paper seeks to elaborate the Competition Model in some slightly different directions. The focus here is on applications to second language learning and the development of a unified model for first language learning, second language learning, and multilingualism. I should state at the outset that, although some of these elaborations are compatible with conceptual developments contributed by Liz and her colleagues in San Diego, Taiwan, Rome, and elsewhere, other aspects of my elaborations go in directions with which she would initially disagree. In particular, the elaboration of the role of linguistic arenas seems that will be developed here may seem to represent a concession to the theory of modularity of mind. In addition, the restatement of the theory of cue cost in terms of chunking and storage may seem like a restatement, rather than a conceptual advance. However, I hope to show that the notion of arenas does not require an acceptance of modularity and that providing a specific characterization of the mechanisms of chunking and storage helps provide additional explanatory power to the model.

CAN WE HAVE A UNIFIED MODEL?

The idea that we could develop a unified model for all forms of language acquisition flies in the face of much of current accepted wisdom and practice. It is relatively easy to point to some core differences between first language learning, second language learning, multilingualism, and language loss in aphasia that would seem to problematize the construction of a unified model. Native language acquisition differs from second language acquisition in several fundamental ways. First, infants who are learning language are also engaged in learning about how the world works. In comparison, second language learners already know a great deal about the world. Second, infants are able to rely on a highly malleable brain that has not yet been committed to other tasks (MacWhinney, Feldman, Sacco, & Valdes-Perez, 2000). Third, infants can rely on an intense system of social support from their caregivers (Snow, 1999). Together, these three differences might suggest that it would make little sense to try to develop a unified model of first and second language acquisition. In fact, many researchers have decided that the two processes are so different that they account for them with totally separate theories. For example, Krashen (1994) sees L1 learning as involving "acquisition" and L2 learning as based instead on "learning." Others (Bley-Vroman, Felix, & Ioup, 1988; Clahsen & Muysken, 1986) argue that Universal Grammar (UG) is available to children up to some critical age, but not to older learners of L2.

On the other hand, even those researchers who have traditionally emphasized the differences between L1 and L2 acquisition have been forced to recognize the fact that L1 learning processes play a large role in L2 learning (Felix & Wode, 1983). For example, the method we use for learning new word forms in a second language is basically an extension of the methods we used for learning words in our first language. Similarly, when we come to combining second language words into sentences, we use many of the same strategies we used as children when learning our first language. Furthermore, the fact that L2 learning is so heavily influenced by transfer from L1 means that it would be impossible to construct a model of L2 learning that did not take into account the structure of the first language. Thus, rather than attempting to build two separate models of L1 and L2 learning, it makes more sense to consider the shape of a unified model in which the mechanisms of L1 learning are seen as a subset of the mechanisms of L2 learning. Although these L1 learning mechanisms are less powerful in the L2 learner, they are still partially accessible (Flynn, 1996). Therefore, it is conceptually simpler to formulate a unified model.

We can use this same logic to motivate the extension of a unified model to the study of both childhood and adult multilingualism. In the case of childhood multilingualism, there is now an emerging consensus (De Houwer, in press) that children acquire multiple languages as separate entities. However, there is also good evidence that these multiple languages interact in children through processes of transfer and code switching (Meuter, in press) much as they do in adults. These processes are best understood within the context of a unified acquisitional model. Similarly, current theories of adult bilingualism have tended to emphasize bilingual competence as a steady state with minimal developmental inputs (La Heij, in press). However, this view fails to consider how dynamic aspects of code switching and interference arise from years of interaction between the languages during the child's development. Furthermore, adult multilinguals continue to develop competence in particular domains such as the skill of simultaneous interpretation (Christoffels & de Groot, in press). These acquisitions depend on many of the same learning mechanisms we see operative in the earliest stages of first language acquisition, as well as other mechanisms evidenced in second language learners.

These initial considerations suggest that we need to at least consider what it might mean to construct a unified model for first language acquisition, childhood multilingualism, second language acquisition, and adult multilingualism. This chapter outlines the first stages of this attempt. It relies on the Competition Model (Bates & MacWhinney, 1982; MacWhinney, 1987a) as the starting point for this new unified model. Although the Competition Model was not originally designed to account for all aspects of second language learning and multilingualism, it has certain core concepts that fit in well with a broader, fuller account. In particular, we can build on the core Competition Model insight that cue strength in the adult speaker is a direct function of cue validity. However, the unified account needs to supplement the theory of cue validity with additional theoretical constructs to deal with what we have come to refer to as "cue cost" and "cue support." Figure 3.1 represents the overall shape of the model that I will develop here. This figure is not to be interpreted as a processing model. Rather, it is a logical decomposition of the general problem of language learning into a series of smaller, but interrelated structural and processing components.

Earlier versions of the Competition Model included the core concept of competition, as well as the three components of arenas, mappings, and storage at the top of the figure. The new aspects of the Unified Competition Model include the components of chunking, codes, and resonance

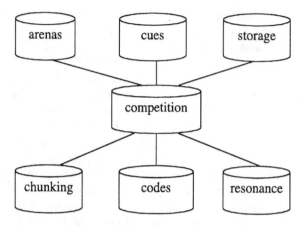

FIG. 3.1. The seven components of the Unified Competition Model.

given at the bottom of the figure. Before examining the operation of the
new model, let us briefly define its seven components.

1. *Competition.* At the core of the model is a processing system that se-
lects between various options or cues on the basis of their relative cue
strength. In the classic version of the model, competition was based on cue
summation and interactive activation. In the unified model, competition is
viewed as based on resonance, as well as cue summation.

2. *Arenas.* The linguistic arenas within which competition occurs are
the four traditional levels recognized in most psycholinguistic processing
models—phonology, lexicon, morphosyntax, and conceptualization. In
production, these arenas involve message formulation, lexical activation,
morphosyntactic arrangement, and articulatory planning. In comprehension, the competitive arenas include auditory processing, lexical activation,
grammatical role decoding, and meaningful interpretation. Processing in
each of these different arenas is subserved by a different combination of
neuronal pathways. In addition to the eight competitive arenas we have
listed, older learners also make use of two arenas of orthographic competition, one for reading and one for writing.

3. *Cues.* At the core of the Competition Model—both in its classical
form and the newer unified form—is a notion of the linguistic sign as a
mapping between form and function. The theory of mappings is similar in
many ways to the theory of linguistic options articulated in Halliday's sys-
temic grammar. In these mappings, forms serve as cues to functions during
comprehension and functions serve as cues to forms during production. In
other words, in production, forms compete to express underlying intentions or functions. In comprehension, functions or interpretations com-

pete on the basis of cues from surface forms. The outcome of these competitions is determined by the relative strength of the relevant cues. For example, in English, the positioning of the subject before the verb is a form that expresses the function of marking the perspective or agent. Or, to give another example, the pronoun "him" is a form that expresses the functions of masculine gender and the role of the object of the verb. The Competition Model focuses primarily on the use of forms as cues to role assignment, coreference, and argument attachment as outlined in MacWhinney (1987a). Mappings are social conventions that must be learned for each of the eight linguistic arenas, including lexicon, phonology, morphosyntax, and mental models.

4. *Storage.* The learning of new mappings relies on storage in both short-term and long-term memory. Gupta & MacWhinney (1997) have developed an account of the role of short-term memory in the construction of memories for the phonological forms of words and the mapping of these forms into meaningful lexical items. Short-term memory is also crucially involved in the online processing of specific syntactic structures (Gibson, Pearlmutter, Canseco-Gonzalez, & Hickok, 1996; MacWhinney & Pléh, 1988). Recently, MacWhinney (1999) has examined how the processes of perspective switching and referent identification can place demands on verbal memory processes during mental model construction. The operation of these memory systems constrains the role of cue validity during both processing and acquisition. For example, the processing of subject-verb agreement for inverted word orders in Italian is not fully learned until about age 8 (Devescovi, D'Amico, Smith, Mimica, & Bates, 1998), despite its high cue validity and high cue strength in adult speakers.

5. *Chunking.* The size of particular mappings depends on the operation of processes of chunking. Work in first language acquisition has shown us that children rely on both combinatorial processing and chunking to build up syllables, words, and sentences. For example, a child may treat learn "what's this" as a single unit or chunk, but will compose phrases such as "more cookie" and "more milk" by combination of "more" with a following argument. MacWhinney (1978, 1982) and Stemberger & MacWhinney (1986) show how large rote chunks compete with smaller analytic chunks in both children and adult learners.

6. *Codes.* When modeling bilingualism and L2 acquisition, it is important to have a clear theory of code activation. The Competition Model distinguishes two components of the theory of code competition. The first component is the theory of transfer. This theory has been articulated in some detail in Competition Model work in terms of predictions for both positive and negative transfer in the various linguistic arenas. The second component is the theory of code interaction, which determines code selection, switching, and mixing. The Competition Model relies on the notion of resonance, discussed below, to account for coactivation processes in both

L2 learners and bilinguals. The choice of a particular code at a particular moment during lexicalization depends on factors such as activation from previous lexical items, the influence of lexical gaps, expression of sociolinguistic options (Ervin-Tripp, 1969), and conversational cues produced by the listener.

7. *Resonance.* Perhaps the most important area of new theoretical development in the Unified Competition Model is the theory of resonance. This theory seeks to relate the Competition Model to research in the area of embodied or embedded cognition, as well as newer models of processing in neural networks.

The seven-component model sketched out above includes no separate component for learning. This is because learning is seen as an interaction between each of the various subcomponents during the processes of competition and resonance. We will now explore each of the seven components of the model in more detail.

Competition

The basic notion of competition is fundamental to most information-processing models in cognitive psychology. In the Unified Model, competition takes on slightly different forms in each of the eight competitive arenas. We think of these arenas not as encapsulated modules, but as playing fields that can readily accept input from other arenas, when that input is made available. In the course of work on the core model and related mechanisms, my colleagues and I have formulated working computational models for most of these competitive arenas.

1. In the auditory arena, competition involves the processing of cues to lexical forms based on both bottom-up features and activation from lexical forms. Models of this process include those that emphasize top-down activation (Elman & McClelland, 1988) and those that exclude it (Norris, 1994). In the Competition Model, bottom-up activation is primary, but top-down activation will occur in natural conditions and in those experimental tasks that promote resonance.

2. In the lexical arena, competition occurs within topological maps (Li, Farkas, & MacWhinney, under review) where words are organized by semantic and lexical type.

3. In the morphosyntactic arena, there is an item-based competition between word orders and grammatical markings centered on valence relations (M. C. MacDonald, Pearlmutter, & Seidenberg, 1994; MacWhinney, 1987b).

4. In the interpretive arena, there is a competition between fragments of mental models as the listener seeks to construct a unified mental model (MacWhinney, 1989) that can be encoded in long-term memory (Hausser, 1999).

5. In the arena of message formulation, there is a competition between communicative goals. Winning goals are typically initialized and topicalized.

6. In the arena of expressive lexicalization, there is a competition between words for the packaging and conflation of chunks of messages (Langacker, 1989).

7. In the arena of sentence planning, there is a competition of phrases for initial position and a competition between arguments for attachment to slots generated by predicates (Dell, Juliano, & Govindjee, 1993).

8. In the arena of articulatory planning, there is a competition between syllables for insertion into a rhythmic phrasal output pattern (Dell et al., 1993).

Cues

Experimental work in the Competition Model tradition has focused on measurement of the relative strength of various cues to the selection of the agent, using a simple sentence interpretation procedure. Subjects listen to a sentence with two nouns and a verb and are asked to say who was the actor. In a few studies, the task involves direct-object identification (Sokolov, 1988, 1989), relative clause processing (MacWhinney & Pléh, 1988), or pronominal assignment (M. MacDonald & MacWhinney, 1990; McDonald & MacWhinney, 1995), but usually the task is agent identification. Sometimes the sentences are well-formed grammatical sentences, such as *the cat is chasing the duck.* Sometimes they involve competitions between cues, as in the ungrammatical sentence **the duck the cat is chasing.* Depending on the language involved, the cues varied in these studies include word order, subject-verb agreement, object-verb agreement, case-marking, prepositional case marking, stress, topicalization, animacy, omission, and pronominalization. These cues are varied in a standard orthogonalized ANOVA design with three or four sentences per cell to increase statistical reliability. The basic question is always the same: what is the relative order of cue strength in the given language and how do these cue strengths interact?

In English, the dominant cue for subject identification is preverbal positioning. For example, in the English sentence *the eraser hits the cat,* we assume that *the eraser* is the agent. However, a parallel sentence in Italian or Spanish would have *the cat* as the agent. This is because the word order cue is not as strong in Italian or Spanish as it is in English. In Spanish, the prepositional object marker "a" is a clear cue to the object and the subject is the noun that is not the object. An example of this is the sentence *el toro mató al torero* (The bull killed to-the bullfighter). No such prepositional cue exists in English. In German, case marking on the definite article is a powerful cue to the subject. In a sentence such as *der Lehrer liebt die Witwe* (The teacher loves the widow), the presence of the nominative masculine article *der* is a sure cue to identification of the subject. In Russian, the subject often has a case suffix. In Arabic, the subject is the noun that agrees with the verb in number and gender and this cue is stronger than the case-marking cue. In French, Spanish, and Italian, when an object pronoun is present, it can help identify the noun that is not the subject. Thus, we see that Indo-European languages can vary markedly in their use of cues to mark case roles. When we go outside of Indo-European to languages like Navajo, Hungarian, or Japanese, the variation becomes even more extreme.

To measure cue strength, Competition Model experiments rely on sentences with conflicting cues. For example, in *the eraser push the dogs* the cues of animacy and subject-verb agreement favor "the dogs" as agent. However, the stronger cue of preverbal positioning favors "the eraser" as agent. As a result, English-speaking adult subjects strongly favor "the eraser" even in a competition sentence of this type. However, about 20% of the participants will choose "the dogs" in this case. To measure the validity of cues in the various languages we have studied, we rely on text counts where we list the cues in favor of each noun and track the relative availability and reliability of each cue. Cue availability is defined as the presence of the cue in some contrastive form. For example, if both of the nouns in a sentence are animate, then the animacy cue is not contrastively available.

By looking at how children, adult monolinguals, and adult bilinguals speaking about 18 different languages process these various types of sentences, we have been able to reach these conclusions, regarding sentence comprehension:

When given enough time during sentence comprehension to make a careful choice, adults assign the role of agency to the nominal with the highest cue strength.

When there is a competition between cues, the levels of choice in a group of adult subjects will closely reflect the relative strengths of the competing cues.

When adult subjects are asked to respond immediately, even before the end of the sentence is reached, they will tend to base their decisions primarily on the strongest cue in the language.

When the strongest cue is neutralized, the next strongest cue will dominate.

The fastest decisions occur when all cues agree and there is no competition. The slowest decisions occur when strong cues compete.

Children begin learning to comprehend sentences by first focusing on the strongest cue in their language.

As children get older, the strength of all cues increases to match the adult pattern with the most valid cue growing most in strength.

As children get older, their reaction times gradually get faster in accord with the adult pattern.

Compared to adults, children are relatively more influenced by cue availability, as opposed to cue reliability.

Cue strength in adults and older children (8–10 years) is not related to cue availability (since all cues have been heavily encountered by this time), but rather to cue reliability. In particular, it is a function of conflict reliability, which measures the reliability of a cue when it conflicts directly with other cues.

This list of findings from Competition Model research underscores the heuristic value of the concept of cue strength.

Storage

One of the core findings of Competition Model research has been that, when adult subjects are given plenty of time to make a decision, their choices are direct reflections of the cumulative validity of all the relevant cues. In this sense, we can say that off-line decisions are optimal reflections of the structure of the language. However, when subjects are asked to make decisions on-line, then their ability to sample all relevant cue is restricted. In such cases, we say that "cue cost" factors limit the application of cue validity. These cue cost factors can involve various aspects of processing. However, the most important factors are those that require listeners to maintain the shape cues in working memory.

Theories of the neural basis of verbal memory view this storage as involving a functional neural circuit that coordinates inputs from Broca's area, lexical storage in the temporal lobe, and additional structures that support phonological memory. Unlike local lexical maps, which are neurologically stable, this functional circuit is easily disrupted and relies heavily on access to a variety of cognitive resources.

At the core of syntactic processing is the learning and use of item-based constructions (MacWhinney, 1975). Item-based constructions open up slots for arguments that may occur in specific positions or that must receive specific morphological markings. Although item-based constructions are encoded in local maps, they specify combinations that must be processed through functional circuits. The importance of item-based constructions has been re-emphasized in a new line of research recently reviewed by Tomasello (2000). The account of MacWhinney (1982) held that children first learn that a verb like *throw* takes three arguments (thrower, object thrown, recipient). Then, by comparing groups of these item-based patterns through analogy, children can then extract broader class-based patterns. In this case, they would extract a pattern that matches the set of transfer verbs that take the double object construction as in *John threw Bill the ball.* By the end of the third year, these new constructions (Goldberg, 1999) begin to provide the child with the ability to produce increasingly fluent discourse. Second language learners go through a similar process, sometimes supported by pattern drills.

By maintaining words and constructions in short-term sentence memory, learners can facilitate a wide range of additional learning and processing mechanisms. Perhaps the most remarkable of these processes is the learning of the skill of simultaneous translation (Christoffels & de Groot, in press). Practitioners of this art are able to listen in one language and speak in the other in parallel, while also performing a complex mapping of the message of the input language to the very different syntax of the output language. The very existence of simultaneous translation underscores the extent to which two languages can be coactivated (Spivey & Marian, 1999) for long periods of time (Meuter, in press).

The problems involved in simultaneous translation nicely illustrate how language can place a heavy load on functional neural circuits. Let us take a simple case to illustrate the problem. Consider a German sentence with a verb in final position. If the German sentence is short, the interpreter will have little problem converting the German SOV order to English SVO. For example, a sentence like *Johannes hat den Mann mit dem dunkele Mantel noch nicht kennengelernt* "John has not yet met the man with the dark coat" will cause few problems, since the interpreter can lag behind the speaker enough to take in the whole utterance along with the verb before starting to speak. The interpreter prepares an utterance with a subject and object already in final form. When the verb comes along, it is simply a matter of translating it to the English equivalent, dropping it into the prepared slot, and starting articulatory output. However, if there is additional material piled up before the verb, the problem can get worse. Typically, simultaneous interpreters try not to lag more than a few words behind the input. To avoid this, one solution would be to store away the short subject and dump out the large object as the head of a passive as in, "The man with the dark coat has not yet been met by John." Another, rather unhappy, solution is topicalization, as in "John, in regard to the man with the dark coat, he hasn't seen him yet." Similar problems can arise when translating from relative clauses in languages with VSO order such as Tagalog or Arabic. Studies of Hungarian (MacWhinney & Pléh, 1988) and Japanese (Hakuta, 1981) show that the stacking up of unlinked noun phrases can be even worse in SOV languages.

If interpreters had access to an unlimited verbal memory capacity, there would be little worry about storing long chunks of verbal material. However, we know that our raw memory for strings of words is not nearly large enough to accommodate the simultaneous interpretation task. In fact, the conventional estimate of the number of items that can be stored in short-term memory is about four. The interpreter's task is made even more difficult by the fact that they must continue to build mental models of incoming material (MacWhinney, 1999) while using previously constructed mental models as the basis for ongoing articulation. In order to do this successfully, the interpreter must be able to delineate chunks of comprehended material that are sufficient to motivate full independent output productions. In effect, the interpreter must maintain two separate conceptual foci centered about two separate points in conceptual space. The first attentional focus continues to take in new material from the speaker in terms of new valence and conceptual relations. The second attentional focus works on the comprehended structure to convert it to a production structure. The location of the production focus is always lagged after that of the comprehended structure, so the interpreter always has a split in conceptual attention. As a result of the load imposed by this attentional split and ongoing activity in two channels, interpreters often find that they cannot continue this line of work past the age of 45 or so.

Interpreters are not the only speakers who are subject to load on their use of functional neural circuits. It is easy to interfere with normal language processing by imposing additional loads on the listener or speaker. Working within a standard Competition Model experimental framework, Kilborn (1989) has shown that even fully competent bilinguals tend to process sentences more slowly than monolinguals. However, when monolinguals are asked to listen to sentences under conditions of white noise, their reaction times are identical to those of the bilinguals. Similarly Blackwell and Bates (1995) and Miyake, Just and Carpenter (1994) have shown that, when subjected to conditions of noise, normals process sentences much like aphasics. Gerver (1974) and Seleskovitch (1976) report parallel results for the effects of noise on simultaneous interpretation.

Chunking

The component of chunking is a recent addition to the Competition Model. However, this idea is certainly not a new one for models of language learning. Chunking operates to take two or more items that frequently occur together and combine them into a single automatic chunk. Chunking is the basic learning mechanism in Newell's general cognitive model (Newell, 1990), as well as in many neural network models. MacWhinney and Anderson (1986) showed how the child can use chunking processes to build up larger grammatical structures and complex lexical forms. Ellis (1994) has shown how chunking can help us understand the growth of fluency in second language learning. Gupta & MacWhinney (1997) show how chunking can also apply to the learning of the phonological shape of individual words for both L1 and L2.

Chunking plays a particularly interesting role in the acquisition of grammar. For second language learners, mastering a complex set of inflectional patterns is a particularly daunting challenge. These problems are a result of the tendency of L2 learners to fail to pick up large enough phrasal chunks. For example, if learners of German would pick up not just that *Mann* means "man", but also learn phrases such as *der alte Mann, meines Mannnes, den junge Männern,* and *ein guter Mann,* then they would not only know the gender of the noun, but would also have a good basis for acquiring the declensional paradigm for both the noun and its modifiers. However, if they analyze a phrase like *der alte Mann* into the literal string "the + old + man" and throw away all of the details of the inflections on "der" and "alte," then they will lose an opportunity to induce the grammar from implicit generalization across stored chunks. If, on the other hand, the learner stores larger chunks of this type, then the rules of grammar can emerge from analogic processing of the stored chunks.

Chunking also leads to improvements in fluency. For example, in Spanish, L2 learners can chunk together the plan for *buenos* with the plan for *dîas* to produce *buenos días.* They can then combine this chunk with *muy* to produce *muy buenos días* "very good morning." Chunking (Ellis, 1994) allows the learner to get around problems with Spanish noun pluralization, gender marking, and agreement that would otherwise have to be reasoned out in detail for each combination. Although the learner understands the meanings of the three words in this phrase, the unit can function as a chunk, thereby speeding production.

Codes and Transfer

Any general model of second language learning must be able to account for interlanguage phenomena such as transfer and code switching. In addition, it must offer an account of age-related learning effects that have been discussed in terms of critical periods and fossilization. Because of space limitations, I will not include a discussion of code-switching theory here, focusing instead on the theory of transfer and its impact on age-related effects.

The basic claim is that whatever can transfer will. This claim is theoretically important for at least two reasons. First, because the competition model emphasizes the interactive nature of cognitive processing, it must assume that, unless the interactions between languages are controlled and coordinated, there would be a large amount of transfer. Second, the model needs to rely on transfer to account for age-related declines in L2 learning ability without invoking the expiration of a genetically programmed critical period (Birdsong, in press).

For simultaneous bilingual acquisition the model predicts code blending in young children only when parents encourage this or when there are gaps in one language that can be filled by "borrowing" from the other. This prediction follows from the role of resonance in blocking transfer. When the child's two languages are roughly similar in dominance or strength, each system generates enough system-internal resonance to block excessive transfer. However, if one of the languages is markedly weaker (Dopke, in press), then it will not have enough internal resonance to block occasional transfer. The situation is very different for L2 learners, since the balance between the languages is then tipped so extremely in favor of L1. In order to permit the growth of resonance in L2, learners must apply additional learning strategies that would not have been needed for children. These strategies focus primarily on optimization of input, promotion of L2 resonance, and avoidance of processes that destroy input chunks.

In the next sections, we briefly review the evidence for transfer from L1 to L2. We will see that there is clear evidence for massive transfer in audition, articulation, lexicon, sentence interpretation, and pragmatics. In the area of morphosyntax and sentence production, transfer is not as massive, largely because it is more difficult to construct the relations between L1 and L2 forms in these areas. Pienemann et al. (in press) have argued that transfer in these areas is less general than postulated by the Competition Model. However, we will see that their analysis underestimates transfer effects in their own data.

Transfer in Audition. Phonological learning involves two very different processes. Auditory acquisition is primary and begins even before birth (Moon, Cooper, & Fifer, 1993). It relies on inherent properties of the mammalian ear (Moon et al., 1993) and early pattern detection through statistical learning. This same statistical learning mechanism is operative in children, adults, and cotton-top tamarins (Hauser, Newport, & Aslin, 2001). Recent research on early auditory processing (Sebastián-Galles & Bosch, in press) has yield three major findings. First, it appears that children begin to separate prosodically distinct languages from the first months. This means, for example, that children who are growing up in a home where Swedish and Portuguese are being spoken will have perhaps 16 months of experience in distinguishing these two languages by the time they come to saying their first words. The fact that these languages are separated in audition so early makes findings of early separation in production less surprising and more clearly understandable in Competition Model terms.

Recent research (Werker, 1995) has also shown that children begin to "lock in" the sounds of their first language(s) by the end of the first year and become relatively insensitive to distinctions in other languages. This commitment to the sounds of L1 can be reversed through childhood. However, for at least some sounds, it is difficult to obtain native-like contrast detection during adulthood. The classic example of this is the difficulty that Japanese adults have in distinguishing /l/ and /r/ in English (Lively, Pisoni, & Logan, 1990). Examples of this type demonstrate the basic claim for generalized transfer effects in the Competition Model. But note that what is transferring here from Japanese is not a contrast, but the L1 tendency to block out a contrast. At the same time, there are other non-L1 distinctions that can easily be perceived by adults. It appears that a full account of which contrasts can be learned and which will be blocked will need to be grounded on a dynamic model of auditory perception that is not yet available.

Finally, work on early audition has shown that children are picking up the auditory shapes of words well before they have their own productive vocabulary. Moreover, they are making the first steps toward classifying words into phrases and combinations on the auditory level even before they understand their meanings. These same mechanisms play an important role in L2 learning, as suggested by the Input Hypothesis. Through exposure to large amounts of auditory input in L2 that echo in a resonant way on the auditory level, L2 learners can also begin acquisition even before they demonstrate much in the way of independent productive ability.

Transfer in Articulation. The major challenge facing the L1 learner is not the acquisition of perceptual patterns, but the development of articulatory methods for reproducing these patterns (Menn & Stoel-Gammon, 1995). The coordination of motor mechanisms for speech output is a relatively late evolutionary emergence (MacWhinney, 2003) and it is not surprising that it is relatively difficult skill for the child to control. However, by age 5, most children have achieved control over articulatory processes.

For the adult L2 learner and the older child, the situation is much different. For them, learning begins with massive transfer of L1 articulatory patterns to L2 (Flege & Davidian, 1984; Hancin-Bhatt, 1994). This transfer is at first successful in the sense that it allows for a reasonable level of communication. However, it is eventually counter-productive, since it embeds L1 phonology into the emergent L2 lexicon. In effect, the learner treats new words in L2 as if they were composed of strings of L1 articulatory units. This method of learning leads to short term gains at the expense of long-term difficulties in correcting erroneous phonological transfer. Older children acquiring a second language can rely on their greater neuronal flexibility to quickly escape these negative transfer effects. In doing so, they are relying on the same types of adolescent motor abilities that allow adolescents to become proficient acrobats, gymnasts, dancers, and golfers. Adults have a reduced ability to rewire motor productions on this basic level. However, even the most difficult cases of negative transfer in adulthood can be corrected through careful training and rehearsal (Flege, Takagi, & Mann, 1995). To do this, adults must rely on resonance, selective attention, and learning strategies to reinvigorate a motor learning process that runs much more naturally in children and adolescents.

Transfer in Lexical Learning.   In the arena of lexical processing, the L2 learner can achieve rapid initial progress by simply transferring the L1 conceptual world *en masse* to L2. Young bilinguals can also benefit from this conceptual transfer. When learners first acquire a new L2 form, such as "silla" in Spanish, they treat this form as simply another way of saying "chair". This means that initially the L2 system has no separate conceptual structure and that its formal structure relies on the structure of L1. L2 relies on L1 forms to access meaning, rather than accessing meaning directly. In this sense, we can say that L2 is parasitic on L1, because of the extensive amount of transfer from L1 to L2. The learner's goal is to reduce this parasitism by building up L2 representations as a separate system. They do this by strengthening the direct linkage between new L2 forms and conceptual representations.

Given the fact that connectionism predicts such massive transfer for L1 knowledge to L2, we might ask why we do not see more transfer error in second language lexical forms. There are three reasons for this.

1. First, a great deal of transfer occurs smoothly and directly without producing error. Consider a word like *chair* in English. When the native English speaker begins to learn Spanish, it is easy to use the concept underlying "chair" to serve as the meaning for the new word *silla* in Spanish. The closer the conceptual, material, and linguistic worlds of the two languages, the more successful this sort of positive transfer will be. Transfer only works smoothly when there is close conceptual match. For example, Ijaz (1986) has shown how difficult transfer can be for Korean learners of English in semantic domains involving transfer verbs, such as *take* or *put.* Similarly, if the source language has a two-color system (Berlin & Kay, 1969), as in Dani, acquisition of an eight-color system, as in Hungarian,

will be difficult. These effects underscore the extent to which L2 lexical items are parasitic on L1 forms.

2. Second, learners are able to suppress some types of incorrect transfer. For example, when a learner tries to translate the English noun *soap* into Spanish by using a cognate, the result is *sopa* or "soup." Misunderstandings created by "false friend" transfers such as this will be quickly detected and corrected. Similarly, an attempt to translate the English form *competence* into Spanish as *competencia* will run into problems, since *competencia* means competition. In laboratory settings, the suppression of these incorrect form relatives is incomplete, even in highly proficient bilinguals. However, this persistent transfer effect is probably less marked in non-laboratory contexts.

3. Third, error is minimized when two words in L1 map onto a single word in L2. For example, it is easy for an L1 Spanish speaker to map the meanings underlying "saber" and "conocer" (Stockwell, Bowen, & Martin, 1965) onto the L2 English form "know." Dropping the distinction between these forms requires little in the way of cognitive reorganization. It is difficult for the L1 English speaker to acquire this new distinction when learning Spanish. In order to control this distinction correctly, the learner must restructure the concept underlying "know" into two new related structures. In the area of lexical learning, these cases should cause the greatest transfer-produced errors.

Transfer in Sentence Comprehension. Transfer is also pervasive in the arena of sentence interpretation. There are now over a dozen Competition Model studies that have demonstrated the transfer of a "syntactic accent" in sentence interpretation (Bates & MacWhinney, 1981; de Bot & van Montfort, 1988; Gass, 1987; Harrington, 1987; Kilborn, 1989; Kilborn & Cooreman, 1987; Kilborn & Ito, 1989; Liu, Bates, & Li, 1992; McDonald, 1987a, 1987b; McDonald & Heilenman, 1991; McDonald & MacWhinney, 1989). Frenck-Mestre (in press) presents a particularly elegant design demonstrating this type of effect during on-line processing. These studies have shown that the learning of sentence processing cues in a second language is a gradual process. The process begins with L2 cue weight settings that are close to those for L1. Over time, these settings change in the direction of the native speakers' settings for L2.

This pattern of results is perhaps most clearly documented in McDonald's studies of English-Dutch and Dutch-English second language learning (McDonald, 1987b). This study shows a linear decline in the strength of the use of word order by English learners of Dutch over increased levels of competence and exactly the opposite pattern for Dutch learners of English. These results and others like them constitute strong support for the Competition Model view of second language learning as the gradual growth of cue strength.

Transfer in Pragmatics. The acquisition of pragmatic patterns is also heavily influenced by L1 transfer. When we first begin to use a second language, we may extend our L1 ideas about the proper form of greetings, questions, offers, promises, expectations, turn taking, topic expansion, face-saving, honorifics, presuppositions, and implications. If the two cultures are relatively similar, much of this transfer will be successful. However, there will inevitably be some gaps. In many cases, the L2 learner will need to eventually reconstruct the entire system of pragmatic patterns in the way they were learned by the child acquiring L1. Much of this learning is based on specific phrases and forms. For example, the L1 learners understanding of greetings is tightly linked to use of specific phrases such as *Guten Morgen* or *bye-bye.* Learning about how and when to use specific speech acts is linked to learning about forms such as *could you? listen,* and *why not?* Learning these forms in a concrete context is important for both L1 and L2 learners. However, pragmatics involves much more than simple speech act units or pairs. We also need to learn larger frames for narratives, argumentation, and polite chatting. By following the flow of perspectives and topics in conversations (MacWhinney, 1999), we can eventually internalize models of how discourse represents reality in both L1 and L2.

Transfer in Morphology. Learning of the morphological marking or inflections of a second language is very different from learning of the other areas we have discussed. This is because, in morphosyntax, it is typically impossible to transfer from L1 to L2. For example, an English learner of German cannot use the English noun gender system as a basis for learning the German noun gender system. This is because English does not have a fully elaborated noun gender system. Of course, English does distinguish between genders in the pronouns ("he" vs. "she") and this distinction is of some help in learning to mark German nouns that have natural gender such as der Vater ("the-MASC father") and die Mutter ("the-FEM mother"). However, one really does not need to rely on cues from English "he" and "she" to realize that fathers are masculine and mothers are feminine. On the other hand, there can be some real transfer effects to German from other languages that have full nominal gender systems. For example, a Spanish speaker might well want to refer to the moon as feminine on the basis of "la luna" in Spanish and produce the erroneous form die Mond in German, rather than the correct masculine form "der Mond."

Similarly, a Spanish learner of Chinese cannot use L1 knowledge to acquire the system of noun classifers, because Spanish has no noun classifers.

Chinese learners of English cannot use their L1 forms to learn the English contrast between definite, indefinite, and zero articles. This is because Chinese makes no overt distinctions in this area, leaving the issue of definiteness to be marked in other ways, if at all.

The fact that morphosyntax is not subject to transfer is a reflection of the general Competition Model dictum that "everything that can transfer will." In the areas of phonology, lexicon, orthography, syntax, and pragmatics, we see attempts to transfer. However, in morphology we see no transfer, because there is no basis for transfer. The exception here is between structurally mapable features, as in the example of gender transfer from Spanish to German.

Although there is no transfer of the exact forms of morphosyntax, and little transfer of secondary mappings such as thinking that the moon is feminine, there is important positive and negative transfer of the underlying functions expressed by morphological devices. Concepts such as the instrumental, locatives, or benefactives often have positive transfer between languages. For example, many languages merge the instrumental "with" and the comitative "with." If L1 has this merger, it is easy to transfer the merged concept to L2. Similarly, semantically grounded grammatical distinctions such as movement towards and movement from can easily be transferred across languages. However in other areas, transfer is less positive. One remarkable area of difficulty is in the learning of article marking in English by speakers of Chinese, Japanese, or Korean. These languages have no separate category of definiteness, instead using classifiers and plurals to express some of the functions marked by the English definite. Moreover, the complexity of the subcomponents of definiteness in English stands as a major barrier for speakers of these languages.

Transfer in Sentence Production.   Pienemann et al. (in press) present evidence that the Competition Model claim that "everything that can transfer will" does not hold in the area of L2 sentence production. Instead, they suggest that "only those linguistic forms that the learner can process can be transferred to L2." Their analysis of this issue is exceptionally detailed and the additional evidence they bring to bear is bound to lead to a very helpful sharpening of the issues at stake. They present the case of the learning of the German V2 rule by speakers of L1 Swedish. The V2 rules in Swedish and German allow speakers to front adverbs like "today" or "now." This produces sentences with the verb in second position with forms such as "Today likes Peter milk." The surprising finding is that Swedes don't produce this order from the beginning, starting instead with "Today Peter likes milk." This finding is only surprising if one believes that what learners transfer are whole syntactic frames for whole sentences. However, the Competition

Model holds that the basic unit of both L1 and L2 acquisition is the item-based pattern. In this case, learners first learn to place the subject before the verb, as in "Peter likes milk". Later they add the adverb to produce "Peter likes milk today." Only in the final stages of learning, do they then pick up the item-based frame that allows adverbs to take the initial slot. The important point here is that in this part of sentence production, much as in morphology, the mapping from L1 to L2 is low-level and conservative. Thus, the failure to see a transfer of the V2 rule from Swedish to German is based on the fact that Swedes are learning German from item-based patterns, not by picking up whole sentence frames at a time. The emphasis on learning from item-based patterns should hold for all beginning L2 learners. For example, we would not expect to see early transfer to Italian of the English cleft structure, although the structure is present in both languages and learners will eventually make the mapping. The problem is that during the first stages of learning, learners are just not working on the sentence level.

The opposite side of this coin is that, when L2 structures can be learned early on as item-based patterns, this learning can block transfer from L1. Pienemann et al. (in press) present the example of learning of Japanese SOV order by speakers of L1 English. These learners almost never generalize English SVO to Japanese. Of course, the input to L2 learners consistently emphasizes SOV order and seldom presents any VO sequences, although these do occur in colloquial Japanese. This learning is best understood in terms of the account of MacWhinney (1982, 1987a). Learners acquire a few initial Japanese verbs as item-based constructions with slots for objects in preverbal position marked by the postposition "o" and topics in initial position marked by the postpositions "wa" or "ga." After learning a few such items, they generalize to the "feature-based" construction of SOV. This is positive learning based on consistent input in L2. If L1 were to have a transfer effect at this point, it would be extremely brief, since L2 is so consistent and these item-based constructions are in the focus of the learner's attention.

What these two examples illustrate is that L1 transfer in the areas of sentence production and morphosyntax is limited by the fact that morphosyntax is the most language-specific part of a target language. Because the mappings are hard to make, transfer in this area is minimized. Once relations between the two languages can be constructed, as in the case of the transfer of the English cleft to Spanish, some positive transfer can be expected. However, we should not expect to see consistent early transfer in this particular area. Thus, the analyses of Pienemann et al. (in press) are remarkably close to those found in the Competition Model, once the importance of item-based patterns is recognized.

Resonance

As we mentioned earlier, the Unified Competition Model includes three new components that were not found in the classic model. These are chunking, codes, and resonance. The theory of chunking is certainly not a new one and could well have been included in the model many years ago. The theory of code relations is also not entirely new, since it incorporates and extends ideas about transfer that have been in development within the Competition Model for nearly 15 years. The component of resonance, on the other hand, is new to the theory. Despite this newness to the model, it plays an important central role in understanding code separation, age-related effects, and the microprocesses of learning and processing.

It is fairly easy to get an intuitive grasp of what resonance means in L1 and L2 learning. Resonance occurs most clearly during covert inner speech. Vygotsky (1962) observed that young children would often give themselves instructions overtly. For example, a two-year-old might say, "pick it up" while picking up a block. At this age, the verbalization tends to guide and control the action. By producing a verbalization that describes an action, the child sets up a resonant connection between vocalization and action. Later, Vygotsky argues, these overt instructions become inner speech and continue to guide our cognition. L2 learners go through a process much like that of the child. At first, they use the language only with others. Then, they begin to talk to themselves in the new language and start to "think in the second language." At this point, the second language begins to assume the same resonant status that the child attains for the first language.

Once a process of inner speech is set into motion, it can also be used to process new input and relate new forms to other forms paradigmatically. For example, if I hear the phrase "ins Mittelalter" in German, I can think to myself that this means that the stem "Alter" must be "das Alter." This means that the dative must take the form "in welchem Alter" or "in meinem Alter." These resonant form-related exercises can be conducted in parallel with more expressive resonant exercises in which I simply try to talk to myself about things around me in German, or whatever language I happen to be learning.

On a mechanistic level, resonance is based on the repeated coactivation of reciprocal connections. As the set of resonant connections grows, the possibilities for cross-associations and mutual activations grow and the language starts to form a coherent co-activating neural circuit. Although this idea of resonance seems so basic and perhaps obvious, it is important to note that modern connectionist models have provided virtually no place for learning in resonant models. This is because current popular neural network models, such as back-propagation, work in only a feed-forward fashion, so resonant links cannot be established or utilized. Self-organizing maps such as the DisLex model of Li et al. (under review) can provide local resonance between sound and meaning, but have not yet been able to model resonance on the syntactic level. Grossberg's (1987) Adaptive Resonance Theory (ART) would seem to be one account that should capture at least some ideas about resonance. However, the resonant connections in that model only capture the role of attentional shifts in motivating the recruitment of additional computational elements.

Perhaps the model that comes closest to expressing the core notion of resonance is the interactive activation (IA) model of the early 1980s. Interactive activation models such as BIA and BIMOLA (Thomas & Van Heuven, in press) have succeeded in accounting for important aspects of bilingual lexical processing. Although these models have not explicitly examined the role of resonance, they are at least compatible with the concept.

We can also use resonance as a way of understanding certain dynamic multilingual processes. For example, variations in the delays involved in code switching in both natural and laboratory tasks can be interpreted in terms of the processes that maintain language-internal resonant activations. If a particular language is being repeatedly accessed, it will be in a highly resonant state. Although another language will be passively accessible, it may take a second or two before the resonant activation of that language can be triggered by a task. Thus, a speaker may not immediately recognize a sentence in a language that has not been spoken in the recent context. On the other hand, a simultaneous interpreter will maintain both languages in continual receptive activation, while trying to minimize resonant activations in the output system of the source language.

I would argue that multilingual processing relies more on activation and resonance than on inhibition (Green, 1988). Of course, we know that the brain makes massive use of inhibitory connections. However, these are typically local connections that sharpen local competitions. Inhibition is also important in providing overt inhibitory control of motor output, as in speech monitoring. However, inhibition by itself cannot produce new learning, coactivation, and inner speech. For these types of processing, resonant activation is more effective.

The cognitive psychology of the 1970s (Atkinson, 1975) placed much emphasis on the role of strategic resonance during learning. More recently, the emphasis has been more on automatic processes of resonance, often within the context of theories of verbal memory. The role of resonance in L1 learning is an area of particular current importance. We know that children can learn new words with only one or two exposures to the new sounds. For this to work successfully, children must resonantly activate the phonological store for that word. In the model of Gupta and MacWhinney (1997), this resonance will involve keeping the phonological form active in short term memory long enough for it to be reliably encoded into the central lexical network (Li et al., under review). This preservation of the auditory form in the phonological buffer is one form of resonant processing.

Resonance can facilitate the sharpening of contrasts between forms. Both L1 and L2 learners may have trouble encoding new phonological forms that are close to words they already know. Children can have trouble learning the two new forms "pif" and "bif" because of their confusability, although they can learn "pif" when it occurs along with "wug" (Stager & Werker, 1997). This same phonological confusability effect can impact second language learners. For example, when I came to learn Cantonese, I needed to learn to pay careful attention to marking with tones, lest I confuse *mother, measles, linen, horse,* and *scold,* as various forms of /ma/. Once a learner has the tonal features right, it is still important to pay attention to each part of a word. For example, when I was learning the Cantonese phrase for "pivoting your foot inward," I initially encoded it as *kau geu,* instead of the correct form *kau geuk.* This is because there is a tendency in Cantonese to reduce final /k/. However, the reduced final /k/ is not totally absent and has an effect on the quality of the preceding vowel. At first, I did not attend to this additional component or cue. However, after my encoding for *kau geu* became automated, my attentional focusing was then freed up enough so that I could notice the presence of the final /k/. This expansion of selective attention during learning is a very general process.

Once the auditory form is captured, the learner needs to establish some pathway between the sound and its meaning. Because few words encode any stable conventional phonological symbolism, pathways of this type must be constructed anew by each language learner. It has been proposed that activation of the hippocampus (McClelland, McNaughton, & O'Reilly, 1995) is sufficient to encode arbitrary relations of this sort. If this were true, second language learners would have virtually no problem picking up long lists of new vocabulary items. Although the hippocampus certainly plays a role in maintaining a temporary resonance between sound and meaning, it is up to the learner to extract additional cues that can facilitate the formation of the sound-meaning linkage.

Resonant mappings can rely on synaesthesia (Ramachandran & Hubbard, 2001), onomatopoeia, sound symbolism, postural associations (Paget, 1930), lexical analysis or a host of other provisional relations. It is not necessary that this symbolism be in accord with any established linguistic pattern. Instead, each learner is free to discover a different pattern of associations. This nonconventional nature of resonant connections means that it will be difficult to demonstrate the use of specific resonant connections in group studies of lexical learning. However, we do know that constructive mnemonics provided by the experimenter (Atkinson, 1975) greatly facilitate learning. For example, when learning the German word

Wasser, we can imagine the sound of water running out of a faucet and associate this sound with the /s/ of *Wasser*. For this word, we can also associate the sound of the German word to the sound of the English word *water*. At the same time, we can associate Wasser with collocations such as *Wasser trinken* which themselves resonate with *Bier trinken* and others. Together, these resonant associations between collocations, sounds, and other words help to link the German word *Wasser* into the developing German lexicon. It is likely that children also use these mechanisms to encode the relations between sounds and meanings. Children are less inhibited than are adults in their ability to create ad hoc symbolic links between sounds and meanings. The child learning German as an L1 might associate the shimmering qualities of *Wasser* with a shimmering aspect of the sibilant; or the child might imagine the sound as plunging downward in tone in the way that water comes over a waterfall. The child may link the concept of *Wasser* tightly to a scene in which someone pours *ein Glas Wasser* and then the association between the sound of *Wasser* and the image of the glass and the pouring are primary. For the first language learner, these resonant links are woven together with the entire nature of experience and the growing concept of the world.

A major dimension of resonant connections is between words and our internal image of the human body. For example, Bailey, Chang, Feldman, & Narayanan (1998) characterize the meaning of the verb "stumble" in terms of the physical motion of the limbs during walking, the encountering of a physical object, and the breaking of gait and posture. As Tomasello (1992) has noted, each new verb learned by the child can be mapped onto a physical or cognitive frame of this type. In this way, verbs and other predicates can support the emergence of a grounded mental model for sentences. Workers in L2 (Asher, 1977) have often emphasized the importance of action for the grounding of new meanings and this new literature in cognitive grammar provides good theoretical support for that approach. Item-based patterns are theoretically central in this discussion, since they provide a powerful link between the earlier Competition Model emphasis on processing and cue validity and the newer theories of grounded cognition (MacWhinney, 1999).

Resonance can make use of analogies between stored chunks, as describe below in the theories for storage and chunking. Gentner & Markman (1997), Hofstadter (1997) and others have formulated models of analogical reasoning that have interesting implications for language acquisition models. Analogies can be helpful in working out the first examples of a pattern. For example, a child learning German may compare *steh auf!* "stand up!" with *er muß aufstehen* "He must get up." The child can see that the two sentences express the same activity, but that the verbal prefix is moved in one. Using this pattern as the basis for further resonant connections, the child can then begin to acquire a general understanding of verbal prefix placement in German.

The adult second language learner tends to rely on rather less imaginative and more structured resonant linkages. One important set of links available to the adult is orthography. When an L2 learner of German learns the word *Wasser*, it is easy to map the sounds of the word directly to the image of the letters. Because German has highly regular mappings from orthography to pronunciation, calling up the image of the spelling of *Wasser* is an extremely good way of activating its sound. When the L2 learner is illiterate or when the L2 orthography is unlike the L1 orthography, this backup system for resonance will not be available. L2 learning of Chinese by speakers of languages with Roman scripts illustrates this problem. In some signs and books in Mainland China, Chinese characters are accompanied by romanized pinyin spellings. This allows the L2 learner a method for establishing resonant connections between new words, their pronunciation, and their representations in Chinese orthography. However, in Taiwan and Hong Kong, characters are seldom written out in pinyin in either books or public notices. As a result, learners cannot learn from these materials. In order to make use of resonant connections from orthography, learners must then focus on the learning of the complex Chinese script. This learning itself requires a large investment in resonant associations, since the Chinese writing system is based largely on radical elements that have multiple resonant associations with the sounds and meanings of word.

Resonance can also play an important role in the resolution of errors. For example, I recently noted that I had wrongly coded the stress on the Spanish word *abanico* "fan" as on the second syllable, as in *abánico*. To correct this error, I spent time both rehearsing the correct stress pattern a few times and then visualizing the word as spelled without the stress mark or with the stress on the second syllable, which is normally not written in Spanish spelling. I also tried to associate this pattern in my mind with the verb *abanicar* "fan" and even the first person singular of this verb that has the form *abanico*. Having rehearsed this form in these various ways and having established these resonant connections, the tendency to produce the only incorrect form was somewhat reduced, although it will take time to fully banish the traces of the incorrect pattern.

Age-Related Effects

At this point, it may be helpful to review how the Unified Competition Model accounts for age-related changes in language learning ability. The default account in this area has been the Critical Period Hypothesis (CPH) which holds that, after some time in late childhood or puberty, second languages can no longer be acquired by the innate language acquisition device, but must be learned painfully and incompletely through explicit instruction. The Unified Competition Model attributes the observed facts about age-related changes to very different sources. The model emphasizes the extent to which repeated use of L1 leads to its ongoing entrenchment. This entrenchment operates differentially across linguistic areas, with the strongest entrenchment occurring in output phonology and the least entrenchment in the area of lexicon, where new learning continues to occur in L1 in any case. To overcome entrenchment, learners must rely on resonant processes that allow the fledgling L2 to resist the intrusions of L1, particularly in phonology (Colomé, 2001; Dijkstra, Grainger, & Van Heuven, 1999). For languages with familiar orthographies, resonance connections can be formed between writing, sound, meaning, and phrasal units. For languages with unfamiliar orthographies, the domain of resonant connections will be more constrained. This problem impacts older learners severely because they have become increasingly reliant on resonant connections between sound and orthography.

Because learning through resonant connections is highly strategic, L2 learners will vary markedly in the constructions they can control or which are missing or incorrectly transferred. In addition to the basic forces of entrenchment, transfer, and strategic resonant learning, older learners will be affected by problems with restricted social contacts, commitments to ongoing L1 interactions, and declining cognitive abilities. None of these changes predict a sharp drop at a certain age in L2 learning abilities. Instead, they predict a gradual decline across the life span.

CONCLUSION

This concludes our examination of the Unified Competition Model. Many of the pieces of this model have already been worked out in some detail. For example, we have a good model of cue competition in syntax for both L1 and L2. We have good models of L1 lexical acquisition. We have good data on phonological and lexical transfer in L2. We have clear data on the ways in which processing load impacts sentence processing in working memory. We are even learning about the neuronal bases of this load (Booth et al., 2001). Other areas provide targets for future work. But the central contribution of the Unified Model is not in terms of accounting for specific empirical findings. Rather, the Unified Model provides us with a high-level road map of a very large territory that we can now fill out in greater detail.

REFERENCES

Asher, J. (1977). Children learning another language: A developmental hypothesis. *Child Development, 48,* 1040–1048.

Atkinson, R. (1975). Mnemotechnics in second-language learning. *American Psychologist, 30,* 821–828.

Bailey, D., Chang, N., Feldman, J., & Narayanan, S. (1998). Expanding embodied lexical development. *Proceedings of the 20th Annual Meeting of the Cognitive Science Society,* 64–69.

Bates, E., Devescovi, A., & Wulfeck, B. (2001). Psycholinguistics: A cross-language perspective. *Annual Review of Psychology, 52,* 369–398.

Bates, E., & MacWhinney, B. (1981). Second language acquisition from a functionalist perspective: Pragmatic, semantic and perceptual strategies. In H. Winitz (Ed.), *Annals of the New York Academy of Sciences conference on native and foreign language acquisition* (pp. 190–214). New York: New York Academy of Sciences.

Bates, E., & MacWhinney, B. (1982). Functionalist approaches to grammar. In E. Wanner & L. Gleitman (Eds.), *Language acquisition: The state of the art* (pp. 173–218). New York: Cambridge University Press.

Berlin, B., & Kay, P. (1969). *Basic Color Terms: Their Universality and Evolution.* Berkeley: University of California Press.

Birdsong, D. (in press). Interpreting age effects in second language acquisition. In J. F. Kroll & A. M. B. DeGroot (Eds.), *Handbook of bilingualism: Psycholinguistic approaches.* New York: Oxford University Press.

Blackwell, A., & Bates, E. (1995). Inducing agrammatic profiles in normals: Evidence for the selective vulnerability of morphology under cognitive resource limitation. *Journal of Cognitive Neuroscience, 7,* 228–257.

Bley-Vroman, R., Felix, S., & Ioup, G. (1988). The accessibility of universal grammar in adult language learning. *Second Language Research, 4,* 1–32.

Booth, J. R., MacWhinney, B., Thulborn, K. R., Sacco, K., Voyvodic, J. T., & Feldman, H. M. (2001). Developmental and lesion effects during brain activation for sentence comprehension and mental rotation. *Developmental Neuropsychology, 18,* 139–169.

Christoffels, I., & de Groot, A. M. B. (in press). Simultaneous interpreting: A cognitive perspective. In J. F. Kroll & A. M. B. DeGroot (Eds.), *Handbook of bilingualism: Psycholinguistic approaches.* New York: Oxford University Press.

Clahsen, H., & Muysken, P. (1986). The availability of UG to adult and child learners: A study of the acquisition of German word order. *Second Language Research, 2,* 93–119.

Colomé, À. (2001). Lexical activation in bilinguals' speech production: Language specific or language independent. *Journal of Memory and Language, 45,* 721–736.

de Bot, K., & van Montfort, R. (1988). 'Cue-validity' in het Nederlands als eerste en tweede taal. *Interdisciplinair Tijdschrift voor Taal en Tekstwetenschap, 8,* 111–120.

De Houwer, A. (in press). Early bilingual acquisition: Focus on morphosyntax and the Separate Development Hypothesis. In J. F. Kroll & A. M. B. DeGroot (Eds.), *Handbook of bilingualism: Psycholinguistic approaches.* New York: Oxford University Press.

Dell, G., Juliano, C., & Govindjee, A. (1993). Structure and content in language production: A theory of frame constraints in phonological speech errors. *Cognitive Science, 17,* 149–195.

Devescovi, A., D'Amico, S., Smith, S., Mimica, I., & Bates, E. (1998). The development of sentence comprehension in Italian and Serbo-Croatian: Local versus distributed cues. In D. Hillert (Ed.), *Syntax and semantics: Vol. 31. Sentence processing: A cross-linguistic perspective* (pp. 345–377). San Diego: Academic Press.

Dick, F., Bates, E., Wulfeck, B., Utman, J., Dronkers, N., & Gernsbacher, M. A. (2001). Language deficits, localization and grammar: Evidence for a distributive model of language breakdown in aphasics and normals. *Psychological Review, 108,* 759–788.

Dijkstra, A., Grainger, J., & Van Heuven, W. J. B. (1999). Recognizing cognates and interlingual homographs: The neglected role of phonology. *Journal of Memory and Language, 41,* 496–518.

Dopke, S. (in press). Generation of and retraction from cross-linguistically motivated structure in bilingual first language acquisition. In F. Genesee (Ed.), *Bilingualism, language, and cognition: Aspects of bilingual acquisition.* Cambridge: Cambridge University Press.

Dussias, P. E. (2001). Bilingual sentence parsing. In J. L. Nicol (Ed.), *One mind, two languages: Bilingual sentence processing* (pp. 159–176). Cambridge, MA: Blackwell.

Ellis, R. (1994). A theory of instructed second language acquisition. In N. C. Ellis (Ed.), *Implicit and explicit learning of language* (pp. 79–114). San Diego: Academic.

Elman, J. L., & McClelland, J. L. (1988). Cognitive penetration of the mechanisms of perception: Compensation for coarticulation of lexically restored phonemes. *Journal of Memory and Language, 27,* 143–165.

Ervin-Tripp, S. (1969). Sociolinguistics. In L. Berkowitz (Ed.), *Advances in experimental social psychology.* New York: Academic Press.

Felix, S., & Wode, H. (Eds.). (1983). *Language development at the crossroads.* Tuebingen: Gunter Narr.

Flege, J., & Davidian, R. (1984). Transfer and developmental processes in adult foreign language speech production. *Applied Psycholinguistics, 5,* 323–347.

Flege, J., Takagi, J., & Mann, V. (1995). Japanese adults can learn to produce English "r" and "l" accurately. *Language Learning, 39,* 23–32.

Flynn, S. (1996). A parameter-setting approach to second language acquisition. In W. C. Ritchie & T. K. Bhatia (Eds.), *Handbook of second language acquisition* (pp. 121–158). San Diego: Academic Press.

Frenck-Mestre, C. (in press). Second language processing: Which theory best accounts for the processing of reduced relative clauses? In J. F. Kroll & A. M. B. DeGroot (Eds.), *Handbook of bilingualism: Psycholinguistic approaches.* New York: Oxford University Press.

Gass, S. (1987). The resolution of conflicts among competing systems: A bidirectional perspective. *Applied Psycholinguistics, 8,* 329–350.

Gentner, D., & Markman, A. (1997). Structure mapping in analogy and similarity. *American Psychologist, 52,* 45–56.

Gerver, D. (1974). The effects of noise on the performance of simultaneous interpreters: Accuracy of performance. *Acta Psychologica, 38,* 159–167.

Gibson, E., Pearlmutter, N., Canseco-Gonzalez, E., & Hickok, G. (1996). Recency preference in the human sentence processing mechanism. *Cognition, 59,* 23–59.

Goldberg, A. E. (1999). The emergence of the semantics of argument structure constructions. In B. MacWhinney (Ed.), *The emergence of language* (pp. 197–213). Mahwah, NJ: Lawrence Erlbaum Associates.

Green, D. M. (1998). Mental control of the bilingual lexico-semantic system. *Language and Cognition, Bilingualism: Language and Cognition* (1).

Grossberg, S. (1987). Competitive learning: From interactive activation to adaptive resonance. *Cognitive Science, 11,* 23–63.

Gupta, P., & MacWhinney, B. (1997). Vocabulary acquisition and verbal short-term memory: Computational and neural bases. *Brain and Language, 59,* 267–333.

Hakuta, K. (1981). Grammatical description versus configurational arrangement in language acquisition: The case of relative clauses in Japanese. *Cognition, 9,* 197–236.

Hancin-Bhatt, B. (1994). Segment transfer: A consequence of a dynamic system. *Second Language Research, 10,* 241–269.

Harrington, M. (1987). Processing transfer: language-specific strategies as a source of interlanguage variation. *Applied Psycholinguistics, 8,* 351–378.

Hauser, M., Newport, E., & Aslin, R. (2001). Segmentation of the speech stream in a non-human primate: Statistical learning in cotton-top tamarins. *Cognition, 78,* B53–B64.

Hausser, R. (1999). *Foundations of computational linguistics: Man-machine communication in natural language.* Berlin: Springer.

Hofstädter, D. (1997). *Fluid concepts and creative analogies: Computer models of the fundamental mechanisms of thought.* London: Allen Lane.

Ijaz, H. (1986). Linguistic and cognitive determinants of lexical acquisition in a second language. *Language Learning, 36,* 401–451.

Kilborn, K. (1989). Sentence processing in a second language: The timing of transfer. *Language and Speech, 32,* 1–23.

Kilborn, K., & Cooreman, A. (1987). Sentence interpretation strategies in adult Dutch-English bilinguals. *Applied Psycholinguistics, 8,* 415–431.

Kilborn, K., & Ito, T. (1989). Sentence processing in Japanese-English and Dutch-English bilinguals. In B. MacWhinney & E. Bates (Eds.), *The crosslinguistic study of sentence processing* (pp. 257–291). New York: Cambridge University Press.

Krashen, S. (1994). The Input Hypothesis and its rivals. In N. C. Ellis (Ed.), *Implicit and explicit learning of languages* (pp. 45–78). San Diego: Academic.

La Heij, W. (in press). Selection processes in monolinguals and bilingual lexical access. In J. F. Kroll & A. M. B. DeGroot (Eds.), *Handbook of bilingualism: Psycholinguistic approaches.* New York: Oxford University Press.

Langacker, R. (1989). *Foundations of cognitive grammar. Vol. 2: Applications.* Stanford: Stanford University Press.

Li, P., Farkas, I., & MacWhinney, B. (under review). The origin of categorical representations of language in the brain. *Cognitive Science.*

Liu, H., Bates, E., & Li, P. (1992). Sentence interpretation in bilingual speakers of English and Chinese. *Applied Psycholinguistics, 13,* 451–484.

Lively, S., Pisoni, D., & Logan, J. (1990). Some effects of training Japanese listeners to identify English /r/ and /l/. In Y. Tohkura (Ed.), *Speech perception, production and linguistic structure.* Tokyo: OHM.

MacDonald, M., & MacWhinney, B. (1990). Measuring inhibition and facilitation from pronouns. *Journal of Memory and Language, 29,* 469–492.

MacDonald, M. C., Pearlmutter, N. J., & Seidenberg, M. S. (1994). Lexical nature of syntactic ambiguity resolution. *Psychological Review, 101*(4), 676–703.

MacWhinney, B. (1975). Pragmatic patterns in child syntax. *Stanford Papers and Reports on Child Language Development, 10,* 153–165.

MacWhinney, B. (1978). The acquisition of morphophonology. *Monographs of the Society for Research in Child Development, 43,* Whole no. 1, pp. 1–123.

MacWhinney, B. (1982). Basic syntactic processes. In S. Kuczaj (Ed.), *Language acquisition: Vol. 1. Syntax and semantics* (pp. 73–136). Hillsdale, NJ: Lawrence Erlbaum.

MacWhinney, B. (1987a). The Competition Model. In B. MacWhinney (Ed.), *Mechanisms of language acquisition* (pp. 249–308). Hillsdale, NJ: Lawrence Erlbaum.

MacWhinney, B. (1987b). Toward a psycholinguistically plausible parser. In S. Thomason (Ed.), *Proceedings of the Eastern States Conference on Linguistics.* Columbus, OH: Ohio State University.

MacWhinney, B. (1989). Competition and lexical categorization. In R. Corrigan, F. Eckman, & M. Noonan (Eds.), *Linguistic categorization* (pp. 195–242). Philadelphia: Benjamin.

MacWhinney, B. (1999). The emergence of language from embodiment. In B. MacWhinney (Ed.), *The emergence of language* (pp. 213–256). Mahwah, NJ: Lawrence Erlbaum.

MacWhinney, B. (2003). The gradual evolution of language. In B. Malle & T. Givón (Eds.), *The evolution of language.* Philadelphia: Benjamin.

MacWhinney, B., & Anderson, J. (1986). The acquisition of grammar. In I. Gopnik & M. Gopnik (Eds.), *From models to modules* (pp. 3–25). Norwood, NJ: Ablex.

MacWhinney, B., & Bates, E. (Eds.). (1989). *The crosslinguistic study of sentence processing.* New York: Cambridge University Press.

MacWhinney, B., Feldman, H. M., Sacco, K., & Valdes-Perez, R. (2000). Online measures of basic language skills in children with early focal brain lesions. *Brain and Language, 71,* 400–431.

MacWhinney, B., & Pléh, C. (1988). The processing of restrictive relative clauses in Hungarian. *Cognition, 29,* 95–141.

McClelland, J. L., McNaughton, B. L., & O'Reilly, R. C. (1995). Why there are complementary learning systems in the hippocampus and neocortex: Insights from the successes and failures of connectionist models of learning and memory. *Psychological Review, 102,* 419–457.

McDonald, J. L. (1987a). Assigning linguistic roles: The influence of conflicting cues. *Journal of Memory and Language, 26,* 100–117.

McDonald, J. L. (1987b). Sentence interpretation in bilingual speakers of English and Dutch. *Applied Psycholinguistics, 8,* 379–414.

McDonald, J. L., & Heilenman, K. (1991). Determinants of cue strength in adult first and second language speakers of French. *Applied Psycholinguistics, 12,* 313–348.

McDonald, J. L., & MacWhinney, B. (1989). Maximum likelihood models for sentence processing research. In B. MacWhinney & E. Bates (Eds.), *The crosslinguistic study of sentence processing* (pp. 397–421). New York: Cambridge University Press.

McDonald, J. L., & MacWhinney, B. J. (1995). The time course of anaphor resolution: Effects of implicit verb causality and gender. *Journal of Memory and Language, 34,* 543–566.

Menn, L., & Stoel-Gammon, C. (1995). Phonological development. In P. Fletcher & B. MacWhinney (Eds.), *The handbook of child language* (pp. 335–360). Oxford: Blackwell.

Meuter, R. (in press). Language selection in bilinguals: Mechanisms and processes of change. In J. F. Kroll & A. M. B. DeGroot (Eds.), *Handbook of bilingualism: Psycholinguistic approaches.* New York: Oxford University Press.

Miyake, A., Carpenter, P., & Just, M. (1994). A capacity approach to syntactic comprehension disorders: Making normal adults perform like aphasic patients. *Cognitive Neuropsychology, 11,* 671–717.

Moon, C., Cooper, R. P., & Fifer, W. P. (1993). Two-day infants prefer their native language. *Infant Behavior and Development, 16,* 495–500.

Newell, A. (1990). *A unified theory of cognition.* Cambridge, MA: Harvard University Press.

Norris, D. (1994). Shortlist: A connectionist model of continuous speech recognition. *Cognition, 52,* 189–234.

Paget, R. (1930). *Human speech.* New York: Harcourt Brace.

Pienemann, M., Di Biase, B., Kawaguchi, S., & Håkansson, G. (in press). Processing constraints on L1 transfer. In J. F. Kroll & A. M. B. DeGroot (Eds.), *Handbook of bilingualism: Psycholinguistic approaches.* New York: Oxford University Press.

Ramachandran, V. S., & Hubbard, E. M. (2001). Synaesthesia: A Window into Perception, Thought and Language. *Journal of Consciousness Studies, 8,* 3–34.

Sebastián-Galles, N., & Bosch, L. (in press). Phonology and bilingualism. In J. F. Kroll & A. M. B. DeGroot (Eds.), *Handbook of bilingualism: Psycholinguistic approaches.* New York: Oxford University Press.

Seleskovitch, D. (1976). Interpretation: A psychological approach to translating. In R. W. Brislin (Ed.), *Translation: Application and Research.* New York: Gardner.

Snow, C. E. (1999). Social perspectives on the emergence of language. In B. MacWhinney (Ed.), *The emergence of language* (pp. 257–276). Mahwah, NJ: Lawrence Erlbaum Associates.

Sokolov, J. L. (1988). Cue validity in Hebrew sentence comprehension. *Journal of Child Language, 15,* 129–156.

Sokolov, J. L. (1989). The development of role assignment in Hebrew. In B. MacWhinney & E. Bates (Eds.), *The crosslinguistic study of sentence processing* (pp. 158–184). New York: Cambridge.

Spivey, M., & Marian, V. (1999). Cross talk between native and second language: Partial activation of an irrelevant lexicon. *Psychological Sciences, 10,* 281–284.

Stager, C. L., & Werker, J. F. (1997). Infants listen for more phonetic detail in speech perception than in word learning tasks. *Nature, 388,* 381–382.

Stemberger, J., & MacWhinney, B. (1986). Frequency and the lexical storage of regularly inflected forms. *Memory and Cognition, 14,* 17–26.

Stockwell, R., Bowen, J., & Martin, J. (1965). *The grammatical structures of English and Spanish.* Chicago: University of Chicago Press.

Thomas, M., & Van Heuven, W. J. B. (in press). Computational models of bilingual comprehension. In J. F. Kroll & A. M. B. DeGroot (Eds.), *Handbook of bilingualism: Psycholinguistic approaches.* New York: Oxford University Press.

Tomasello, M. (1992). *First verbs: A case study of early grammatical development.* Cambridge: Cambridge University Press.

Tomasello, M. (2000). The item-based nature of children's early syntactic development. *Trends in Cognitive Sciences, 4,* 156–163.

Vygotsky, L. (1962). *Thought and language.* Cambridge: MIT Press.

Werker, J. F. (1995). Exploring developmental changes in cross-language speech perception. In L. Gleitman & M. Liberman (Eds.), *An Invitation to Cognitive Science. Language Volume 1* (pp. 87–106). Cambridge, MA: MIT Press.

Chapter 4

Cues, Constraints, and Competition in Sentence Processing

Jeffrey L. Elman
University of California, San Diego

Mary Hare
Bowling Green State University

Ken McRae
University of Western Ontario

INTRODUCTION

One of the hallmarks of human behavior is that it reflects the rapid integration of constraints from an often large number of sources, in a manner that is flexible, responsive to novel situations, and apparently effortless. This is true in virtually every sensorimotor activity in which we engage, whether it be vision, motor activity or audition, and is also particularly evident in the domain of language. There is now abundant evidence suggesting that processing of language requires the integration of information at a variety of levels: grammatical structure, meaning, discourse, world-knowledge, and so on (Bates & MacWhinney, 1989; Clifton, 1993; Jurafsky, 1996; McClelland, St. John, & Taraban, 1989; MacDonald, Pearlmutter, & Seidenberg, 1994; Spivey-Knowlton & Sedivy, 1995; Spivey-Knowlton, Trueswell & Tanenhaus, 1993; Swinney, 1979; Tanenhaus & Trueswell, 1995).

In the case of comprehension, the information a listener or reader has access to is rarely completely transparent. Rather, it is useful to think of the input as providing cues to structure and meaning. Some of these cues may be highly reliable. Others are only weakly informative. Some are frequent; others are rare. Sometimes the cues converge, but they may also conflict. Successful comprehension requires that all this information be computed, integrated, reconciled, and resolved. Furthermore, this is a dynamic process in which different interpretations may prevail at different points in time.

111

But how does this occur? The challenge for those who strive to understand such behaviors is that the complexities of multivariable systems—particularly those that exhibit nonlinear interactions and temporal dynamics—are formidable. Moreover, the standard computational metaphor that has traditionally been invoked in analyses of human behavior (viz., the human brain as a digital computer) does not lend itself to modeling such systems.

Because of this, over the past several decades there have emerged a number of alternative frameworks that appear to offer more promise for understanding human behavior. One of the earliest and most influential has been the Competition Model of Bates and MacWhinney (1989; see also MacWhinney, this volume). The Competition Model (henceforth, CM) explicitly recognizes the fundamental importance in behavioral analyses of identifying the informational value of cues—distinguishing between their availability and reliability—and the potential of such cues to interact in complex ways. Although elegantly simple, the CM provides a rich conceptual framework not only for understanding behaviors in their (putative) end-state, but has also generated insights into their ontogeny as well as causes for variation, both at the level of individuals as well as across languages and cultures. One reason that the CM has had such an impact on language research is that it was one of the first models to focus on multiple cues and competition among them, countering a popular view at the time which focused instead on syntactic variables and a modular grammar.

Of course, there are many issues that remain to be resolved, and in domains such as sentence processing, significant controversies remain over the nature of the underlying mechanisms by which language is produced and processed. Indeed, one of the deepest divides in psycholinguistics concerns the degree to which sentence processing involves an autonomous component that is sensitive to only to syntactic relations and major grammatical categories, or whether the sorts of interactions that are posited by the CM (and others of its class) potentially occur at all stages in processing.

In sentence comprehension research, one of the most influential of the former theories is the two-stage serial model (sometimes also known as the "garden path" model) of Frazier and colleagues (Frazier, 1979, 1995; Frazier & Rayner, 1982; Rayner, Carlson, & Frazier, 1983). The two-stage theory assigns primary importance to syntactic considerations. Access to lexically-specific information, including structural information associated with specific words, detailed lexical semantics, discourse, and world knowledge, is assumed not to be available at this stage. With only impoverished information to guide the comprehender, it is assumed that she employs a set of heuristics to parse the incoming words (e.g., attach the new word to the syntactic tree in a way that minimizes number of nodes; or create an attachment that—all things being equal—is to a currently open phrase, rather than create a new phrase). These heuristics may not always work in the long run, and during a subsequent "second pass", when additional information becomes available to the comprehender, revision of the initial parse may be necessary. However, the heuristics have the advantage that they are often correct and are quick and easy to employ.

In recent years, an alternative has emerged challenging the assumptions of the two-stage serial account of sentence processing. This contrasting approach, often termed the constraint-based (henceforth, CB) or expectation-driven model, emphasizes the probabilistic and context-sensitive aspects of sentence processing and assumes that comprehenders use idiosyncratic lexical, semantic, and pragmatic information about each incoming word to determine an initial structural analysis (Altmann, 1998, 1999; Altmann & Kamide, 1999; MacDonald, 1993; MacDonald et al., 1994; St. John & McClelland, 1990; Tanenhaus & Carlson, 1989; Trueswell, Tanenhaus, & Garnsey, 1994). On this account, a much broader range of information is assumed to be available and used at very early stages of processing. This information is often fine-grained and word-specific (McRae, Ferretti, & Amyote, 1997; McRae, Spivey-Knowlton, & Tanenhaus, 1998), may reflect lexical (MacDonald, 1994) and context-contingent frequency information (Allen & MacDonald, 1995; Juliano & Tanenhaus, 1993), and may contribute to the immediate computation of semantic plausibility (Garnsey, Pearlmutter, Meyers, & Lotocky, 1997; Pickering & Traxler, 1998; Trueswell, Tanenhaus, & Kello, 1993).

Clearly, there is a close relationship, theoretically as well as historically, between the CB-approaches and the CM. The two approaches share core assumptions: (1) all sources of information matter; (2) these sources of information become available as soon as possible, but can differ in their timecourse of availability; (3) information is used as soon as it becomes available; and (4) the influence of the various information sources depends on their strength and the relative strengths of other cues/constraints. In practice, the two approaches have tended to focus on different domains (CM on acquisition, cross-linguistic differences, and aphasia; CB on syntactic ambiguity resolution, the role of lexically-specific information in processing, and syntax-semantics interactions) and the approaches have also differed somewhat in methodologies. But there is considerable overlap, and the differences are historical more than theoretical.

One frequent criticism of CM/CB models has been that with so many free parameters and with no constraints on the nature of interactions, virtually any pattern of behavior might be explained. The criticism is not entirely fair, because an explicit goal of both CM and CB models has been to articulate precisely the conditions under which information becomes available, the factors that determine the informativeness and use of cues, and the principles that determine how multiple cues interact. Nonetheless, it is true that as CM/CB models increase in complexity, the ability to predict the fine detail of their behavior based only on first principles is severely limited (particularly when it is assumed that cue interactions involve nonlinearities). Furthermore, as the debate between two-stage and CM/CB models heated up, the role of differences in predictions regarding the time course of processing became increasingly significant. Often, experimental outcomes that differ by only a few hundred milliseconds are taken as discriminating between the two classes of models. With so much resting on such small differences, any sloppiness in the accuracy of a model's predictions can not be tolerated.

What was needed, then was an implemented CM/CB model. Fortunately, at about the same time as the CM/CB models were being developed, there was a dramatic development on the computational front. The advent of neurally-inspired models of computation, in the form of connectionist simulations, provided a natural framework for understanding exactly the issues that the CM/CB models had pushed to the fore: What information is used in sentence processing, when it becomes available, and the nature of the (often nonlinear) interactions between information sources. These simulations furthermore made it possible to make precise predictions about the temporal dynamics of the interactions—predictions that were sometimes not what intuition might have predicted in the absence of simulation.

The family of connectionist models of language is large, and includes a variety of frameworks (see Bechtel & Abrahamsen, 2002; Christiansen & Chater, 2001; Reilly & Sharkey, 1992; and Smolensky, 2001 for recent overviews). In the remainder of this chapter, we focus on a specific architecture that comes closest in its explicit form to embodying the principles of the CM and related CB approaches: the Competition-Integration Model (McRae, Spivey-Knowlton, & Tanenhaus, 1998; McRae, Hare, & Elman, 2002; Spivey-Knowlton, 1996; Tanenhaus, Spivey-Knowlton, & Hanna, 2000). We begin by presenting the model in general terms, describe a set of empirical data involving the resolution of a syntactic ambiguity, and then show how the model implements the principles of the CM and CB framework.

THE COMPETITION-INTEGRATION MODEL

The Competition-Integration Model (Spivey-Knowlton, 1996; henceforth, CIM) had as its central principle that multiple constraints provide probabilistic support for possible syntactic alternatives. These cues thus compete in a manner that is analogous to Bates and MacWhinney's (1989) conception of a competition model. The model has matured over the years. Further developments included a mechanism for processing multiple words or regions of text, thus enabling simulations of reading time throughout the critical regions of sentences. Spivey-Knowlton and Tanenhaus (1998) incorporated an additional critical feature of the model in that they determined the strength of the various constraints using off-line norms and corpora analyses, so that these parameters were determined in a principled manner rather than being free. In both of these initial implementations, the influence of each constraint was determined by a weight connecting it to the possible interpretations. A critical issue left unresolved by these implementations, however, was constraint weighting: What determines the weight associated with a constraint? If left a free parameter, the constraint-based model itself becomes unconstrained.

Spivey-Knowlton and Tanenhaus dealt with this issue by equally weighting each constraint, but the reason for doing so was that it seemed least biased alternative. McRae et al. (1998) provided a solution to this problem, in that not only were all constraints determined by independent means, but in addition, the weight on each constraint was set by fitting the output of the model to human off-line completion norms, thus reducing the degrees of freedom in the model in a principled manner. The McRae et al. model is shown in Fig. 4.1.

The goal of this model was to account for experimental data that had been collected in an attempt to understand how readers resolve the syntactic ambiguity that arises temporarily in sentences such as *The man arrested* . . . At the point when the verb is encountered, two possible continuations might be expected: One in which *arrested* is the main verb (MV) in its past tense form (*The man arrested the criminal*), and the other in which it is a past participle in a reduced relative (RR) construction (*The man arrested by the police was found guilty*).

The experimental data indicated that a number of constraints influenced readers' preference for either the MV or RR interpretation as the sentence was read. These included the overall likelihood of such fragments being a main clause, given language-wide statistics; the relative frequencies with which specific verbs occur in their past participle versus past tense form; the constraining effect that a subsequent *by* has on the MV versus RR interpretation; and finally, the goodness of fit of the initial noun as a potential agent as opposed to patient of the specific verb being read (thematic fit). The data showed that readers are sensitive to the thematic fit of the noun to each of these roles, and that this influenced their ability to resolve the ambiguity, as all target sentences in this study contained the RR construction. For example, *The cop arrested* . . . favored a MV reading whereas *The crook arrested* . . . favored the RR reading.

McRae et al. (1998) used both corpus analyses (for the first three constraints) and off-line data from role/filler typicality ratings (for the thematic fit constraint) to estimate the degree to which each constraint sup-

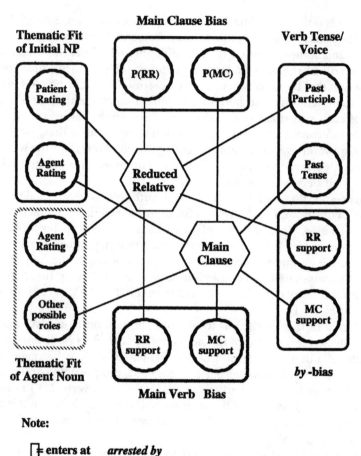

Note:

⊐≠ **enters at**   *arrested by*

⊰≠ **enters at**   *the detective*

◻≠ **enters at**   *was guilty*

FIG. 4.1.   A schematic of the Competition-Integration Model. Thematic fit of the initial NP, the main clause bias, the *by* bias, and the verb tense/voice constraint become operative at the verb+*by* region. The thematic fit of the agent NP comes into play at the agent NP region and the main verb bias becomes operative at the main verb region. From McRae, Spivey-Knowlton, and Tanenhaus (1998).

ported each of the two interpretations. (Details of the implementation are given in the next section when we discuss a CIM implementation of another phenomenon.) Because the model could be given information incrementally, in the same way that the readers viewed successive pairs of words in the actual experiment, it was possible to measure the model's changing interpretation of the sentence on a moment-by-moment basis. Moreover, a simple change in the model—the delay in availability of thematic-fit and lexically-specific structural information, so that only the configurational constraint operated initially—made it possible to simulate a two-stage serial account, and then contrast these predictions with those of a CM/CB model that allows all information to be made available and used as the words relevant to each constraint are read. Impressively, this latter condition provided a close quantitative fit to the reading time data from human subjects, whereas the two-stage serial version deviated significantly from the empirical data.

The MV/RR structural ambiguity is only one of several structural ambiguities that have been studied in the psycholinguistic literature. Another ambiguity arises when the nature of a verb's complement (Direct Object or Sentential Complement) is temporarily unclear. As is true in the MV/RR ambiguity, this ambiguity affords a rich testing ground for probing comprehenders' sensitivity to various sources of information, and the time course with which that information is brought to bear. In the next section, we summarize previous work showing that interacting sources of information play a significant and early role in the resolution of this ambiguity, then turn to a series of studies that we have carried out that demonstrate that both discourse context and meaning have a significant effect as well. We then show how these effects are well-modeled by a CIM.

THE DIRECT OBJECT/SENTENTIAL COMPLEMENT AMBIGUITY

Some verbs occur in only one syntactic frame, for example, with only one type of possible complement (*She devoured hamburgers by the dozen*; **She devoured*; **She devoured that he would soon leave*; etc.). However, many other verbs can be used in multiple frames (*She believed John; She believed that John was telling the truth*). Under certain circumstances, this fact may result in temporary ambiguity as a sentence is being read or heard. Consider, for example, the sentence *The woman heard the dog had barked all night*. The argument of the verb *heard* turns out to be a sentential complement (SC). However, if the sentence is read incrementally, at the point where the postverbal noun phrase (NP), *the dog*, is read, it is possible that rather than being the subject of the SC (as it turns out to be), *the dog* is the direct object (DO) of the verb (as it would be if the sentence ended at that point, e.g., *The woman heard the dog.*). Thus, the role of the NP is temporarily ambiguous. Of course, the ambiguity can be avoided if the complementizer *that* occurs (*The woman heard that the dog* . . . unambiguously signals that the NP is the subject of a SC). But in practice, the omission of the complementizer is common. In that case, the true structure is not revealed until the reader encounters the verb in the SC (*had barked* in the sentence above). This is referred to as the disambiguation region.

Resolving the DO/SC Ambiguity: The Role of Verb Bias and DO Plausibility

Although some verbs occur in both SC and DO constructions with equal likelihood, many exhibit a bias toward one structure or the other. The notion that such differences (also referred to as subcategorization preferences) might play a role in sentence processing has been considered by a number of researchers (Clark & Clark, 1977; Connine, Ferreira, Jones, Clifton, & Frazier, 1984; Ferreira & McClure, 1997; Fodor, 1978; Fodor & Garrett, 1967; Ford, Bresnan, & Kaplan, 1983). Some researchers, such as Ford et al. (1983), have suggested that comprehenders use their knowledge of the relative probability with which a verb occurs with different subcategorizations to guide syntactic analysis. Others, such as Frazier (1987) and Ferreira and Henderson (1990), have claimed that lexically-specific knowledge of this sort is used only in the second stage of processing.

The role of verb bias in comprehension has been the focus of a number of studies involving the DO/SC ambiguity. Although some studies report late or no effects of verb bias (Mitchell, 1987; Ferreira & Henderson, 1990), more recent work has shown early effects (though see Kennison, 2001). Trueswell et al. (1993) contrasted sentence pairs that were structurally ambiguous at the postverbal NP, and differed only in the bias of the main verb. These sentences were then contrasted with the reading time for structurally unambiguous versions (i.e., containing the complementizer *that*). The additional time taken to read the ambiguous version was referred to as the ambiguity effect. In a self-paced reading time experiment, Trueswell et al. found a large ambiguity effect for sentences containing DO-biased verbs at the point following the disambiguation toward a SC. In sentences involving SC-biased verbs, on the other hand, reading times for ambiguous sentences were similar to unambiguous controls.

In the Trueswell et al. study, the same sentence frame (with the same postverbal NP) was used for both a DO- and a SC-biased verb. This NP was always a plausible DO for the DO-biased verbs (e.g. *The waiter confirmed the reservation was made yesterday . . .*) but rarely or never plausible as DO for the SC-biased verbs (*The waiter insisted the reservation was made yesterday . . .*). As a result, bias was confounded with DO plausibility, and the results may have been influenced by the degree of commitment to a semantically plausible or implausible parse (cf. Pickering & Traxler, 1998).

Garnsey et al. (1997) addressed this issue in an eyetracking study in which both verb bias and DO plausibility were separately manipulated.

Verbs of each bias type (including a third, equi-biased condition) appeared in sentences in which the post-verbal NP was either plausible or implausible as a DO. Thus for the implausible conditions, the NP was syntactically ambiguous, but semantically anomalous if interpreted as a DO. An effect of verb bias was found nonetheless: At the disambiguation, reading times were longer in the ambiguous than the unambiguous conditions for DO-biased, but not SC-biased verbs. In addition, with DO-biased verbs, sentences with plausible DOs yielded a significant ambiguity effect whereas the effect for those with implausible DOs was not statistically reliable. Finally, the clearest influence of plausibility was found when verbs were relatively equi-biased in terms of subcategorization preferences. Together, then these two studies offer compelling evidence that both verb bias and DO plausibility play a role in guiding the interpretation of ambiguous sentences.

Resolving the DO/SC Ambiguity:
The Role of Verb Meaning

The studies reviewed above assume (as do many computational models) that subcategorization bias is computed across all instances of a verb. But verb bias effects, in our view, reflect the relationship between verb meaning and verb subcategorization (e.g., Fisher, Gleitman, & Gleitman, 1991), If this is true, then subcategorization bias should be sensitive to verb meaning—and thus for many verbs with multiple senses, the verb's subcategorization bias may vary depending on which sense is intended. For example, the verb *find* must take a DO when it is used to mean 'locate', but when it is used to mean 'understand', a SC structure is more common. This follows logically from the different requirements that the two meanings impose on the arguments in each case. When one performs a concrete action (*He found the book on the table*), a patient is likely to be specified and to be realized as a DO. However, mental events or expressions of mental attitude are more typically followed by a proposition that describes the event or situation (*He found the plane had left without him*), and this is naturally realized by a SC (although note that a DO can sometimes be used as well: *He found nothing but confusion*). If the relevant relationship is between structure and a specific sense of a verb, not structure and the verb in the aggregate, then patterns of verb bias would be better described by considering the specific sense that is used.[1]

Linguistic research (e.g., Argaman & Pearlmutter, 2002: Grimshaw, 1979; Levin, 1993; Pesetsky, 1995; Pinker, 1989) has detailed a complex re-

---

[1]In what follows we follow the standard practice of referring to different meanings of a polysemous word as *senses* of the word, to distinguish them from the distinct meanings of homonyms like *bank*.

lationship between verb meaning and verb subcategorization. Thus, although earlier studies have assumed that the bias of the verb overall helps guide comprehension, we argue that subcategorization preferences are best measured with respect to specific senses of the verb. This view has been corroborated by corpus analyses (Hare, McRae, & Elman, in press; Roland & Jurafsky, 2002). Hare et al. demonstrated that a large set of individual verbs show significant differences in their subcategorization profiles across three corpora, but that cross-corpus bias estimates are much more stable when sense is taken into account. In addition, they showed that consistency between sense-specific subcategorization biases and experimenters' classifications largely predicts results of recent experiments on the resolution of the DO/SC ambiguity.

Hare et al. (in press) and Roland and Jurafsky (2002) establish that there are systematic relations between verb sense and subcategorization preferences. Hare et al.'s results demonstrating the correspondence between sense-specific subcategorization preferences and the success of various experiments in obtaining an influence of verb subcategorization information suggested that comprehenders might learn and exploit meaning-form correlations at the level of individual verb senses, rather than the verb in the aggregate. However, these results did not directly demonstrate this.

In what follows, we present such a demonstration. We begin with a close examination of the relationships that exist between verb meaning and structure for a specific set of verbs. We find that a reliable correlation exists for these verbs in corpus analyses, and that comprehenders make use of such relationships in off-line sentence completion norms when verb sense is biased by preceding context. Next, we demonstrate that this knowledge plays a role in how readers resolve the DO/SC ambiguity in an on-line reading task. All of this sets the stage for the final section, in which we use the CIM architecture described above to simulate and understand the precise mechanism by which multiple constraints interact in order to resolve the DO/SC ambiguity.

Sense and Structure

How might one evaluate whether or not verb sense plays a role in a reader's expectations regarding which syntactic frame is likely (and by extension, how DO/SC ambiguities are resolved)? Two steps are involved. First, we need to know what the pattern of usage is for the various senses of a set of candidate verbs, and the syntactic structures that are typically used with each sense. This can be determined through analysis of large-scale corpora. Second, a set of experimental stimuli are needed in which, for each verb, the same initial sentence fragment may be preceded by different contexts, one which biases toward the sense associated with a DO structure, and the other which biases toward the sense associated with a SC structure. The question then becomes whether, in an on-line task (such as reading), there is evidence that comprehenders process the same sentence fragments differently, depending on the prior sense-biasing context.

Corpus Analyses. We began with 20 verbs that could occur with both DO and SC arguments, and which were categorized in WordNet (Miller, Beckwith, Fellbaum, Gross, & Miller, 1993) as having more than one sense. Typically, the DO associated sense involved a concrete event (e.g., an action) and the SC associated sense involved a more abstract one (e.g., a mental event or statement making). All sentences containing these verbs were extracted from three written and one conversational corpora: the Wall Street Journal (WSJ), Brown Corpus (BC), WSJ87/Brown Laboratory for Linguistic Information Processing (BLLIP), and Switchboard (SWBD), respectively. All corpora are available from the Linguistic Data Consortium at the University of Pennsylvania.

Because these corpora were parsed, we were able to classify each sentence according to 20 subcategorization frames expanded from the set used by Roland and Jurafsky (2002). The fine-grained parse categories were then collapsed into the more general categories of DO, SC, and Other (see Hare et al., 2003, for details). This analysis provided information about the overall frequency of occurrence with which each verb occurs in the DO, SC, and Other frames. We then computed sense-contingent bias counts to test whether these would differ from the overall probabilities. For each of the 20 verbs, we identified two senses that appear to be sufficiently distinct, that we believe are known to undergraduates, and that allow different subcategorization frames according to WordNet. We searched WordNet's Semantic Concordance for the two senses of each target verb. The Concordance consists of a subset of the Brown corpus, with all content words tagged for sense. This allowed us to extract all sentences containing the relevant verb senses. The result of this analysis demonstrated a probabilistic relationship between a verb's sense and its subcategorization preferences.

Experimental Results. But are comprehenders sensitive to such differences, and does a verb's sense affect how a comprehender will interpret the DO/SC ambiguity? To test this, we constructed a set of items based on the 20 polysemous verbs. Each item consisted of a context sentence intended to promote either the SC-biased or DO-biased sense (as determined by the corpus analyses), followed by a target sentence that contained the verb and continued with a SC. For example, the verb *admit* occurred in the same sentence but preceded by two different contexts (all target sentences were identical to at least one word past the postdisambiguation region):

1. SC-biasing:
   The intro psychology students hated having to read the assigned text
   because it was so boring.
   They found (that) the book was written poorly and difficult to understand.

2. DO-biasing:
   Allison and her friends had been searching for John Grisham's new
   novel for a week, but yesterday they were finally successful.
   They found (that) the book was written poorly and were annoyed that
   they had spent so much time trying to get it.

In (1), the context biases toward the 'become aware of' sense of *found*,
which is highly associated with an SC structure; in (2) the context biases toward the DO associated 'discover' sense. To verify that the two contexts did
in fact promote the desired senses of each verb, a series of norming studies
were carried out in which subjects completed various sentence fragments
(with the postverbal noun, without the postverbal noun, and with and without the prior context).

In a final study, subjects read target sentences, presented one word at a
time on a computer screen, and preceded (for any given subject) by one of
the two contexts. After reading each word, subjects pressed a key that revealed the next word. In order to assess the specific difficulty introduced by
the ambiguity, some subjects saw versions in which the complementizer *that*
was present, and others saw the ambiguous version without the complementizer. Differences in reading times between these two conditions provided a measure of the ambiguity effect.

The results are shown graphically in Fig. 4.2. There are no effects of either context (DO versus SC biasing) or ambiguity (presence or absence of
that) up through the first word of the disambiguating region (*was* in the example shown). At the second word of the disambiguating region (*written*),
there is a significant interaction between context and ambiguity. This occurs because in the DO-biasing context, reading times are longer for ambiguous sentences than for unambiguous sentences (i.e., there is a significant
ambiguity effect); but no such effect occurs in the SC-biasing context.
There are also main effects for context (reading times in the SC-biasing
context are shorter than in the DO-biasing context) and for ambiguity (longer reading times for ambiguous sentences than for unambiguous sentences).
But by the first word of the post-disambiguating region (*poorly*), the context
by ambiguity interaction disappears, and there is no longer a significant
main effect of either ambiguity or context.

Our interpretation of the context by ambiguity interaction in the disambiguating region is that the DO-biasing contexts led readers to expect the
sense of the verb that typically occurred with DOs; SC-biasing contexts had

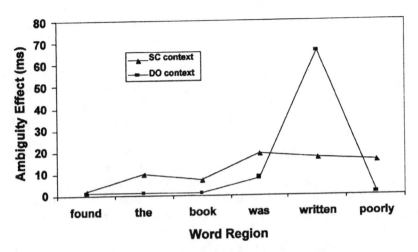

FIG. 4.2.   Results of the sense-biasing experiment. Ambiguity effect from the verb through the first word of the postdisambiguating region.

exactly the opposite effect. In the SC condition, therefore, subjects were primed to expect a sentential complement, whether or not the complementizer was present. When subjects encountered the disambiguating words indicating that in fact there was a sentential complement, these were consistent with their expectations. However, in the DO condition, the absence of the complementizer reinforced the expectation that the postverbal NP was a DO. The inconsistency between this interpretation and the evidence provided by the words disambiguating toward an SC led to elevated reading times, relative to when the complementizer was present as an early warning of an SC structure.

Modeling the DO/SC Ambiguity Resolution

We have implemented a CIM to evaluate whether the experimental results of Hare et al. (2003) are consistent with the predictions one might make, given the CM/CB approaches described at the outset of this chapter. We have already described one such model; here we give a more detailed explanation of the model that we used to account for the effects that sense and other constraints have on resolving the DO/SC ambiguity. A graphical depiction of the model is shown in Fig. 4.3. After describing the model's architecture, we present results of its behavior when it was used to simulate the actual stimuli used in the human experiment. We then provide our interpretation of how the model's behavior captures the principles of the CM/CB framework.

Architecture. As Fig. 4.3 shows, we assumed there are at least seven constraints that interact and contribute to the relative strength of a DO versus
SC interpretation in Hare et al.'s (2003) experimental items. The two octa-
gons in the center, marked "DO" and "SC", are metaphorical interpretation
nodes that have associated activation values ranging between 0.0 and 1.0.
These activations are intended to indicate the model's confidence in a DO
or SC interpretation; these interpretations change over time as new input is
received and as different constraints interact.

The seven constraints themselves are shown as rectangles surrounding
the interpretation nodes. Each constraint has a strength that was estimated
in a manner appropriate to it. (1) The **sense-specific subcategorization bias**
reflects the influence of the context sentences in promoting each of the two
targeted senses of each verb, where one sense is used predominantly with a
DO, and the other is used predominantly with an SC. The strength of this
constraint was estimated from completion norms in which subjects completed a sentence fragment that included only the subject and verb and was

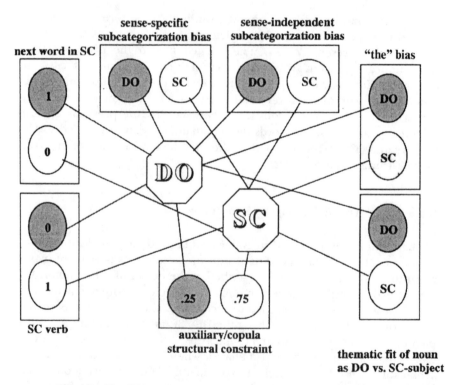

FIG. 4.3. The CIM used to model the effects of sense on the DO/SC ambiguity.

preceded by one of the two context sentences. The completions were scored for the sense of the verb, regardless of the actual syntactic structure the subject used, and the percentage of times that subjects used each target sense of the verb was then used as the value of the constraint. As shown in Table 4.1, on average, the SC-context promoted the SC-correlated verb sense for 89% of the completions, and the DO-context promoted the DO-correlated sense 76% of the time. This constraint varies by verb and by context. (2) The **sense-independent subcategorization bias** was estimated for each verb from the Brown Corpus, and reflected the verb's overall frequency of usage—regardless of sense—with DO and SC arguments. We assume that the over-all usage of a verb might influence a comprehender's expectations of its usage in any given context, independent of its likely sense in that context. Thus, this constraint varies by verb, but not by context. (3) The *the* bias was taken from completion norms out of context (i.e., subjects saw only fragments of the form *She admitted*). We counted the number of times a postverbal *the* was used in DO versus SC completions. Other work involving corpus analyses (Roland, Elman, & Ferreira, 2003) had indicated that the presence of a postverbal *the* (in the absence of a complementizer) is a strong predictor that the postverbal noun is a DO. Consistent with that research, the *the* bias strongly supported a DO-interpretation on average. This constraint varied by verb, but not by context. (4) The **thematic fit of noun as DO vs. SC subject** allowed the model to take into account the goodness of fit of the postverbal noun as either a DO or SC subject. For example, *goals* can be either a DO or SC subject in the sentence fragment *She realized her goals . . .* , whereas *shoes* is a very implausible DO and thus might be expected to promote a SC interpretation (cf. Garnsey et al., 1997; Pickering & Traxler, 1998). Thematic fit was estimated based on a combination of completion norms, WordNet semantic representations, and Resnik's (1993) measure of selection association. Thematic fit varied by both verb and context, although Hare et al. purposely did not manipulate this variable and avoided using highly plausible or implausible NPs. (5) The **structural bias of SC auxiliary or copula** was estimated in the following manner. This word was the first in what is usually termed the disambiguation region because the words in this region provide strong structural cues that a SC is being read. The most obvious possibility is to provide full support to the SC interpretation. However, in 16 of the 20 target sentences, the first word of the disambiguation was an auxiliary or copula, which carries no semantic content, and is the short type of word that is often skipped (not fixated) in free reading (as measured by eyetracking studies). In contrast, in 15 of 20 cases, the second word of the disambiguation region was a content word such as the main verb of the SC, a predicate adjective, predicate nominal, or adverb. Because of these facts, the **structural bias of SC auxiliary or copula** provided 75% of its support to the SC, and 25% to the

DO interpretation. (6) and (7) The influence of both the **structural bias of SC main verb** and the **structural bias of next word in SC** was estimated as fully supporting the SC interpretation.

Normalized Recurrence. Constraints were integrated using a three-step normalized recurrence mechanism developed by Spivey-Knowlton (1996). First, each of the c informational constraints (two for fragments that ended at the verb) was condensed into its normalized probabilistic support for the a relevant competing alternatives (i.e., SC and DO).

$$S_{c,a}(\text{norm}) = S_{c,a} / \Sigma \ S_{c,a} \tag{1}$$

$S_{c,a}$ represents the activation of the cth constraint that is connected to the ath interpretation node. $S_{c,a}(\text{norm})$ is $S_{c,a}$ normalized within each constraint. Constraints were then integrated at each interpretation node via a weighted sum based on Equation 2.

$$I_a = \Sigma \ [w_c * S_{c,a}(\text{norm})] \tag{2}$$

I_a is the activation of the ath interpretation node. The weight from the cth constraint node to interpretation node I_a is represented by w_c. Equation 2 was applied to each interpretation node and summed across all constraint nodes that supported it. Finally, the interpretation nodes sent positive feedback to the constraints commensurate with how responsible the constraints were for the interpretation node's activation, as in Equation 3.

$$S_{c,a} = S_{c,a}(\text{norm}) + I_a * w_c * S_{c,a}(\text{norm}) \tag{3}$$

These three steps (Equations 1, 2, then 3) comprised a single cycle of competition. On the basis on these equations, as competition cycles progress, the difference between the two interpretation nodes gradually increases. For example, when the verb is presented, we assume that information from the sense-specific and sense-independent subcategorization biases becomes available. The DO/SC values within a constraint are normalized so that internal to each constraint they sum to one. This normalization produces competition; for example, for the DO value to become larger, the SC value must decrease. Each of these two constraints then sends input to the interpretation nodes: This input is equal to the relevant (DO or SC) value of the constraint times the strength of the weight that connects it to the interpretation node. The value of each interpretation node is now the sum of its two current inputs. Finally, each interpretation node sends positive feedback to the sense-specific and sense-independent bias constraints; this is equal to its current activation times the strength of the relevant weight times the current relevant constraint strength. This changes the values of those constraints, so that incoming information on the next cycle of competition will differ.

Estimating Weights. The **sense-general verb bias** and **sense bias of context** weights were determined by fitting the weights to off-line data (sentence completion norms) in the same manner as McRae et al. (1998). For simulating completions, because the basic model stops processing only when the activation of one interpretation node reaches 0 and the other reaches 1, we halted competition after various numbers of cycles and sampled the interpretation nodes' activations. Because it is not clear how to determine the number of cycles that best simulate subjects' behavior in the completion task, we simulated completions given the context plus verb using 20 to 40 cycles, with a step size of 2 (i.e., 20, 22, 24, . . . 40).[2] For each number of cycles, to estimate the weights for the two constraints, we varied each weight from .01 to .99 using a step size of .01. The activation of the SC interpretation node was used to estimate the proportion of human subject SC completions. For each simulation, we calculated root mean square error between the activation of the interpretation nodes and the proportion of SC completions. As in McRae et al., we averaged the weights over 110 simulations; the best-fitting ten models at each number of cycles. This process provided weights of .512 for the **sense-independent subcategorization bias** and .488 for the **sense-specific subcategorization bias**. These same weights were fixed and used in the simulation of the reading time experiment. Because all other constraints entered into processing one at a time at each subsequent word (e.g., *the, book, was, written, poorly*), the weight associated with each of them was fixed at 1.0.

Simulating On-Line Reading Times. To simulate reading time data, competition continued at each word, beginning at the verb, until one of the interpretation nodes reached a criterion level of activation. All activations were retained as the initial state for competition at the following word. The criterion within a region was dynamic and was a function of the cycle of competition, according to Equation 4.

$$dynamic\ criterion = 1 - \Delta crit * cycle \qquad (4)$$

The constant controlling the rate of change of the dynamic criterion is represented by $\Delta crit$. The current cycle of competition in a certain region is represented by *cycle*. According to Equation 4, as the duration of competi-

---

[2]This range of cycles was chosen following McRae et al. (1998), where it was shown to produce reasonable behavior.

tion in a particular region increases, the criterion for stopping competition and moving to the next region becomes more lenient. Competition necessarily terminates in a region when the dynamic criterion becomes .5 because the activation of at least one of the interpretation nodes must be greater than or equal to .5. For example, if $\Delta crit$ = .005, the maximum number of competition cycles is .5/$\Delta crit$ = .5/.005 = 100. A dynamic criterion is necessary for modeling reading across multiple regions of a sentence because fixation durations are partially determined by a preset timing program (Rayner & Pollatsek, 1989; Vaughan, 1983). In other words, a reader will spend only so long on a fixation before making a saccade. Presumably, this same logic holds for self-paced reading in that readers attempt to resolve competition at each one-word segment for only so long before pressing the space bar for more information. It does not make sense for readers to expect ambiguity to be fully resolved at each point in a sentence; reading processes are presumably sensitive to the fact that language contains numerous local ambiguities that are typically disambiguated by subsequent input.

In the simulation, for a specific value of $\Delta crit$, competition began at the verb (*found*), where only the first two constraints, **sense-independent subcategorization bias** and **sense-specific subcategorization bias** were involved. At *the*, the *the* **bias** entered competition and the three weights were normalized. At the noun (*book*), the **thematic fit of noun as DO vs. SC subject** entered competition and the weights were again normalized. This continued through the third word of the disambiguation region. Because it is not entirely obvious what $\Delta crit$ is the most appropriate, 40 simulations were conducted in which this parameter was varied from .005 to .0089 in steps of .0001. This range of $\Delta crit$ provides reasonable behavior in the model because competition is not halted too quickly nor allowed to go on for long periods of time. The mean number of cycles of competition were mapped onto differences in reading times between the versions of the SC target sentences that included versus excluded the postverbal *that*, under the assumption that the versions with *that* provide the proper baseline against which to measure competition effects. Thus reading time differences due to processes not simulated by the model are factored out, so there is no need to incorporate variables such as word length and frequency. The activation of the DO and SC interpretation nodes were also recorded.

Results.   The results of the model's performance are shown in Fig. 4.4 (left axis); to facilitate comparison with the sense-biasing experiment, human data from Fig. 4.2 are reproduced (right axis). As is obvious, there is a close quantitative match between the human data and the performance of the model. Why does this occur?

In this framework, available constraints combine in a nonlinear fashion to produce competition among alternative interpretations. Differences be-

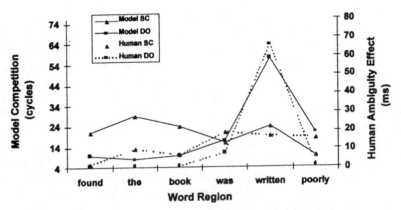

FIG. 4.4.   Comparison of human reading times from sense-biasing experiment (right axis) with model completion times (left axis).

tween ambiguous and unambiguous versions of sentences are considered to result from competition among constraints that support alternative interpretations. When the constraints strongly support a single interpretation, this interpretation is activated highly and there is little competition among alternatives, corresponding to the prediction of little or no ambiguity effects. At the other extreme, when the constraints are balanced among different alternatives, the activation levels of those interpretations are more equal and there is a great deal of competition. This produces large ambiguity effects. Let us consider now these effects in more detail, taking into account the sources of constraint that are active at each word, and what their net effect is. At each region, we consider the constraints that are operative and the ways in which their interactions are different in the two contexts.

At the point when the verb (e.g. *found*) is read, two sources of information are available to combine and influence the interpretation. The **sense-independent subcategorization bias** of the verb amounts to a weak transitivity bias because most of our verbs—and arguably, most in the language as a whole—tend to occur somewhat more often in DO structures. This is the same for both the DO- and the SC-biasing contexts. The **sense-specific subcategorization bias** of each verb in each context promoted a DO interpretation in the DO-biasing contexts, and an SC interpretation in the SC-biasing contexts. Therefore, for DO-biasing contexts, both constraints support the DO interpretation so that there is little competition at the verb and the DO interpretation node is highly activated (.87; i.e., on average, the model is 87% sure that a DO will follow these items). For SC-biasing contexts, the sense-specific bias tend to dominate, producing a small amount of competition on average with an SC interpretation being favored (SC node activation of .66; i.e., on average, the model is 66% sure an SC will follow these items).

When *the* is encountered, it tends to strongly support a DO interpretation for virtually all items. Therefore, for DO-biasing contexts, the model strongly tends to reinforce a DO interpretation (resulting mean DO interpretation node activation of .92), and little competition occurs. For the SC-biased items, because the *the* **bias** is contrary to the current SC interpretation, some competition results and the mean activation of the SC interpretation node is lowered (.41). When the noun, *book*, is encountered, the **thematic fit of noun as DO vs. SC subject** becomes relevant. Because it was computed taking sense into account, it overall supports the DO interpretation for the DO-biased items and SC interpretation for the SC-biased items. This provides yet more reinforcement for the (eventually incorrect) DO interpretation for the DO-biased items, and little competition results (DO interpretation node activation of .94). On the other hand, the SC-biased items receive support for the (eventually correct) SC interpretation, and the mean activation is raised back over .5 (SC interpretation node activation of .56).

From this point forward, for all items, evidence accumulates that strongly supports an SC interpretation. Because the SC-biased items already show, on average, an SC interpretation in the model, competition is relatively minimal, properly predicting the small ambiguity effects obtained in the human data (the activation of the SC interpretation node is .63 at *was*, 84 at *written*, and 94 at *poorly*). However, this information is contradictory for the DO-biased items for which the model has constructed a strong DO interpretation up to the postverbal noun *book* (i.e., the SC interpretation was activated only at .06). The first word of the disambiguation (*was*, **auxiliary/copula structural constraint**) causes somewhat increased competition for the DO-biased items, as in the human data. However, the model continues to reflect a DO-interpretation (SC interpretation node activated only at .13). This inconsistency is intensified when the second word of the disambiguation (*written*) is encountered because of the presence of this additional word that is an extremely strong cue for a SC. The competition between alternative interpretations produces large competition effects in the model that are similar to the ambiguity effects found in the human data (this is the point at which the crucial interaction occurred). Due to this competition, the activation of the SC interpretation node for DO-biased items jumps over .5 to .62 on average. Because the model has now interpreted even the DO-biased items as a SC (albeit without a great deal of confidence, on average), the **next word in SC** simply provides a further strong cue for a SC structure, and there is little competition even for these items (as mirrored in the lack of an ambiguity effect in the human data at *poorly*). By the end of competition at *poorly*, the activation of the SC interpretation is now .86 on average.

CONCLUSIONS

There is no question that the Competition Model of Bates and MacWhinney has played a pivotal role in re-thinking the mechanisms of language processing. At the time when the theory was first proposed, many psycholinguists, following the lead of theoretical linguists who argued for autonomous syntactic and semantic components in the grammar, believed that processing was highly modular, and that there were minimal interactions between processing components. On this account, interactions between meaning and structure were not to be expected.

The Competition Model challenged this assumption, and led to a program of research that revealed a far richer view of language processing in which a myriad of cues compete to constrain interpretation. To be sure, there are patterns of behavior that may primarily reflect constraints having to do with structure, and others that primarily affect meaning. But there is no firewall that prohibits interactions between constraints from different domains.

In the time that has followed, the empirical evidence in favor of this view has become increasingly compelling. A number of new accounts have been proposed in response to these data. But although the names and details many differ, the Competition Model stands as probably the earliest and most influential of such accounts. With a richer understanding of the empirical phenomena, it has also become apparent that a more precise and detailed description of the processing mechanism is desirable. This role has been filled by computational simulations, most often using connectionist networks, of the sort we have described here. These computational models make possible detailed and precise predictions about human behavior. One lesson of such models is that the verbal description of a model often does not lead to clear or reliable predictions about what behavior should be expected. The models may be conceptually simple, but their behavior is not. A second role played by such computational models is that they lay the foundation for a more formal analysis of the deeper principles that underlie processing. Finally, simulations make it possible to explore a broader space of possibilities than may have been revealed by existing empirical data, and can serve to generate hypotheses regarding human behavior that has yet to be studied. They thus lay the groundwork for future research.

What are questions that remain to be answered? With regard to the specific phenomenon we have considered here—viz., the interpretation of sentences that are temporarily ambiguous—the model suggests that the following issues should be pursued.

Plausibility.   As we described earlier, several studies have found evidence that the plausibility of the postverbal NP as a potential DO versus SC subject may play affect how comprehenders interpret these NPs. But at least two questions can be asked.

First, what are the conditions under which plausibility matters? The empirical results are unclear. Some studies report have reported that plausibility does play a role in resolving temporary syntactic ambiguities (e.g., Pickering & Traxler, 1998), but the effect may be complex. Garnsey et al. (1997) found that, with DO-biased verbs, ambiguity effects (i.e., difficulties in processing that arise when the complementizer is absent) occur only when the postverbal NP is a plausible DO. Implausible DOs, on the other hand, did not generate ambiguity effects (as if the absence of the complementizer were compensated for by the implausibility of the NP). In the experiment we carried out to study the effect of verb sense on subcategorization expectations, we attempted to hold the plausibility of the NP constant. In the modeling these data, plausibility plays a role only with respect to context. But the model provides a powerful tool for asking what effect differences in plausibility might have on the DO/SC ambiguity. That is, one can easily manipulate plausibility as a variable that is crossed with the other cues, in order to generate predictions about the cue effects and cue interactions that would be predicted of human data.

A second question concerns exactly what is meant by plausibility. Although it is often invoked in the experimental literature, this is a term that remains somewhat fuzzy. Many studies use off-line data to operationalize the measure of DO plausibility. However, differences in the precise nature of the off-line tasks may yield very different estimates. For example, if one asks subjects to judge the plausibility of a sentence—in its entirety—it is possible that different subjects may focus on different aspects of the sentence. If a subject judges the sentence *The Pope deveined the shrimp* to be implausible, is this because the Pope is an unlikely agent of this activity? Or because the activity itself is rare? Or because it is unusual to devein shrimp (as opposed to something else)? The problem here is that although the sentence as a whole may in fact be implausible, the postverbal NP itself is an excellent direct object for this verb. Thus, despite the off-line characterization of this as an implausible sentence, one might expect that in an on-line reading experiment, reading times to *shrimp* would be consistent with the NP being a very plausible DO.

For these reasons, we believe that, at least in the context of the DO/SC ambiguity, it is more fruitful to think of the postverbal NP plausibility in terms of the NP's goodness of fit to the competing thematic roles of patient or agent (realized in this case as DO or SC subject). In that case, it makes more sense to use sentence completion, role-filler judgments, or corpus data to directly assess the degree to which the NP is a likely filler of the two roles. However, this remains an area that is yet to be fully explored.

The Importance of Other Cues?   At present, the model incorporates seven cues that we believe play a role in resolving the DO/SC ambiguity. We believe these are important cues, but we do not imagine they are the only cues that are relevant. There is good reason to suspect that other cues play a role as well.

The main verb subject itself is probably one such cue. Several empirical findings lead us to this conclusion. First, we have observed from corpus analyses (Hare et al., 2003; in press) that the animacy of the subject of some verbs is highly correlated with the sense of the verb. For example, the verb *worry* can mean 'to cause concern in' (as in *The illness worried her mother*) as well as 'to be concerned about' (as in *The daughter worried her mother was sick*). When the subject is inanimate, only the first sense is possible. When the two senses are also correlated with different subcategorization frames, as is the case with *worry*, the subject animacy then might be interpreted as a cue to verb sense, which in turn will influence the interpretation of the postverbal noun when there is a DO/SC ambiguity.

Second, in a related vein, we know from experimental work studying the MV/RR ambiguity (e.g., *The man arrested . . .*) that comprehenders are sensitive to the thematic fit of the subject to either the agent or patient roles (McRae et al., 1998). When the subject is a good agent (e.g., *The cop arrested . . .*), readers tend initially to prefer a MV reading of the verb. When the subject is a good patient (*The crook arrested . . .*), the RR relative interpretation is preferred.

We believe that the same kinds of considerations regarding verb-specific thematic role filler expectations may interact with the sense/structure relationship that plays a role in the DO/SC ambiguity. This is because senses of the same verb often have different preferred fillers for the same thematic role. The verb *admit* has multiple senses, including 'let in' and 'acknowledge.' These two senses generate different expectations about what are likely fillers of the agent role: *doorman* is a good agent for the 'let in' sense, whereas *criminal* is a better agent for the 'acknowledge' sense. The subject may potentially provide a source of information about which sense of the verb was intended, and this in turn could lead to different expectations about whether a DO or SC will follow. If this is true, then we predict that *The doorman admitted the man had spoken . . .* would lead to larger ambiguity effects at *had spoken* than would *The criminal admitted the man had spoken. . . .*

Nor does this exhaust the potential sources of cues that might be used in resolving the DO/SC ambiguity. Corpus analyses of sentences that contain DO/SC ambiguities have revealed a strong correlation between the length of the postverbal NP and a DO structure (Roland et al., 2003). Other analyses suggest that there are conventional expressions that are highly associated with specific senses of some verbs (*Mr. & Mrs. Smith proudly announce*

. . . is highly predictive of a DO, whereas other usages predict an SC). It has yet to be demonstrated that comprehenders use such correlations as a cue to structure, and if they do, what the strength of the cues might be. This is all fertile ground for future empirical work as well as modeling.

THE FINAL FRONTIER: CAN WE LEARN THE CONSTRAINTS?

Finally, we turn to what we see as a longer-term challenge (or, more optimistically, opportunity) for the CIM: Can models be devised that are able to learn the constraints from scratch? The goal of the model we have described, and the broader class of models like it, is to understand in detail the ways in which constraints affect outcomes. As our empirical knowledge of domains such as sentence processing has deepened, we have gained a richer appreciation of the multiplicity of the constraints that effect processing and of the complexity of their interactions. Being able to simulate these effects has become a crucial tool in developing and testing our theoretical accounts.

Identifying the constraints that apply in a domain has largely occurred through the process of hypothesis-and-test, often by carrying out off-line experiments in order to independently motivate the existence and strength of a candidate constraint. But can one imagine a model whose goal is to simultaneously identify constraints, and then to learn their effects? This is not simply a matter of trying to short-cut the modeling process; it is actually the task that confronts novices in any domain. We would argue that the two-year old who is learning language does not bring to the task the full set of constraints as an adult with many years of experience as a language user. (Obviously, we part company here with those who believe that the significant core of constraints relevant to language is in fact part of a child's innate endowment.) Being able to model the acquisition of constraints, as well as their effect, would thus allow us to study a number of developmental phenomena that are currently not easily modeled by the current version of the CIM.

There is good reason to believe that such a goal can be achieved. To a large extent, this is precisely what has fueled the interest in learning within the connectionist community. We now know, as a result of this work, that there is much more information in the environment than may at first be obvious, and that there are relatively simple learning mechanisms that are able to extract this information. This in turn has led to a re-evaluation of the so-called 'poverty of the stimulus' arguments in favor of linguistic nativism (e.g., Lewis & Elman, 2002).

But another lesson of this work is that as knowledge domains increase in complexity, so too must the architecture of the mechanisms that process them. A model that is architecturally homogenous is no more likely to be able learn language than would a brain that is architecturally homogenous. It is for good reason, therefore, that models such as the CIM build complexity into their architecture at the outset. In those models, the structure of constraint knowledge is directly reflected in the structure of the models. The challenge, if one wants to model the process by which those constraints are learned, thus in part becomes the challenge of modeling the developmental process by which initially simple mechanisms architectures become more complex over time as a result of experience. We believe this can be done, and represents the next significant advance in constraint-based models. But it is, as we have said, a challenge.

ACKNOWLEDGMENTS

This work was supported by NIH grant MH6051701A2 to all three authors, NSERC grant OGP0155704 to the second author, and NFS DBSS92-09432 to the third author. We would like to thank Doug Roland for helpful discussions and comments, and for assistance with the corpus analyses.

REFERENCES

Allen, J., & MacDonald, M. C. (1995). *Semantic and structural contingencies in syntactic ambiguity resolution.* Presented at the Eighth Annual CUNY Conference on Human Sentence Processing, Tucson.

Altmann, G. T. M. (1998). Ambiguity in sentence processing. *Trends in Cognitive Sciences, 2,* 146–152.

Altmann, G. T. M. (1999). Thematic role assignment in context. *Journal of Memory and Language, 41,* 124–145.

Altmann, G. T. M., & Kamide, Y. (1999). Incremental interpretation at verbs: restricting the domain of subsequent reference. *Cognition, 73,* 247–264.

Argaman, V., & Pearlmutter, N. J. (2002). Lexical semantics as a basis for argument structure frequency biases. In P. Merlo & S. Stevenson (Eds.), *Sentence processing and the lexicon: Formal, computational and experimental perspectives.* Amsterdam: John Benjamins.

Bates, E., & MacWhinney. B. (1989). Competition, variation, and language learning. In B. MacWhinney (Ed.), *Mechanisms of Language Learning* (pp. 157–193). Hillsdale, NJ: Erlbaum.

Bechtel, W., & Abrahamsen, A. (2002). *Connectionism and the Mind.* Malden, MA: Blackwell.

Christiansen, M. H., & Chater, N. (2001). Connectionist psycholinguistics in perspective. In M. H. Christiansen & N. Chater (Eds.), *Connectionist psycholinguistics* (pp. 19–75). Westport, CT: Ablex.

Clark, H., & Clark, E. (1977). *Psychology and language.* New York: Harcourt Brace Jovanovich.

Clifton, C. (1993). Thematic roles in sentence parsing. *Canadian Journal of Experimental Psychology, 47,* 222–246.

Connine, C., Ferreira, F., Jones, C., Clifton, C., Jr., & Frazier, L. (1984). Verb Frame preferences: Descriptive norms. *Journal of Psycholinguistic Research, 13,* 307–319.

Ferreira, F., & McClure, K. (1997). Parsing of garden-path sentences with reciprocal verbs. *Language and Cognitive Processes, 12,* 273–306.

Ferreira, F., & Henderson, J. M. (1990). Use of verb information in syntactic parsing: Evidence from eye movements and word-by-word self-paced reading. *Journal of Experimental Psychology: Learning, Memory, and Cognition, 16,* 555–568.

Fisher, C., Gleitman, H., & Gleitman, L. R. (1991). On the semantic content of subcategorization frames. *Cognitive Psychology, 23,* 331–392.

Fodor, J. D. (1978). Parsing strategies and constraints on transformations. *Linguistic Inquiry, 9,* 427–474.

Fodor, J. A., & Garret, M. (1967). Some syntactic determinants of sentence complexity. *Perception & Psychophysics, 2,* 289–296.

Ford, M., Bresnan, J., & Kaplan, R. M. (1982). *A competence-based theory of syntactic closure.* Cambridge, MA: MIT Press.

Frazier, L. (1979). *On comprehending sentences: Syntactic parsing strategies.* Bloomington, IN: Indiana University Linguistics Club.

Frazier, L. (1987). *Sentence processing: a tutorial review.* Hillsdale, NJ: Erlbaum.

Frazier, L. (1995). Constraint satisfaction as a theory of sentence processing. *Journal of Psycholinguistic Research, 24,* 434–468.

Garnsey, S. M., Pearlmutter, N. J., Meyers, E., & Lotocky, M. A. (1997). The contribution of verb-bias and plausibility to the comprehension of temporarily ambiguous sentences. *Journal of Memory and Language, 37,* 58–93.

Grimshaw, J. (1979). Complement Structure and the Lexicon. *Linguistic Inquiry, 10,* 279–326.

Hare, M., McRae, K., & Elman, J. L. (2003). Sense and structure: Meaning as a determinant of verb subcategorization preferences. *Journal of Memory and Language, 48,* 281–303.

Hare, M., McRae, K., & Elman, J. L. (in press). Admitting that admitting verb sense into corpus analyses makes sense. *Language and Cognitive Processes.*

Juliano, C., & Tanenhaus, M. K. (1993). Contingent frequency effects in syntactic ambiguity resolution. In *Proceedings of the 15th Annual Conference of the Cognitive Science Society* (pp. 593–598). Hillsdale, NJ: Erlbaum.

Jurafsky, D. (1996). A probabilistic Model of Lexical and Syntactic Access and Disambiguation. *Cognitive Science, 10,* 137–194.

Kennison, S. M. (2001). Limitations on the use of verb information during sentence comprehension. *Psychonomic Bulletin & Review, 8,* 132–138.

Klein, D. E., & Murphy, G. (2001). The representation of polysemous words. *Journal of Memory and Language, 45,* 259–282.

Lakoff, G. (1987). *Women, fire, and dangerous things.* Chicago: University of Chicago Press.

Levin, B. (1993). *English Verb Classes and Alternations, A preliminary investigation.* Chicago: University of Chicago Press.

Lewis, J., & Elman, J. (2002). Learnability and the statistical structure of language: Poverty of the stimulus arguments revisited. In *Proceedings of the 26th Annual Boston University Conference on Language Development.*

MacDonald, M. C. (1993). The interaction of lexical and syntactic ambiguity. *Journal of Memory and Language, 32,* 692–715.

MacDonald, M. C. (1994). Probabilistic constraints and syntactic ambiguity resolution. *Language and Cognitive Processes, 9,* 157–201.

MacDonald, M. C., Pearlmutter, N. J., & Seidenberg, M. S. (1994). Lexical nature of syntactic ambiguity resolution. *Psychological Review, 101,* 676–703.

McClelland, J. L., St. John, M., & Taraban, R. (1989). Sentence comprehension: A parallel distributed approach. *Language and Cognitive Processes, 4*, 287–335.

McRae, K., Ferretti, T. R., & Amyote, L. (1997). Thematic roles as verb-specific concepts. *Language and Cognitive Processes, 12*, 137–176.

McRae, K., Spivey-Knowlton, M. J., & Tanenhaus, M. K. (1998). Modeling the influence of thematic fit (and other constraints) in on-line sentence comprehension. *Journal of Memory and Language, 38*, 283–312.

Miller, G. A., Beckwith, R., Fellbaum, C., Gross, D., & Miller, K. J. (1990). Introduction to WordNet: An on-line lexical database. *International Journal of Lexicography, 3*, 235–244.

Mitchell, D. C. (1987). Lexical guidance in human parsing: Locus and processing characteristics. In M. Coltheart (Ed.), *Attention and Performance XII: The psychology of reading* (pp. 601–618). Hillsdale, NJ: Erlbaum.

Pesetsky, D. (1995). *Zero Syntax*. Cambridge, MA: MIT Press.

Pickering, M., & Traxler, M. J. (1998). Plausibility and recovery from garden-paths: An eye-tracking study. *Journal of Experimental Psychology: Learning, Memory, & Cognition, 24*, 940–961.

Pinker, S. (1989). *Learnability and cognition*. Cambridge, MA: MIT Press.

Rayner, K., Carlson, M., & Frazier, L. (1983). The interaction of syntax and semantics during sentence processing. *Journal of Verbal Learning and Verbal Behavior, 22*, 358–374.

Rayner, K., & Pollatsek, A. (1989). *The Psychology of Reading*. Englewood Cliffs, NJ: Prentice Hall.

Reilly, R. G., & Sharkey, N. E. (1992). *Connectionist Approaches to Natural Language Processing*. Hillsdale, NJ: Lawrence Erlbaum Associates.

Resnik, P. (1996). Selectional constraints: an information-theoretic model and its computational realization. *Cognition, 61*, 127–159.

Rice, S. A. (1992). Polysemy and lexical representation: The case of three English prepositions. In *Proceedings of the Fourteenth Annual Conference of the Cognitive Science Society* (pp. 89–94). Hillsdale, NJ: Erlbaum.

Rodd, J., Gaskell, M. G., & Marslen-Wilson, W. D. (1999). Semantic competition and ambiguity disadvantage. In *Proceedings of the Twenty-first Annual Conference of the Cognitive Science Society*. Hillsdale, NJ: Erlbaum.

Roland, D., Elman, J. L., & Ferreira, V. (2003). *Signposts along the garden path.* Presented at the Sixteenth Annual CUNY Conference on Human Sentence Processing, Boston MA.

Roland, D., & Jurafsky, D. (2002). Verb sense and verb subcategorization probabilities. In P. Merlo and S. Stevenson (Eds.), *The Lexical Basis of Sentence Processing: Formal, computational, and experimental issues* (pp. 303–324). Philadelphia: Benjamins.

Schwanenflugel, P. J., Harnishfeger, K. K., & Stowe, R. W. (1988). Context availability and lexical decisions for abstract and concrete words. *Journal of Memory and Language, 27*, 499–520.

Smolensky, P. (2001). Connectionist approaches to language. In R. A. Wilson & F. C. Keil (Eds.) *The MIT Encyclopedia of the Cognitive Sciences*. Cambridge, MA: MIT Press.

Spivey-Knowlton, M. J. (1996). *Integration of visual and linguistic information: Human data and model simulations*. Unpublished doctoral dissertation. University of Rochester, Rochester, NY.

Spivey-Knowlton, M. J., & Sedivy, J. (1995). Resolving attachment ambiguities with multiple constraints. *Cognition, 55*, 227–267.

Spivey-Knowlton, M. J., Trueswell, J. C., & Tanenhaus, M. K. (1993). Context effects in syntactic ambiguity resolution: Discourse and semantic influences in parsing reduced relative clauses. *Canadian Journal of Experimental Psychology, 37*, 276–309.

St. John, M., & McClelland, J. L. (1990). Learning and applying contextual constraints in sentence comprehension. *Artificial Intelligence, 46*, 217–257.

Swinney, D. A. (1979). The resolution of indeterminacy during language comprehension: Perspectives on modularity in lexical, structural, and pragmatic processing. In G. B. Simpson (Ed.), *Understanding word and sentence.* Amsterdam: North Holland.

Tanenhaus, M., & Carlson, G. (1989). Lexical structure and language comprehension. In W. D. Marslen-Wilson (Ed.) *Lexical representation and process* (pp. 505–528). Cambridge, MA: MIT Press.

Tanenhaus, M. K., Spivey-Knowlton, M. J., & Hanna, J. E. (2000). Modeling thematic and discourse context effects on syntactic ambiguity resolution within a multiple constraints framework: Implications for the architecture of the language processing system. In M. Pickering, C. Clifton, & M. Crocker (Eds.), *Architecture and Mechanisms of the Language Processing System* (pp. 90–118). Cambridge: Cambridge University Press.

Tanenhaus, M. K., & Trueswell, J. C. (1995). Sentence comprehension. In J. Miller & P. Eimas (Eds.), *Handbook of Cognition and Perception.* San Diego, CA: Academic Press.

Trueswell, J. C., Tanenhaus, M. K., & Garnsey, S. M. (1994). Semantic influences on parsing: Use of thematic role information in syntactic disambiguation. *Journal of Memory and Language, 33,* 285–318.

Trueswell, J. C., Tanenhaus, M. K., & Kello, K. (1993). Verb-specific constraints in sentence processing: Separating effects of lexical preference from garden-paths. *Journal of Experimental Psychology: Learning, Memory, and Cognition, 19,* 528–553.

Vaughan, J. (1983). Control of fixation duration in visual search and memory search: Another look. *Journal of Experimental Psychology: Human Perception and Performance, 8,* 709–723.

Williams, J. N. (1992). Processing polysemous words in context: Evidence for interrelated meanings. *Journal of Psycholinguistic Research, 21,* 193–218.

Part III

GRAMMAR

Chapter 5

Words and Grammar

Virginia A. Marchman
The University of Texas at Dallas

Donna J. Thal
San Diego State University and University of California, San Diego

INTRODUCTION

Since the 1970s, an extensive body of scholarly work by Elizabeth Bates has addressed significant and important questions facing the cognitive sciences. In numerous articles and books, Bates and colleagues have tackled core issues in the debate about the origins of grammar, and in so doing, have helped to clarify many issues in the well-known struggles between nativism vs. empiricism and domain-specificity vs. domain-generality. Through accessible prose, clever metaphors and apt analogies, her contributions have helped the field to tighten contrasts and clarify thinking on these classic debates. Her perspective has also helped us to move beyond the "same old" arguments by illuminating other important distinctions such as, content vs. process, heterotypic vs. homotypic continuity, emergence vs. learning, hard vs. soft constraints, and universals vs. individual differences (to name only a few). Beginning in the early 1970s, Bates and colleagues from around the world took their "hunches about how to conduct and interpret crosslinguistic studies of language learning" (Thelen & Bates, 2003, p. 384), and built an extensive research machine that continues to amass an impressive body of knowledge about the nature of language and language learning.

In this chapter, we provide a necessarily brief overview of work focused on the acquisition of words and grammar by children. We highlight a theme that is core to Bates' work in this area; specifically, that grammars are built using the same set of domain-general learning mechanisms that guide the child's developing lexical knowledge (see also reviews in Bates & Goodman, 1997, 1999). It would be impossible in the space allotted to offer a comprehensive review of the relevant issues or even to do justice to all of Bates' contributions. Instead, we give the reader a feel for three areas of work by Bates that, in our view, have been and continue to be particularly innovative, significant and influential: (1) language as a domain-general system, (2) the study of individual differences, and (3) evidence for relationships between the lexicon and grammar.

DOMAIN GENERALITY: BUILDING A NEW SYSTEM OUT OF OLD PARTS

Elizabeth Bates was intrigued by the puzzle of "how the mind works and how we use language" from early on in her career (Thelen & Bates, 2003, p. 383). And, like many students of this issue, Bates soon realized that the answers were not likely to be simple. A quick perusal of the world's languages reveals that the end-state of language acquisition (i.e., grammars of any and all of the world's languages) is extraordinarily complex. For those interested in understanding how grammars come to be mastered, such complexity is particularly disheartening, especially in light of the prevailing view that the environment fails to provide much of what children need to learn a rich system of linguistic representations on their own (e.g., information about what is *not* permitted in the target language). In conjunction with a relatively simplistic view of the mechanisms available to the language learning child (e.g., Gold's all-or-none learner), a minimal role for input is core to the traditional view that the acquisition of grammar depends on innate, domain-specific mental structures (a "mental organ") that must be triggered by specifically linguistic input (e.g., Chomsky, 1975). In other words, the indeterminacy of the input to children (i.e., the "poverty of the stimulus") and the richness of the end-product seemingly *force* the conclusion that grammars cannot be learned. Since most children successfully begin to use the key aspects of grammar within the first few years of life, it is quite logical to assume that children must get a running start via a rich system of innately-specified rules and representations (i.e., Universal Grammar) that enable them to zero-in on the particular set that characterizes their own native language.

Yet, Bates and colleagues have consistently reminded us over the last 30 years that although it might be *hard* to envision how grammar could be anything else but encoded innately in this "representational" sense (Elman et al., 1996), it will be well worth the effort to look elsewhere for an alternative. Bates ends *The emergence of symbols* (1979) with the following passage:

There is a very, very old joke about a drunk who loses his keys in the bushes late one night. A passerby finds him on his hands and knees, searching a bare piece of pavement directly under a streetlight. "What happened?" asks the stranger. "I lost my keys in the bushes," replied the drunk. "Then why are you looking here?" the stranger asked in bewilderment. The response was one we can all sympathize with: "Because it's so much easier to look out here in the light." We are engaged in a very difficult enterprise thrashing about in the darkness for the causes of the human capacity for symbols. *It may be easier to look in the light, but we will have to do what we are doing if we are going to find the key* (emphasis added, p. 370).

The alternative that Bates and colleagues proposed is that an intricate and complex grammatical system is neither prespecified nor triggered. Instead, it *emerges*, constructed by the child over the course of development. Incorporating important ideas from Piagetian epistemology (e.g., 1962), linguistic functionalism (e.g., Li & Thompson, 1976) and biological and evolutionary theory (e.g., Thompson, 1942; Gould, 1977), Bates argued that learning language becomes a task of integrating and coordinating multiple sources of information in the service of communicative goals (a "functionalist approach") (e.g., Bates & MacWhinney, 1978, 1987; Bates, Camaioni & Volterra, 1975, Bates et al., 1979). This conceptualization ran directly counter to the prevailing view (i.e., the standard theory) that acquisition is the relatively quick and straight-forward process of selecting among predetermined linguistic parameters. More significantly, it transformed the notion of a static all-or-none triggering process that is responsible for language development into a considerably more dynamic, and inherently developmental idea that language learning is the process of children "discovering *for themselves* the constraints that determine the form of the grammar" (Bates & MacWhinney, 1979, p. 168). More specifically, in this approach,

the child's acquisition of grammar is guided, not by abstract categories, but by the pragmatic and semantic structure of communications interacting with the performance constraints of the speech channel . . . [grammars] are *emergent solutions* to the problem of communicating non-linear meanings onto a linear speech channel (Bates & MacWhinney, 1979, p. 168–169, emphasis added).

But how is this possible? Bates and colleagues proposed that children can create their own grammatical systems by harnessing an impressive array of domain-general skills and mechanisms, e.g., linguistic, communicative, perceptual and cognitive. All of this is done in real time, during real-life interactions with the physical and social world. Some of these skills may appear at first blush to have only an indirect relationship to the final end product. Others may be perceived to fall well outside the domain of language proper. The important point is that children are able to construct the phylogenetically new system of language by borrowing component parts from the well-warn and highly robust mechanisms and products that comprise the core human cognitive and social repertoires. In other words,

> Nature is a miser. She clothes her children in hand-me-downs, builds new machinery in makeshift fashion from sundry old parts, and saves genetic expenditures whenever she can by relying on high-probability world events to insure and stabilize outcomes. Looking at the beauty of her finished products, we often fail to see that they are held together with tape and safety pins . . . (Bates et al., 1979, p. 1, emphasis added).

> Nature builds many new systems out of old parts. . . . human language may be just such a jerrybuilt system, with human infants *discovering and elaborating their capacity for symbolic communication by a route similar to the one that led our ancestors into language* (Bates et al., 1979, p. 20).

Bates and colleagues put these ideas forward in the 1970s along with a few others who were frustrated with the prevailing approach in which grammar is innate and autonomous from the rest of linguistic and non-linguistic cognition (e.g., Bloom, 1973, Slobin, 1973). Over the subsequent 30 years, there has been much deliberation regarding the wisdom of abandoning the power and security of autonomous grammars (e.g., Pinker, 1999). All the while, Bates and colleagues have garnered extensive empirical support for the viability of an emergentist theory of language acquisition and processing on multiple fronts, with multiple techniques and across multiple populations (e.g., Bates, Bretherton & Snyder, 1988; Bates et al, 1997; Bates & Goodman, 1997; Bates & Wulfeck, 1989; Dick, Bates, Wulfeck, Utman, Dronkers & Gernsbacher, 2001; Elman et al., 1996; MacWhinney & Bates, 1989). While some remain unconvinced, what is certain is that this work endowed the field with key logical and empirical tools for re-thinking nativist assumptions about the nature of language and language learning.

Before discussing further details of these endeavors, it should be underscored that both emergentist and nativist views share the appreciation that the acquisition of grammar is a very complex and special human accomplishment. In the nativist view, however, children are special because they "have" something (i.e., an innate domain-specific endowment for particular kinds of representations with particular kinds of computational properties). In an emergentist view, in contrast, children are special because what they have enables them to *do something*, i.e., they construct an impressive system of grammar using domain-general skills in the context of doing everyday, ordinary things. As Bates notes:

> . . . we can be overwhelmed . . . at the complexity and perfection of a symbol-using mind. But if we trace this marvel to its beginning in human infancy, we will see that this particular work of art is a collage, put together out of a series

of old parts that developed quite independently. *This does not make the achievement any less wonderful. But it does begin to make it understandable* (Bates et al., 1979, p. 1, emphasis added).

INDIVIDUAL DIFFERENCES: SAME GOAL, MANY ROUTES

The proposal that language is constructed, rather than triggered, does not come without a price. In particular, it moves the developmental psycholinguist out of the comfortable position of "knowing" that language learning will be characterized by an inevitable and highly predictable set of events. Placing the responsibility of building grammar squarely into the hands of the child unleashes the disheartening possibility that many things could, and probably will, go wrong along the way. Fortunately for the field, Bates and others have turned this apparent disadvantage into an advantage by embracing the study of individual differences in acquisition as a rich source of information about how the system is put together in the first place (e.g., Bates et al., 1988).

Most students of child language are taught a set of general facts about acquisition that do not necessarily provide an accurate representation of the process for all children. These "facts" include the following:

- Typically-developing children demonstrate systematic signs of word comprehension around 9–10 months of age, producing first words sometime around their first birthday.
- Early expressive vocabularies expand in size over the next several months at a steady and relatively slow pace, but after reaching about 50–75 words, the rate of word learning increases dramatically (i.e., there is a vocabulary "burst").
- First word combinations appear as strings of content words that are "telegraphic" and lacking in explicit morphological marking (e.g., *mommy go*).
- By the beginning of the third year, function words and inflectional morphemes are added to two- or three-word phrases as children begin to fill in the morphosyntactic structure of their language (i.e., "like ivy among the bricks," Brown, 1973).

However, from her earliest work Bates has consistently pointed out that this description does not reflect what really goes on. Although it may characterize the timing and sequence of events *on the average* ("the modal child"; Fenson et al., 1994, p. 1), the reality is that there is massive variation in both *when and how* children move through these important language milestones

(Bates et al., 1988; 1994; Bloom, Lightbown, & Hood, 1975; Fenson et al., 1994; Goldfield & Snow, 1985; Nelson, 1973, Nelson, Baker, Denninger, Bonvillian, & Kaplan, 1985; Peters, 1977, 1983). For example, although some 18-month-olds have already built up a 50–75 word vocabulary, other children do not use recognizable words until 22 months or later. Some of these "late talkers" will catch up in vocabulary a few months down the road, while others will remain late and continue to be at risk for language or learning disorders. Some children tend to adhere to the standard agenda (i.e., referential" style) preferring names for common objects and telegraphic combinations (e.g., Nelson, 1973; Pine & Lieven, 1990). Other children (i.e., "expressive" style) have more heterogeneous vocabularies as well as multiword phrases and formulae, jumping right into long sentence-like utterances that contain function words and morphologically complex forms (e.g., Peters, 1977, 1983). Yet the vast majority of these children are in the process of learning language in a normal manner.

Individual differences in language acquisition have been well-documented in behavioral studies since the mid-1970s. However, the mapping of the limits and extent of the variation was facilitated by the more recent development of parent report instruments like the MacArthur Communicative Development Inventories (CDI, Fenson et al., 1994; see Dale & Goodman, this volume) and the Language Development Survey (Rescorla, 1989). The currently available versions of the CDIs are direct descendants of interviews designed by Bates and colleagues for use in longitudinal studies of the transition from gestures to first words (Bates et al., 1975; 1979) and then later from first words to grammar (Bates et al., 1988). Bates continued to develop these easy-to-administer paper-and-pencil checklists, making it feasible to assess communicative behaviors in larger samples than those typically used in child language research. Further, a range of communicative behaviors were sampled, allowing a broad-based look at *patterns* of variation both within and across domains (e.g., lexical comprehension vs. production, communicative vs. symbolic gestures, lexical production vs. grammar).

While there are clearly some limitations to the parent report methodology (e.g., Mervis & Tomasello, 1994), this technique facilitated the documentation of general facts about acquisition for all children (i.e., universals), as well as the substantial variation that characterizes the "normal" population (i.e., children who do not have any obvious risk factors for language or developmental delay). The development of parallel instruments in other languages has also created the opportunity for examination of this variation from a crosslinguistic perspective (e.g., in Italian by Caselli, Casadio & Bates, 1995, 1999; in Mexican Spanish by Jackson-Maldonado, Thal, Marchman, Newton, Fenson, & Conboy, 2003; in Hebrew by Maitel, Dromi, Sagi & Bornstein, 2000), as well as in children learning two languages simultaneously (e.g., Pearson, Fernández & Oller, 1993; Marchman & Martínez-Sussmann, 2002; Conboy, 2002). Of course, characteristics of individual languages must have an impact on many features of early acquisition (e.g., Caselli et al., 1999; Choi & Bowerman, 2001; Tardif, Gelman & Xuan, 1999; Tardif, Shatz & Naigles, 1997), however, crosslinguistic research has consistently demonstrated remarkable similarities in the extent of the variation that is observed.

Examples of individual differences in two important domains are presented in Figs. 5.1 and 5.2, based on the original norming of the English CDI: Words & Sentences (from Fenson et al., 1994). Looking first at word production (Fig. 5.1) in children 16–30 months of age, the median line representing the 50th percentile indicates that, not unexpectedly, about half of the children in the sample are reported to produce at least 50–75 words at 18 months. However, some 18-months-olds produce considerably more than that (approximately 250 words) and some children say hardly anything at all (fewer than 20 words). At 24 months, the range is even greater. Twenty-four-month-old children at the 10th percentile are reported to produce fewer than 50 words, whereas, other children (90th percentile) are reported to produce nearly 600 words. That this variability in vocabulary development persists at all ages measured by the CDI underscores the fact that the variation is characteristic over a broad age range. A similar degree of variability is seen in grammar (Fig. 5.2), as measured by the complexity section of the CDI (number of times the parent indicated that their child produced the more complex of two example phrases, e.g., "kitty sleep" vs. "kitty sleeping"). Some children are reported to produce many complex constructions by 24 months, whereas, other children use no complex constructions at that age.

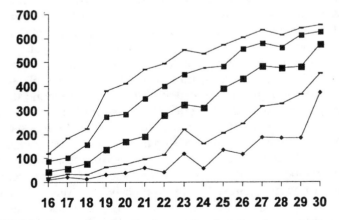

FIG. 5.1.   Reported word production as a function of age in months (based on data from Fenson et al., 1994). Redrawn from Bates & Goodman (1999).

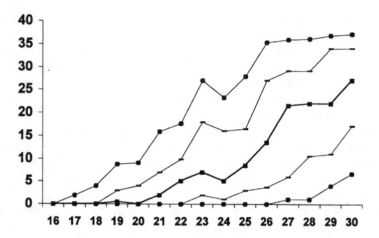

FIG. 5.2. Reported grammatical complexity as a function of age in months (based on data from Fenson et al., 1994)

So, what do these individual differences tell us about the mechanisms underlying acquisition? At first glance, it would seem that variation is everywhere. However, as it turns out, variation tends to be remarkably consistent *across* domains of acquisition (Nelson, 1981; Goldfield & Snow, 1985; Peters, 1977, 1983; Bates et al., 1988; Lieven, Pine, & Barnes, 1992; Pine & Lieven, 1990; Snow, 1983; Fenson et al., 1994; Bates, Dale & Thal, 1994; Thal, Bates, Goodman & Jahn-Samilo, 1997). For example, in the norming study of the CDI: Words & Gestures (8–16 months), Fenson et al. (1994) report that receptive and expressive vocabulary were moderately correlated ($r = .65$), yet, receptive vocabulary was even more strongly correlated with early gesture use ($r = .73$). In slightly older children (16- to 30-months), data from the CDI: Words & Sentences provided evidence for another cross-domain relationship, in that size of production vocabulary was strongly correlated with grammatical complexity score ($r = .85$). Figure 5.3 (from Fenson et al., 1994) presents this latter finding, plotting grammatical complexity score as a function of vocabulary size. Again, both median values and percentile scores are shown in order to highlight the extent of the variation around the central tendency. In contrast to the "fan effect" that is seen when word production and grammatical complexity are each plotted separately by age (see Figs. 5.1 and 5.2), the variance in the relationship between these two domains of language is considerably more narrow and even across most vocabulary levels (see Bates & Goodman, 1999, for more discussion). Note that there is little variability in grammar scores at the earliest vocabulary levels, with changes in the shape of the function later on. The true strength of this non-linear relationship is thus likely to be underestimated by the linear correlation statistics that are reported above (Dale et al., 2000).

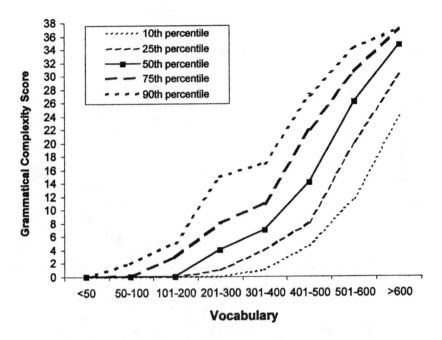

FIG. 5.3.   The relationship between vocabulary and grammar within each vocabulary level (based on data from Fenson et al., 1994).

Where does this variation come from and why is it that some parts of the
process hang together and others do so to a lesser degree? Clearly, variation
in acquisition must, to some extent, have its origins in the nature of talk to
the child (e.g., Huttenlocher, Bryk, & Seltzer, 1991, Huttenlocher, Vasilyeva,
Cymerman, Levine, 2002; Hart & Risely, 1995) or social variables (e.g., birth
order, socioeconomic status, maternal style or quality of mother-child attachment, Bates et al., 1988). The source of these differences could also be based
on "preferences" in processing style; for example, the tendency to select analyzed vs. unanalyzed units (e.g., "analytical" vs. "holistic") (Peters, 1983), segmentation strategies which orient to small "word-sized" vs. larger "phrase-
sized" units (Plunkett, 1992; Bates et al., 1994), or a propensity for "imitative-
ness" (Bloom et al., 1974). Although many interesting proposals have been
explored, the search for a *single* culprit has been elusive (see Bates et al., 1988
for review), with evidence suggesting that many factors probably conspire to
bring about the individual differences that are observed.

    An important insight offered by Bates and colleagues in this regard is
that differences across individuals can emerge as a consequence of the
complex interaction of domain-general "waves" of skill that mix and mingle
in various ways over the course of learning. A way to visualize this is presented in Fig. 5.4, redrawn from *The emergence of symbols* (Bates et al., 1979)

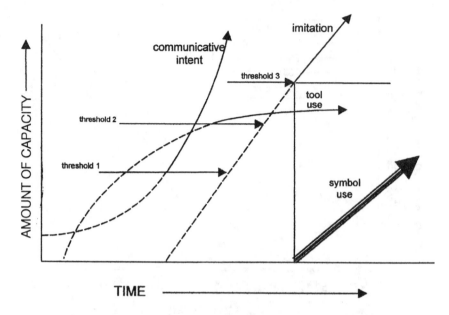

FIG. 5.4. Redrawn from Figure 7.4 (p. 368) Bates, Benigni, Bretherton, Camaioni, & Volterra (1979).

(Figure 7.4, p. 368). The candidate "old parts" leading to first words depicted here are imitation, tool use, and communicative intent. Note that each has its own independent developmental time course, with each coming online and reaching "threshold" levels at different points in time. The resulting system (i.e., symbol use) is, in this view, the consequence of these three "precursors" coming together in the service of building a working system of communication.

Our point here is not to debate the evidence for these particular component parts. Instead, we would like to highlight the insight that language learning can be viewed as a complex and dynamic process in which various components emerge at various levels, to various degrees, and at various times. Individual differences are a natural consequence of learning within such a framework because of the dynamic and multi-faceted nature of the emergent system. Slight differences in the relative rate, strength or timing (chronotopic constraints) of the component achievements can result in relatively significant differences between individuals in behavioral outcomes (Bates et al., 1979, 1988, 1994; Elman et al., 1994). This is in stark contrast to proposals in which differences in language level are due to variation in the nature or efficiency of domain-specific, dedicated components that comprise the language-building machinery (i.e., individuals are "missing" key knowledge, e.g., Rice, 1997; Gopnik & Crago, 1991). Instead, from an emergentist view, children differ in language learning skill not because of domain-specific knowledge that they either have or don't have, but because of variations in how and when the pieces of the process were *put together* during learning. As Bates states:

> ... we remain convinced that the *patterns of variation shown by individual children* contain rich information about universal mechanisms of language learning. By looking at the way that things come apart, under normal or abnormal conditions, we can see more clearly how they were put together in the first place (Bates et al., 1988, pp. 298–299, *emphasis added*).

LEXICON AND GRAMMAR: A LARGE MUNICIPAL ZOO . . .

As mentioned above, research on individual differences provides evidence that acquisition is characterized by continuities that do not necessarily align themselves within the traditional domains of language (e.g., lexical-semantics, phonology, syntax). Instead, patterns of variation tend to be stable across domains (e.g., between language and gesture). One particularly significant finding is the strong *interdependence* of the lexicon and grammar. The interdependence of vocabulary and grammar is consistent with the emergentist perspective of Bates and colleagues, specifically the claim that the mechanisms that underlie the emergence of language are homologous across a host of communicative and representational tasks, whether they be learning words or learning grammatical rules. In other words,

> ... the native speaker learns to map phrasal configurations onto propositions, using the *same learning principles and representational mechanisms* needed to map single words onto their meanings (Bates & MacWhinney, 1987, p. 163, emphasis added).

Interestingly, over the years, enhanced sentiment for domain-general continuity has been incorporated into several approaches to modern-day linguistics (e.g., Bresnan, 2001; Croft, 2001; Goldberg, 1995; Langacker, 1987). There has also been an increased integration of linguistic structures even within traditional generative grammar, the school of thought that originally advocated a domain-specific distinction between grammar and the lexicon (Chomsky, 1995). And, these assumptions have evolved to be at the core of much of the work in developmental psycholinguistics within a connectionist and dynamical systems framework (e.g., Rumelhart & McClelland, 1987; Elman et al., 1996; Port & van Gelder, 1995; Thelen & Smith, 1994; van Geert, 1998). Bates & Goodman (1999) help us visualize this situation with yet another apt metaphor:

Lexically-based grammars can be likened to a large municipal zoo, with many different kinds of animals. To be sure the animals vary greatly in size, shape, food preference, lifestyle, and the kind of handling they require. But they *live together in one compound, under common management* (p. 38, emphasis added).

Research continues to provide empirical support for strong associations between the lexicon and grammar in development. In addition to data from the CDI norming study presented earlier (see Figure 5.3), several other studies can be briefly mentioned. In the ground-breaking longitudinal study of 27 children, Bates et al. (1988) reported that the best predictor of grammatical sophistication (as measured by mean length of utterance, MLU) was lexical development (size of vocabulary) 10 months earlier. Bates & Goodman (1997) cite similar relationships in another longitudinal sample in which children were followed monthly using the CDIs from 12–30 months. Looking at a specific aspect of morphosyntax, Marchman and Bates (1994) found that size of verb vocabulary strongly predicted number of verb overregularization errors (e.g., *daddy goed*). These "mistakes" are typically viewed as a major milestone in the development of grammatical rule-based knowledge.

More recently, links between lexical and grammatical milestones have been reported in a number of other populations. Several researchers have targeted children at the extremes in acquisition (e.g., late vs. early talkers) and the long-term consequences of variation in early language achievements has become a rich topic of research. Late talkers have been defined by delay in vocabulary development when the children were around two years of age. Results from studies of three different longitudinal cohorts, using different measures, and carried out in different parts of the United States, have shown that the majority of children who were delayed in vocabulary production moved into the normal range of lexical development when they were 3 to 4 years old, but remained delayed in use of grammatical forms (Paul, 1996, 1997; Rescorla & Schwartz, 1993; Rescorla, Roberts & Dahlsgaard, 1997, 2000; Thal & Tobias, 1994; Thal & Katich, 1996). At 4 to 5 years of age, they scored within the normal range on measures of expressive grammar, including MLU, Developmental Sentence Scoring (Lee, 1974), and standardized language tests (Rescorla et al., 1997; Paul, 1996, 1997; Thal & Tobias, 1994). The pattern of developmental growth was not different from that of typically developing children, with vocabulary moving into a particular range before grammatical development was measurable. In two more recent studies, a more direct test of the relation between lexicon and grammar in late talkers was carried out. In the first study, lexical-grammatical continuities were consistently stronger than other within-domain relationships (e.g., lexical production vs. comprehension), although there was some evidence to suggest that this link may be weaker in some late-learning populations (e.g., Ellis Weismer, Marchman & Evans,

2001). In the second study, clear unidirectional effects of lexical development on grammatical development were observed, but at later ages (30 months of age to 42 months of age and 42 months of age to 54 months of age) than in typically developing children (Jones, Ellis Weismer, Evans, & Hollar, 2003). These results are consistent with the critical mass hypothesis, suggesting delayed execution of the critical mass event in late talkers.

We are aware of only one study in which the relation between lexicon and grammar has been specifically examined in early talkers. Thal, Bates, Zappia, & Oroz (1996) describe two case studies of children with precocious language development (both were above the 99th percentile in vocabulary production compared to children their age on the MacArthur CDI (Fenson et al., 1994)). The first child was 17 months old and had a vocabulary of 603 words. She also had a mean length of utterance (MLU) of 2.13 which is commensurate with what is expected for her vocabulary level. The second was 21 months old with a vocabulary of 696 words and an MLU of 1.12. On the face of it, this appears to be evidence that contradicts the critical mass hypothesis, since this child had just begun to combine words despite her unusually large vocabulary. A closer look at the child's corpus, however, disabuses the reader of this conclusion. Her spontaneous utterances contained single words with contrasting inflections (e.g., talk, talking), a phenomenon seen in typical children who are learning highly inflected languages such as Turkish (Slobin, 1985). When productive use of morphological inflections was considered (using the Brown, 1973 criteria) this child was found to be comparable to a 30 month old child, a level that is commensurate with her vocabulary level.

In addition to these studies of children at the extremes of the normal range, Bates has participated in additional research in which similar patterns have been observed in populations of children with clinically defined disorders. For example, studies find no evidence for a selective dissociation between lexical and grammatical development in children with focal brain injury (e.g., Bates, Thal, Trauner, Fenson, Aram, Eisele, & Nass, 1997; Marchman, Miller, & Bates, 1991; Marchman, Saccuman, & Wulfeck, 2004; Thal, Marchman, Stiles, Aram, Trauner, Nass, & Bates, 1991), or in Williams syndrome (e.g., Singer-Harris, Bellugi, Bates, Jones, & Rossen, 1997).

All of these findings provide empirical support for the view that lexical and grammatical development "hang together" during language learning, and offer evidence for Bates' suggestion that these traditionally distinct domains are actually an emergent property of the same domain-general component "old parts." As these ideas have evolved over the years, several important theoretical claims have been made regarding how these seemingly different types of systems (i.e., words and rules) could travel so tightly together over the course of acquisition (see Bates & Goodman, 1999; Dale et al., 2000; Marchman, Martínez-Sussmann, & Dale, 2004). In some proposals, lexical learning provides the foundation for later grammar learning. That is, grammatical analysis requires some minimum quantity of exemplars of lexical forms (within a range) in order to abstract the regularities and irregularities that yield the productive mastery of grammar (e.g., the "critical mass hypothesis," Marchman & Bates, 1994). Once lexical size reaches a particular level, the luxury of item-based storage is no longer feasible, and the child's linguistic system takes on a different organizational structure due to the constraints on storage and information processing. Thus, as in the Competition Model (Bates & MacWhinney, 1989), the learning mechanisms and representational formats that underlie lexical and grammar acquisition are similar, if not identical.

At the same time, others have proposed that grammatical knowledge, like words, is built up on a case-by-case basis. Early word combinations are often highly routinized and situation-specific. Learning grammar is thus characterized by processes that are item-specific and frequency dependent in the same way that words are mapped to their referents. It is only later that grammatical structures become encoded in terms of their abstract syntactic form (e.g., Akhtar, 1999; Lieven, Pine, & Baldwin, 1997; Tomasello, 2003). Yet another view suggests that the relationship between lexical and grammatical development operates in the reverse direction. For example, those who propose a syntactic bootstrapping approach argue that the process of analyzing sentences into their constituent grammatical parts facilitates the further acquisition of lexical-semantic knowledge. Here, lexical-grammatical continuities exist because grammatical analysis is a driving force behind word learning (Anisfeld, Rosenberg, Hoberman, & Gasparini, 1998; Naigles, 1990; 1996).

As Bates and Goodman (1997) have pointed out, these proposals are not necessarily mutually exclusive and there are likely to be others that either have yet to be proposed or that we have inadvertently neglected to mention. The important point here, however, is that each of these proposals makes very explicit claims regarding how lexical and grammatical learning feed into each other in terms of the representations and/or acquisition mechanisms that they share. Unfortunately, before we can rest assured that associations between lexical and grammatical development are really telling us about fundamental core properties of the acquisition system, other more global explanations for this relationship must be ruled out. In other words, it must be acknowledged that strong lexical-grammatical associations are also consistent with a view of language learning in which lexical and grammatical development are not actually linked in any meaningful way. That is, the lexical-grammar associations that Bates and others have reported could simply reflect an *indirect* relationship between the two domains, a by-product of their individual relationship to some third factor that has a parallel impact on each individual system.

One possible candidate would be general cognitive or information processing ability. There is growing evidence to suggest that speed and accuracy of online spoken language understanding is associated with growth in productive language (Fernald, Swingley & Pinto, 2001; Zangl, Klarman, Thal, Fernald & Bates, in press; Perfors, Fernald, Magnani & Marchman, submitted). If these links reflect global characteristics of a child's information processing system, it is certainly reasonable to propose that processing speed or efficiency could impact a child's progress in both learning words and learning grammar in the absence of any specific links between the two.

Another possibility is that something in the input to children also mediates progress in both domains. It is well-known that the quantity and quality of talk to children influences the rate and overall progress that children will make in lexical and grammatical development (e.g., Huttenlocher et al., 1991, 2002; Hart & Risely, 1995, Reznick, Corley & Robinson, 1997). Without more specific understanding of how these factors operate in the language learning child, it remains a viable possibility that lexicon-grammar relationships are simply an artifact of the fact that they both happen to be housed within the same language learning child (with a particular global information processing capacity) and within the same language learning environment (with a particular "diet" of linguistic input). If evidence for these global mechanisms is found, it would undermine the claim that the lexicon and grammar hang together due to a common set of core parts that determine their system of representational requirements or learning mechanisms.

A recent series of behavioral genetic studies have provided useful insights into the degree to which lexical grammatical relationships are specifically linked, as opposed to being attributable to more global exogenous or endogenous factors that exert a "shared" influence on both factors. Dale et al. (2000) report a study of language development in approximately 5000 monozygotic (MZ) and dizygotic (DZ) two-year-old twins. Language abilities were assessed using a short version of the MacArthur CDI, consisting of a 100-item expressive vocabulary checklist and a 12-item grammar scale. First, univariate behavior genetic modeling was used to investigate the extent to which vocabulary and grammar outcomes were attributable to shared genetic, shared environmental, or nonshared environmental factors. Results indicated that genetic influences were moderate for both vocabulary (28% of the variance accounted for) and grammar (39% of the variance accounted for). In both cases, a greater proportion of variance was accounted for by shared environmental factors (69% for vocabulary and 48% for grammar), consistent with results from several recent studies suggesting an important role for the environment in promoting language development (e.g., Reznick et al., 1997; Huttenlocher et al., 2002).

However, as Dale and colleagues point out, this type of analysis does not address which of these factors (genetic, shared environmental, nonshared environmental) accounts for the relationship *between* lexical and grammatical development. That is, it could be the case that the heritability of the lexicon and grammar is relatively small (i.e., a small overall genetic contribution compared to that which is attributable to shared environment), yet the same genetic factors account for development in both domains. Multivariate analyses are needed to assess the environmental and genetic contribution to the association between the two traits (e.g., the variance that accounts for the correlation between lexical and grammatical accomplishments). Dale et al. (2000) report a significant multivariate genetic correlation (a measure of the genetic contribution to the relationship between lexical and grammatical growth) as well as a strong impact of shared environmental features. In other words, while genetic factors made a relatively weak contribution to each aspect of language when they were assessed individually, the genetic factors that influence lexical growth were the same as those that influenced grammatical growth. It is still possible that this effect is attributable to some endogenous factor that operates outside the lexical and grammatical systems *per se.* To explore one such possible factor, nonverbal cognitive skills were also assessed in this population using a parent-administered test of non-verbal intelligence (Parent Report of Children's Abilities, PARCA, Saudino, Dale, Oliver, Petrill, Richardson, Rutter, Simonoff, Stevenson & Plomin, 1998). The non-verbal abilities were only weakly related to either lexical or grammatical level.

Taken together, these results indicate that there is indeed substantial genetic influence on the relationship between vocabulary and grammar, providing evidence that strong vocabulary-grammar links that have been observed in other studies are not likely to be reducible to common environmental influences on learning in both domains. Further, the weak correlation that was observed between the language skills and non-verbal cognitive abilities suggests that general abilities that do not have a strong verbal component are also not likely to be responsible for pacing the developments in both domains.

While these data are important for ruling out general explanations for the link between lexical and grammatical development, it is also possible that this conclusion is only applicable during a particular time window of development. Studies that examine concurrent relationships between vocabulary and grammar cannot rule out the possibility that the two domains may look more or less associated or autonomous depending on the particular period being assessed. In a recent follow-up study, Dionne, Dale, Boivin, & Plomin (2003) used two samples of MZ and DZ same-sexed twins assessed at both 2 and 3 years of age. This study replicated the findings of the 2 year sample reported in Dale et al. (2000) and further noted that the association was stable across the 2 to 3 year time period. That is, variance in the relationship between lexicon and grammar was attributable to shared genetic, as well as shared environmental, factors. These results suggest that whatever mechanisms operate in determining how lexicon and grammar relate to each other are underpinned by the same endogenous individual differences factors and rely on a similar set of exogenous features of the environment. In addition, the study used a cross-lagged technique to determine the directionality of the effects. Here, the findings indicated that lexical knowledge was related to grammatical level, as well as grammatical level facilitating lexical learning (i.e., syntactic bootstrapping).

There is yet another hypothesis that could explain an impact of global effects on lexicon-grammar relationships. It is possible that individual differences are due to variability in global language learning skill, i.e., individual differences in the efficiency or effectiveness in abstracting linguistic information from the surrounding environmental input. Facility in this global skill would enable an individual to process linguistic information more efficiently at both the lexical and grammatical levels, but not necessarily imply that lexical and grammatical development are related in any tight-knit way.

Recent studies with children learning both English and Spanish have shed some light on this issue (Marchman et al., 2004; Conboy, 2002). Since general levels of language learning skill are confounded with direct relationships between lexicon and grammar in a child who is learning only one language, the study of children who are learning two languages provides an interesting way to tease apart the contribution of various child-based and input-based factors to the course of acquisition (Pearson et al., 1994). Presumably a child who is better at processing linguistic input might be able to do more with a given linguistic environment than other individuals with less skill. In those cases, we might expect to see "spill over" from one language to the other in terms of grammatical accomplishments more than one would expect given the particular level of exposure. On the other hand, if grammatical accomplishments are tightly yoked to the specific lexical accomplishments that are observed in a given language, then one would expect that lexicon-grammar associations would be stronger within than across languages.

In Marchman et al. (2004), caregivers of children learning Spanish and English ($n = 113$) completed the MacArthur Communicative Development Inventory: Words and Sentences (CDI) in English and the Inventario del Desarrollo de Habilidades Comunicativas: Palabras y Enunciados (Inventario II) in Spanish. All of the children had regular exposure to both languages and all of the children had some reported words in both English and Spanish, although not unexpectedly, there was considerable variation in how many words children were reported to use in the two languages. At the same time, the children were learning the two languages to different degrees, in that the correlation between reported Spanish and reported English production vocabulary was moderate ($r = .35$). Results indicated that grammatical accomplishments were indeed strongly tied to specific developments in the lexical domain in each language. Further, the strength of the within-language cross-domain relationships ($Rs = .78–.80$) were considerably stronger overall than the within-domain, cross-language relationships ($Rs = .13–.26$). Multiple regression analyses indicated that the lexicon-grammar links were not attributable to other factors that may have been guiding the child's general progress in that language. The best unique predictor of grammar in English was the child's lexical level in English, accounting for 36% unique variance, over and above other possible co-contributors such as age, mother's years of education, relative proportion of exposure, and lexical and grammatical accomplishments in Spanish. Analogously, lexical level in Spanish accounted for 25% unique variance in Spanish grammatical level, over and above other possible predictors (age, mother's years of education, exposure level, and English lexical and grammatical level). Similar patterns were seen using naturalistic language samples, indicating that these findings were not an artifact of the parent report technique. In addition, these language-specific lexicon to grammar relationships have been replicated in a different cohort of children learning Spanish and English (Conboy, 2002).

Interestingly, this lexical-grammatical relationship appears to take on the characteristic non-linear shape that has been observed in monolingual speakers of several languages. Figures 5.5 and 5.6 (from Marchman et al., 2004) present reported grammar as a function of lexical level in English and Spanish, respectively. Comparing these trajectories to those reported for monolingual speakers (Figure 5.3, above, based on English-speaking children, Bates & Goodman, 1997; see also Figure 9 in Caselli et al., 1999), it is striking that we see the same characteristic shape in both monolingual and bilingual populations.

In general, these results suggest that links between lexicon and grammar are not an artifact of a global ability that exerts influence on two separate processes or mechanisms. Instead, it is suggested that lexical and grammatical accomplishments are tied together in a very precise way for children and that the associations that we see emerge in the context of solving a very precise problem. Thus, consistent with a domain-general, functionalist approach to acquisition, the child requires a variety of learning principles and representational mechanisms in order to learn language. What the evidence has consistently shown is that those principles and mechanisms are shared across many different levels of the linguistic system, in particular, the process of mapping various types of linguistic entities on to communicative functions.

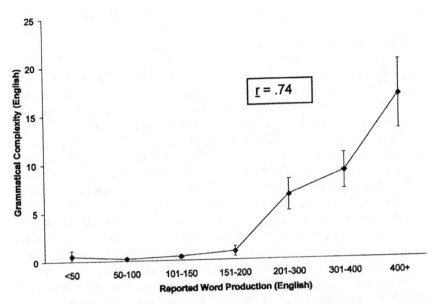

FIG. 5.5. Reported English grammatical complexity as a function of English vocabulary size in children who are learning both English and Spanish (from Marchman et al., 2004).

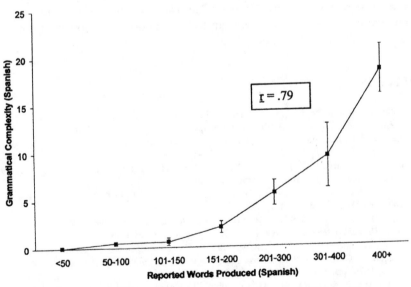

FIG. 5.6. Reported Spanish grammatical complexity as a function of Spanish vocabulary size in children who are learning both English and Spanish (from Marchman et al., 2004).

SOME FINAL THOUGHTS. . .

As Bates and Goodman (1999) point out, strong claims about the domain-general character of human language, and in particular about lexically-based grammars, require considerable evidence beyond the developmental story. That is, it is perfectly possible that the lexicon and grammar may be part of the same system in the developing organism, but in the proficient and highly automatized language processing that is observed in the adult, the systems operate for their own purposes and with their own requirements. We must leave it to other contributors to this volume to address this issue. Within the domain of acquisition, however, it is clear that Bates has provided several influential and innovative ideas about how such a domain-general view of language can account for what is universal as well as what is variable across the course of learning. In particular, the evidence for strong relationships between lexicon and grammar is strikingly robust across studies that examine a variety of populations and adopt several different methodologies. Further, recent studies appear to rule out what these lexical-grammatical links are not—i.e., a reflection of common environmental influences or a general cognitive or language learning skill that reduce lexicon-grammar continuities to a methodological artifact. There is still much to be learned of course. Yet, we believe that Elizabeth Bates has brought us a long way from those early "hunches" and we are closer to finding the key to how the amazing system of grammar is an emergent property of the human cognitive and social enterprise.

REFERENCES

Anisfeld, M., Rosenberg, E. S., Hoberman, M. J., & Gasparini, D. (1998). Lexical acceleration coincides with the onset of combinatorial speech. *First Language, 18,* 165–184.
Akhtar, N. (1999). Acquiring basic word order: Evidence for data-driven learning of syntactic structure. *Journal of Child Language, 26,* 339–356.
Bailey, T. M., Plunkett, K., & Scarpa, E. (1999) A cross-linguistic study in learning prosodic rhythms: Rules, constraints and similarity. *Language and Speech, 42*(1), 1–38.
Bates, E., Benigni, L., Bretherton, I., Camaioni, I., & Volterra, V. (1979). *The emergence of symbols.* New York: Academic Press.
Bates, E., Bretherton, I., & Snyder, L. (1988). *From first words to grammar: Individual differences and dissociable mechanisms.* New York: Cambridge University Press.
Bates, E., Camaioni, L., & Volterra, V. (1975). The acquisition of performatives prior to speech. E. Ochs & B. Schieffelin (Eds.), *Developmental pragmatics.* New York: Academic Press, 1979, pp. 111–128.
Bates, E., Dale, P., & Thal, D. (1994). Individual differences and their implications for theories of language development. In P. Fletcher and B. MacWhinney (Eds.), *Handbook of Child Language.* Oxford: Blackwell.
Bates, E., & Goodman, J. (1997). On the inseparability of grammar and the lexicon: Evidence from acquisition, aphasia and real-time processing. In G. Altmann (Ed.), Special issue on the lexicon, *Language and Cognitive Processes, 12*(5/6), 507–586.

Bates, E., & Goodman, J. (1999). On the emergence of grammar from the lexicon. In B. MacWhinney (Ed.), *The emergence of language* (pp. 29–79). Mahwah, NJ: Lawrence Erlbaum.

Bates, E., & MacWhinney, B. (1979). A functionalist approach to the acquisition of grammar. In E. Ochs & B. Schieffelin (Eds.), *Developmental pragmatics.* New York: Academic Press, 167–209.

Bates, E., & MacWhinney, B. (1987). Competition, variation and language learning. In B. MacWhinney (Ed.), *Mechanisms of language acquisition.* Hillsdale, NJ: Erlbaum, 157–194.

Bates, E., Marchman, V., Thal, D., Fenson, L., Dale, P., Reznick, J. S., Reilly, J., & Hartung, J. (1994). Developmental and stylistic variation in the composition of early vocabulary. *Journal of Child Language, 21*(1), 85–124.

Bates, E., Thal, D., Trauner, D., Fenson, J., Aram, D., Eisele, J., & Nass, R. (1997). From first words to grammar in children with focal brain injury. In D. Thal & J. Reilly (Eds.), Special issue on Origins of Communication Disorders, *Developmental Neuropsychology, 13*(3), 275–343.

Bloom, L. (1973). *One word at a time: The use of single word utterances before syntax.* Cambridge, MA: MIT Press.

Bloom, L., Lightbown, L., & Hood, L. (1975). Structure and variation in child language. *Monographs for the Society for Research in Child Development, 40, Serial No. 160.*

Bresnan, J. (2001). *Lexical functional syntax.* Malden, MA: Blackwell.

Brown, R. (1973). *A first language: The early stages.* Cambridge, MA: Harvard University Press.

Caselli, M. C., Casadio, P., & Bates, E. (1999). A comparison of the transition from first words to grammar in English and Italian. *Journal of Child Language, 26,* 69–111.

Choi, S., & Bowerman, M. (2001). Learning to express motion events in English and Korean: The influence of language-specific lexicalization patterns. *Cognition, 41*(1–3), 83–121.

Chomsky, N. (1975). *Reflections on language.* New York: Pantheon Books.

Chomsky, N. (1995). *The Minimalist Program.* Cambridge, MA: MIT Press.

Conboy, B. (2002). Patterns of language processing and growth in early English-Spanish bilingualism. Unpublished doctoral dissertation, University of California, San Diego and San Diego State University.

Croft, W. (2001). *Radical construction grammar: Syntactic theory in typological perspective.* Oxford: Oxford University Press.

Dale, P. S., Dionne, G., Eley, T. C., & Plomin, R. (2000). Lexical and grammatical development: A behavioral genetic perspective. *Journal of Child Language, 27,* 619–642.

Dick, F., Bates, E., Wulfeck, B., Utman, J., Dronkers, N., & Gernsbacher, M. (2001). Language deficits, localization and grammar: Evidence for a distribute model of language breakdown in aphasics and normals. *Psychological Review, 108* (4), 759–788.

Dionne, G., Dale, P. S., Boivin, M., & Plomin, R. (2003). Genetic evidence for bidirectional effects of early lexical and grammatical development. *Child Development, 74*(2), 394–412.

Ellis Weismer, S., Marchman, V. A., & Evans, J. (2001). Continuity of Lexical-Grammatical Development in Typical and Late-Talking Toddlers. Poster presented at the Early Lexicon Acquisition Conference, Lyon, France (December 2001).

Elman, J., Bates, E., Johnson, M., Karmiloff-Smith, A., Parisi, D., & Plunkett, K. (1996). *Rethinking innateness: A connectionist perspective on development.* Cambridge, MA: MIT Press/ Bradford Books.

Fernald, A., Swingley, D., & Pinto, J. (2001). When half a word is enough: Infants can recognize spoken words using partial phonetic information. *Child Development, 72*(4), 1003–1015.

Fenson, L., Dale, P. A., Reznick, J. S., Bates, E., Thal, D., & Pethick, S. J. (1994). Variability in early communicative development. *Monographs of the Society for Research in Child Development, Serial No. 242, Vol. 59, No. 5.*

Goldberg, A. (1995). *Constructions: A construction grammar approach to argument structure.* Chicago: University of Chicago Press.

Goldfield, B., & Snow, C. (1985). Individual differences in language acquisition. In J. Gleason (Ed.), *Language development.* Columbus, OH: Merrill Publishing Co.

Gopnik, M., & Crago, M. B. (1991). Familial aggregation of a developmental language disorder. *Cognition, 39*(1), 1–50

Gould, S. J. (1977) *Ever since Darwin: reflections in natural history.* New York: Norton

Hart, B., & Risley, T. (1995). *Meaningful differences in the everyday experience of young American children.* Baltimore: P.H. Brookes.

Hirsh-Pasek, K., Golinkoff, R., & Hollich, G. (2000). An emergentist coalition account of word learning: Mapping words to objects is a product of the interaction of multiple cues. In R. M. Golinkoff, K. Hirsh-Pasek, N. Akhtar, L. Bloom, G. Hollich, L. Smith, M. Tomasello, & A. Woodward, *Becoming a word learner.* N.Y.: Oxford University Press.

Huttenlocher, J., Haight, W., Bryk, A., Seltzer, M. (1991) Early Vocabulary Growth: Relation to Language Input and Gender. *Developmental Psychology, 27,* 236–248.

Huttenlocher, J., Vasilyeva, M, Cymerman, E., & Levine, S. (2002). Language input and child syntax. *Cognitive Psychology, 45,* 337–374.

Jackson-Maldonado, D., Thal, D. J., Marchman, V., Newton, T., Fenson, L., & Conboy, B. (2003). *El Inventario del Desarrollo de Habilidades Comunicativas: User's Guide and Technical Manual.* Brookes Publishing Co.

Jones, M., Ellis Weismer, S., Evans, J., & Hollar, C. (2003). Longitudinal relationships between lexical and grammatical development in typical and late-talking children. Poster presented at the Symposium on Child Language Disorders, Madison, WI, June.

Langacker, R. (1987). *Foundations of cognitive grammar.* Stanford: Stanford University Press.

Li, C. N., & Thompson, S. A. (1976). Strategies for signaling grammatical relations in Wappo. Papers from the Regional Meetings, Chicago Linguistic Society, 12, 450–458.

Lieven, E., Pine, J. M., & Barnes, H. D. (1992). Individual differences in early vocabulary development: Redefining the referential-expressive distinction. *Journal of Child Language, 19,* 287–310.

Lieven, E., Pine, J. M., & Baldwin, G. (1992). Lexically-based learning and early grammatical development. *Journal of Child Language, 24*(1), 187–219.

MacWhinney, B., & Bates, E. (Eds.) *The crosslinguistic study of sentence processing.* New York: Cambridge University Press.

Maitel, S. L., Dromi, E., Sagi, A., & Bornstein, M. H. (2000). The Hebrew Communicative Development Inventory: Language specific properties and cross-linguistic generalizations. *Journal of Child Language, 27,* 43–67.

Marchman, V., & Armstrong, E. (2003). Productive use of inflectional morphology by "late-blooming" and typically-developing toddlers: A follow-up at 3 1/2 years. Poster presented at the Biennial Meeting of the Society for Research in Child Development (SRCD), Tampa, FL (April 2003).

Marchman, V., & Bates, E. (1994). Continuity in lexical and morphological development: A test of the critical mass hypothesis. *Journal of Child Language, 21*(2), 339–366.

Marchman, V., & Martínez-Sussmann, C. (2002). Concurrent validity of caregiver/parent report measures of language for children who are learning both English and Spanish. *Journal of Speech, Language, & Hearing Research, 45*(5), 983–997.

Marchman, V., Martínez-Sussmann, C., & Dale, P. S. (2004). The language-specific nature of grammatical development: Evidence from bilingual language learners. *Developmental Science, 7*(2), 212–224.

Marchman, V., Miller, R., & Bates., E. (1991). Babble and first words in infants with focal brain injury. *Applied Psycholinguistics, 12*(1), 1–22.

Marchman, V., Saccuman, C., & Wulfeck, B. (2004). Productive language use in children with early focal brain injury and specific language impairment. *Brain & Language, 88,* 202–214.

Mervis, C., & Tomasello, M. (1994) The instrument is great, but measuring comprehension is still a problem. In Fenson, L., Dale, P. A., Reznick, J. S., Bates, E., Thal, D., & Pethick, S. J.

(Eds). Variability in early communicative development. *Monographs of the Society for Research in Child Development, Serial No. 242, Vol. 59, No. 5.*

Naigles, L. G. (1990). Children use syntax to learn verb meanings. *Journal of Child Language, 17,* 357–74.

Naigles, L. G. (1996). The use of multiple frames in verb learning via syntactic bootstrapping. *Cognition, 58(2),* 221–251.

Nelson, K. (1973). Structure and strategy in learning to talk. *Monographs of the Society for Research in Child Development, 38, Serial No. 149.*

Nelson, K. E., Baker, N., Denninger, M., Bonvillian, J., & Kaplan, B. (1985). "Cookie" vs. "do-it-again": Imitative-referential and personal-social-syntactic-initiating styles in young children. *Linguistics, 23, 3,* 433–454.

Ogura, T., Yamashita, Y., Murase, T., & Dale, P. S. (1993). Some findings from the Japanese Early Communicative Development Inventories. Memoirs of the Faculty of Education, Shimane University, 27, 26–38. (In English).

Paul, R. (1996). Clinical implications of the natural history of slow expressive language development. *American Journal of Speech-Language Pathology, 5,* 5–21.

Paul, R. (1997). Understanding language delay: A response to van Kleek, Gillam, and Davis. American *Journal of Speech-Language Pathology, 6,* 40–49.

Pearson, B. Z., Fernández, S. C., & Oller, D. K. (1993). Lexical development in bilingual infants and toddlers: Comparison to monolingual norms. *Language Learning, 43,* 93–120.

Peters, A. M. (1977). Language learning strategies: Does the whole equal the sum of the parts? *Language, 53,* 560–573.

Perfors, A., Fernald, A. Magnani, K., & Marchman, V. (submitted). Picking up speed in understanding: How increased efficiency in on-line speech processing relates to lexical and grammatical development in the second year.

Peters, A. M. (1983). *The units of language acquisition.* Cambridge: Cambridge Univ. Press.

Piaget, J. (1962). *Play, dreams and imitation in childhood.* New York: Norton.

Pine, J. M., & Lieven, E. (1990). Referential style at 13 months: Why age-defined cross-sectional measures are inappropriate for the study of strategy differences in early language development. *Journal of Child Language, 17,* 625–631.

Pinker, S. (1999) *Words and Rules: The Ingredients of Language.* New York: Basic Books.

Plunkett, K. (1992). The segmentation problem in early language acquisition. *Journal of Child Language, 20(1),* 43–60.

Plunkett, K., Sinha, C. G., Möller, M. F., & Strandsby (1992) Symbol grounding or the emergence of symbols? Vocabulary growth in children and a connectionist net. *Connection Science, 4,* 293–312.

Port, R., & van Gelder, T. J. (1995) *Mind as Motion: Explorations in the Dynamics of Cognition.* Cambridge MA: MIT Press.

Rescorla, L. (1989) The Language Development Survey: a screening tool for delayed language in toddlers. *Journal of Speech and Hearing Disorders, 54(4),* 587–99.

Rescorla, L., & Schwartz, E. (1990). Outcome of toddlers with specific expressive language delay. *Applied Psycholinguistics, 11,* 393–407.

Rescorla, L., Roberts, J., & Dahlsgaard, K. (1997). Late talkers at 2: Outcome at age 3. *Journal of Speech, Language, and Hearing Research, 40,* 556–566.

Rescorla, L., Roberts, J., & Dahlsgaard, K. (2000). Late talkers: MLU and IPSyn outcomes at 3;0 and 4;0. *Journal of Child Language, 27,* 643–664.

Reznick, J. S., Corley, R., & Robinson, J. (1997). A longitudinal twin study of intelligence in the second year. *Monographs of the Society for Research in Child Development, 62(1),* 1–154.

Rice, M. (1997). Specific language impairments: In search of diagnostic markers and genetic contributions. *Mental Retardation & Developmental Disabilities Research Reviews, 3(4),* 350–357.

Rumelhart, D., & McClelland, J. L. (1987). Learning the past tenses of English verbs: Implicit rules or parallel distributed processing. In B. MacWhinney (Ed.), *Mechanisms of Language Acquisition.* Hillsdale, NJ: Erlbaum.

Saudino, K. J., Dale, P. S., Oliver, B., Petrill, S. A., Richardson, V., Rutter, M., Simonoff, E., Stevenson, J., & Plomin, R. (1998). The validity of parent-based assessment of the cognitive abilities of two-year-olds. *British Journal of Developmental Psychology, 16,* 349–63.

Singer-Harris, N., Bellugi, U., Bates, E., Jones, W., & Rossen, M. (1997). Contrasting profiles of language development in children with Williams and Down syndromes. In D. Thal & J. Reilly (Eds.), Special issue on Origins of Communication Disorders. *Developmental Neuropsychology, 13*(3), 45–370.

Slobin, D. I. (1973). Cognitive prerequisites for the development of grammar. In C. Ferguson & D. I. Slobin (Eds). *Studies of child language development.* New York: Holt, Rinehart & Winston.

Slobin, D. I. (Ed.) (1985). *The crosslinguistic study of language acquisition, Vols. 1 and 2.* Hillsdale, NJ: Erlbaum.

Smith, L. B. (1999). Children's noun learning: How general processes make specialized learning mechanisms. In MacWhinney, B. (Ed.) *The emergence of language.* Mahwah, NJ: Erlbaum.

Snow, C. (1983). Saying it again: The role of expanded and deferred imitations in language acquisition. In K. E. Nelson (Ed.), *Child Language (Vol. 4).* Hillsdale, NJ: Erlbaum.

Tardif, T., Shatz, M., & Naigles, L. (1997). Caregiver speech and children's use of nouns versus verbs: a comparison of English, Italian, and Mandarin. *Journal of Child Language 24,* 535–65.

Tardif, T., Gelman, S. A., & Xuan, F. (1999). Putting the "noun bias" in context: A comparison of English and Mandarin. *Child Development, 70,* 620–635.

Thal, D., & Katich, J. (1996). Does the early bird always catch the worm? Predicaments in early identification of specific language impairment. In K. Cole, P. Dale, and D. Thal (Eds.), *The measurement of communication and language: Vol 6, Assessment.* pp. 1–28. Baltimore, MD: Brookes Publishers.

Thal, D., & Tobias, S. (1994). Relationships between language and gesture in normally developing and late-talking toddlers. *Journal of Speech and Hearing Research, 37,* 157–170.

Thal, D., Bates, E., Goodman, J., & Jahn-Samilo, J. (1997). Continuity of language abilities: An exploratory study of late- and early-talking toddlers. *Developmental Neuropsychology, 13*(3), 239–274.

Thal, D., Bates, E., Zappia, M., & Oroz, M. (1996). Ties between lexical and grammatical development: Evidence from early talkers. *Journal of Child Language, 23*(2), 349–368.

Thal, D., Marchman, V., Stiles, J., Aram, D., Trauner, D., Nass, R., & Bates, E. (1991). Early lexical development in children with focal brain injury. *Brain & Language, 40,* 491–527.

Thelen, E., & Bates, E. (2003). Connectionism and dynamical systems: Are they really different? *Developmental Science, 6*(4), 378–391.

Thelen, E., & Smith, L. B. (1994). *A dynamic systems approach to the development of cognition and action.* Cambridge, MA: Bradford Books/MIT Press.

Thompson, D'Arcy W. (1942). *On growth and form.* Cambridge: The University Press.

Tomasello, M. (2003). *Constructing a language: A usage-based theory of language acquisition.* Cambridge, MA: Harvard University Press.

Van Geert, P. (1998). A dynamic systems model of basic developmental mechanisms: Piaget, Vygotsky, and beyond. *Psychological Review, 105,* 634–677.

Zangl, R., Klarman, L., Thal, D. J., Fernald, A., & Bates, E., (in press). Dynamics of word comprehension in infancy: Development in timing, accuracy, and resistance to acoustic degradation. *Journal of Cognition and Development.*

Chapter 6

The Competition Model: Crosslinguistic Studies of Online Processing

Antonella Devescovi
Simonetta D'Amico
University of Rome La Sapienza

The purpose of psycholinguistic research is to identify universal processes that govern the development, use, and breakdown of language. There is a large agreement in considering crosslinguistic studies essential to uncover similarities and differences across languages in the order in which specific structures are acquired by children, the sparing and impairment of those structures in aphasic patients, and the structures that normal adults rely upon most heavily in real-time word and sentence processing.

In the late eighties Bates and MacWhinney developed the *Competition Model*—an interactive activation approach to language processing—to account for qualitative and quantitative differences in processing by child and adult speakers of different language and by different clinical population (Bates and MacWhinney, 1987; MacWhinney and Bates, 1989). The term *competition* reflects a central assumption of the model: different sources of information (i.e., cues) converge, compete, and/or conspire to determine the outcome of language processing, with different outcomes, depending on the relative strength of cues from one language to another.

Two organizing principles operate within the model: *cue validity*, which refers to the information value of a given phonological, lexical, morphological, or syntactic form within a particular language, and *cue cost*, which refers to the amount and type of processing associated with the activation and use of that form. The Competition Model assumes a dynamic process of form–function mapping, in which alternative interpretations of the input are activated in parallel; the ensuing competition between these mappings is resolved through a computational process in which the cue validities for each form-function mapping are combined (working from left to right) until a "winner" emerges. The Model makes strong predictions about the processing and acquisition of cues within a given language: rules and structures that are high in cue validity should be the ones that normal adults attend to and rely upon most in real time processing, and should be the ones acquired earlier by children and preserved in aphasic patients. Variation in cue cost may reduce or amplify the effect of cue validity, especially in children and aphasics.

In order to verify the model's prediction, researchers working within the Competition Model applied the same experimental design in two or more languages to determine how specific linguistic differences affect subject's performance. The first studies involved tasks which make use of *offline* (untimed) procedures. For example, children or adults were tested in an acting-out task, where they were asked to indicate their interpretation of a given sentence by moving toy models (for summaries see Li, Bates & MacWhinney, 1993; MacWhinney & Bates, 1989). These methods made it possible to verify the assumptions of the Competition Model and consistently improved our knowledge about universal and/or language-specific mechanisms for learning and processing languages. Moreover, they highlight cognitive domains—such as perception, attention, motor planning, and memory—that are critical for language but are not unique to language.

However, these methods focusing on post-sentence performance did not tap real-time properties of natural language processing. In order to understand the complex mechanisms underlying language representation and processing, new *online*, computer-controlled tasks were developed to yield real time information about the temporal dynamics of word and sentence processing, monitoring the response time of subjects' performance on specific task. Introducing online techniques opened new perspective in exploring the predictive power of the Competition Model in relation to lexical and sentential processing and the interaction between these different linguistic levels.

The cue validity principles of the Competition Model generate four predictions for response time within this paradigm: (1) Strong cues lead to faster reaction times than weak cues; (2) converging information speeds reaction times; (3) competing information slows reaction times; (4) if a competition or convergence involves a very strong cue, reaction times may be so close to ceiling that competition and convergence effects are difficult to observe (i.e. the "enough is enough" principle).

The purpose of this chapter is to review the online research related to language processing within the Competition Model framework. We will describe the experimental methods and the principal findings coming from three major research lines: word processing out of context, influence of semantic/syntactic context on lexical access, processing at the sentence level.

Due to the specific crosslinguistic perspective of the Competition Model, a large number of languages have been involved in the research programs. Specifically, we will refer on research regarding: Bulgarian, Chinese, English, German, Hungarian, Kiswahli, Italian, Spanish, and Russian. These languages challenge the Competition Model's predictions, due to their powerful lexical and grammatical contrasts, with implications for cue validity and cue cost in word retrieval.

First of all the languages come from different families: Hungarian is a Uralic language (from the Finno-Ugric subclass) and is one of the few non-Indo-European languages in Europe. Chinese is a Sino-Tibetan language with strikingly different features from all of the other languages (e.g., lexical tone, a very high degree of compounding, and no inflectional paradigms). The other languages are Indo-European, although they have different historical roots: Bulgarian is a Slavic language, Italian and Spanish are Romance languages, German is the prototypical Germanic language, and English shares history and synchronic features with both Germanic and Romance languages.

Moreover these languages display striking differences along several dimensions that are known or believed to affect real-time language perception and production. These include *Grammar*: syntax-degree of word order flexibility (e.g., how many different orders of subject, verb and object are permitted in each language) and the range of contexts in which subjects and/or objects can be omitted; morphology—availability of morphological cues to the identity of an upcoming word, including nominal classifiers (in Chinese) and elements that agree in grammatical gender (in Spanish, Italian, German, Bulgarian, Russian) or case (in German and Hungarian). *Word structure*: variations in word length, (i.e. in English monosyllabic content words are common, whereas are rare in Italian), use of compounding (in Chinese, more than 80% of all content words are compounds, that are relatively uncommon in Spanish or Italian). *Sound system*: Phonological features that also assist in word retrieval and recognition include lexical tone (in Chinese), vowel harmony (in Hungarian), and stress (except Chinese). Because of length limitation this review is restricted to research on monolinguals, however a large set of studies has been conducted inside the Competition Model framework related to the three major research line.

WORD PROCESSING OUT OF CONTEXT

Despite the well-known cross-language differences in the shape of words (i.e. *dog* in English, *perro* in Spanish, *cane* in Italian are the different names for the same animal), it is generally assumed that people access their mental lexicon in the same way in every natural language, based on a universal architecture for word comprehension and production. This belief rests crucially on the assumption that the relationship between meaning and form is arbitrary: word forms have no effect on the process by which speakers move from concept to lexical selection, and meanings have no effect on the shape of words or on the kind of processing required to map a selected concept onto its associated sound.

This theoretical point is hardly questioned by the Competition Model assumption that features that are relevant for lexical access vary *qualitatively and quantitatively* according to language. *Qualitatively*, languages can vary in the presence/absence of specific aspect implied in lexical access (e.g., Chinese has lexical tone, Hungarian has nominal case markers, and English has neither). *Quantitatively*, differences between languages are in the shape and magnitude of the lexical, phonological, and grammatical challenges posed by equivalent structures for real-time processing and learning. For example, the "same" lexical item (translation equivalents, names for the same pictures) may vary in frequency from one language to another. Holding frequency constant, equivalent lexical, phonological and/or grammatical structures can also vary in their reliability (*cue validity*) and processibility (*cue cost*).

From this concept a large number of specific questions arise: Are there are significant differences across languages in "ease of naming," and/or in the particular items that are hard or easy to name? Will such differences reflect cultural variations in the accessibility of concepts and/or linguistic variations in the properties of target names? Will crosslinguistic differences reflect the linguistic distance that separates languages (e.g., Germanic, Romance, and Slavic variants of Indo-European; Uralic; Sino-Tibetan)? Do the relationships between word structure and lexical access hold in every language (e.g., effects of frequency on naming latency) or are some of them language-specific?

Another interesting window on lexical access is comparing different tasks (i.e. naming a picture, reading a word, and repeating a word) to asses the nature and the processing involved (i.e., word recognition, word retrieval, and word production).

Timed picture naming is one of the oldest techniques in psycholinguistics, used around the world for the assessment of the amount of time required for a speaker to find the right name ("lexical retrieval," also called "lemma selection") and produce the required motor response ("lexical production," also called "word form production"). Word reading and picture naming both require the same motor response (word form production), and both involve visual processing (written words vs. black-and-white drawings), but they differ in the input processes applied to the visual stimulus (letter or graphemic processing in reading; object identification in picture naming) and in the amount and kind of memory retrieval involved (recognition only in word reading; retrieval from long-term memory in picture naming). Cued shadowing (auditory word production) provides an interesting control condition for both word reading and picture naming. Like word reading, cue shadowing involves recognition rather than retrieval from long-term memory, indeed cue shadowing can be viewed as the auditory analogue to word reading.

Several studies have addressed lexical retrieval of nouns for common objects and simple actions. In some of them, pictures have been named out of context by monolingual adults (Iyer, Saccuman, Bates, & Wulfeck, 2001; Szekely & Bates, 2000; Szekely et al., 2003, in press), by young children (D'Amico et al., 2001), and by Spanish-English bilinguals across the lifespan (Hernandez, Dapretto, Mazziotta, & Bookheimer, 2001; Hernandez, Martinez, & Kohnert, 2000; Kohnert, 2000; Kohnert, Bates, & Hernandez, 1999; Kohnert, Hernandez, & Bates, 1998), comparing different tasks in behavioral studies and in functional neural imaging paradigms (D'Amico et al. 2003).

Because the crosslinguistic comparisons were limited by the absence of comparable naming norms across a large set of languages, Bates launched a huge international project (the IPNP International Picture Naming Project, see Table 6.1) to obtain timed picture-naming norms across a wide range of languages.

Object-naming norms, including both naming and latency, have been obtained for 520 black-and-white drawings of common objects, in seven different languages: American English, Spanish, Italian, German, Bulgarian, Hungarian, and Mandarin Chinese. Action-naming norms are also avail-

TABLE 6.1.
Language and Research Groups Participating in the IPNP Project

English	Elizabeth Bates, Kara Federmeier, Dan Herron, Gowri Iyer
	University of California, San Diego
German	Thomas Jacobsen, Thomas Pechmann
	University of Leipzig
Italian	Simonetta D'Amico, Antonella Devescovi
	University of Rome "La Sapienza"
Spanish	Nicole Wicha, Araceli Orozco-Figueroa
	University of California, San Diego & Universidad Autonóma de Baja California
Spanish-English Bilinguals	Kathryn Kohnert, Gabriel Gutierrez
	San Diego State University & University of California, San Diego
Chinese	ChingChing Lu, Daisy Hung, Jean Hsu, Ovid Tzeng
	Yang Ming University, Taipei
Bulgarian	Elena Andonova, Irina Gerdjikova, Teodora Mehotcheva
	New Bulgarian University, Sofia
Hungarian	Anna Székely, Csaba Pléh
	Eotvos Lorand University, Budapest & University of Szeged

able (or nearly complete) for 275 drawings of transitive and intransitive actions, in English, Spanish, Bulgarian, Italian, and Chinese. In addition, both object and action norms have been collected for Spanish-English bilinguals, in both their languages. The same methodology, number of participant, apparatus, procedure, and data scoring was used by each research group. The response time and the names produces by subjects for each pictures, presented on a computer screen, were recorded and scored to determine (a) the target name (defined as the name produced by the largest number of speakers), (b) morphophonological variants of that name, (c) synonyms of the target name, and (d) all other responses (including visual errors).

To supplement these norms, ratings were collected in English, Italian, Chinese, and Spanish for "goodness of depiction," subjective familiarity, and estimated age-of-acquisition (AOA) for the target names. Ancillary information about target names in each language, including objective frequency counts, age-of-acquisition, and familiarity ratings (where available), semantic properties (e.g., animacy and other semantic categories for nouns, argument structure for verbs), phonological properties (various measures of length, initial phoneme; sonority), and (where relevant) language-specific grammatical features (e.g., noun gender; verb conjugation class) were calculated over items. Based on the analysis of the object naming results for seven languages, language-universal and language-specific contributions to timed picture naming were revealed. Specifically, universal effects include word frequency, the age at which a word is acquired, and subjective ratings of goodness-of-depiction (there were no effects in any language based on the objective visual complexity of the pictures themselves). Crosslinguistic differences were found in the effects of word length and word complexity. However, our findings suggest strong similarities in the factors that influence retrieval and production of words within this paradigm. The most surprising and important finding to date for adults is that word frequency in one language predicts efficiency (speed and accuracy) of naming in another language. So, for example, the frequency of a word in Hungarian predicts speed of reaction time in Italian, and the strength of the Hungarian Frequency → Italian RT effects is just as large as the strength of the Hungarian Frequency → Hungarian RT effect. This finding is important because it shows, for the first time, that frequency effects on picture naming do not (as usually supposed) reflect frequency of the word form itself, but rather, universal facts about the frequency and/or accessibility of the concept represented in the picture. We also discovered that cross-language correlations are much higher for reaction times than for any other measure of naming behavior. This result underscores the value of a timed picture-naming paradigm, which appears to be sensitive to universal stages and/or processes that we could not detect with off-line naming measures.

Similarities and differences in the characteristics of the target names that emerged in each language proved to be largely independent of picture characteristics. As expected, we found substantial cross-language differences in word structure, however, there were also significant correlations across languages, suggesting that target names that are frequent, long, or fricative-initial in one language tend to have the same characteristics in other languages as well. The frication effect reflects the presence of cognates across all of these languages (including unrelated languages like English and Hungarian). The length-frequency confound within languages reflects a well-known tendency for languages to assign shorter words to more frequent concepts (i.e., Zipf's Law). Our cross-language results show that Zipf's Law manifests itself both within and across languages, reflecting crosslinguistic similarities in the frequency, familiarity and/or accessibility of the concepts illustrated by our picture stimuli.

The qualitative look at the items that proved to be especially "hard" or "easy" within or across languages highlighted that crosslinguistic differences tended to be smaller for "natural kinds" (e.g., body parts or animals) and larger for artifacts that often take a different form from one culture to another (e.g., people in uniforms depicting particular roles; foods; manmade objects of various kinds and sizes).

The large crosslinguistic study of action naming with adults, that is currently underway, contribute to the lively debate on the role of grammatical categories especially the noun-verb distinction in lexical access. Comparing results for action naming with previews published results for object naming (Szekely et al., research in progress) reveals a huge verb disadvantage in picture naming for verbs, in every language studied to date (English, Italian, Spanish, Bulgarian, Hungarian and Chinese). Previous analysis conducted on English showed a massive difference between object and action naming, both in response time and name agreement. A reaction time disadvantage for action naming remains even after controlling for picture properties, target word properties, and name agreement itself (reflecting the differential ambiguity of nouns and verbs), as well as a measure of conceptual or psychological complexity based on the number of relevant objects in the scene.

Developmental studies replicated the same verb disadvantage: in a pioneer study comparing action and object naming in 5-year-old children and adults, all Italians native speakers, D'Amico et al. (2003) note that, although child and adult performance were highly correlated in analyses over items, children showed substantially less name agreement and slower reaction times than adults; and for both age groups, action naming was slower and resulted in less agreement. Moreover for object naming, target names (the names given by the majority of participants) were the same for children and adults on 92% of the items; for action naming, children and adults agreed on only 48% of the items. However, even for those items on which children and adults produced the same target name, children showed a significantly greater RT disadvantage for verbs. This developmental disadvantage for verbs remained significant even after multiple attributes of the target names were controlled (e.g., frequency, age of acquisition, length, complexity, initial frication).

It appears that the verb disadvantage lies primarily in decisions about how to lexicalize or package an action or scene for verbal expression. This is specially hard for children, who take a more concrete stance in the action-naming task; in fact they often produce scene descriptions (e.g., "He is tying his shoe") despite instructions to produce a single name, and favor third-person singular over verbs in the infinitive. Following claims by Gentner (1982), the authors suggested that the verb disadvantage in lexical retrieval involves a great difficulty in mapping from concept to sound, because there is so much more variation within and across languages in the ways that the same action can be interpreted and "packaged" for lexical expression, compared with the more straightforward and predictable mappings that link objects with their names. The debate on noun-verb differences is also addressed with regard to potential differences in brain organization for nouns (object names) and verbs (action names). In this view the studies of object and action naming in Chinese aphasics have led to new ideas about the neural structure of the lexicon (Chen & Bates, 1998; Bates et al., 1993, 2000). Because Chinese has no inflectional morphology of any kind (Hung, D., & Tzeng, O., 1996; Lu, C.-C. et al., in press), this finding helps to rule out the hypothesis that verbs are more difficult for Broca's aphasics because of their inflectional demands. But it also yields important new information about the locus of this effect, demonstrating dissociations at the sublexical as well as the lexical level. More than 80% of Chinese words are compounds. A word that is a noun or verb at the whole-word level may contain a combination of nominal and verbal elements at the sublexical level (e.g., the word for 'read' is literally 'look-book'—see Methods for further details). A double dissociation between nouns and verbs occurs for Chinese patients at both levels: Broca's have more difficulty with whole verbs, and with the verbal element in compound words; Wernicke's have more difficulty with whole nouns, and with the nominal element in compound words. The authors' interpretation is that the noun-verb dissociations in patients and in imaging studies of adults may reflect dynamic and long-standing developmental differences in how these items are produced, rather than a localization in separate part of the brain (a common explanation for dissociations in adults—see Chen & Bates 1998 for a review).

The above studies concentrated on relatively simple words, in their citation form for the languages in question (the unmarked form or "zero" form used in dictionaries). We say "relatively simple" because languages vary significantly in the average length, phonological and morphological complexity of words, even in their citation form.

Studies that focused on morphological cues to lexical access included the role of nominal grammatical gender and the verbs morphologies.

The role of grammatical gender in real-time language processing has increased in interest in recent years, and for several reasons this is an important topic for testing the Competition Model's explanatory power (Akhutina et al., 1999; Akhutina et al., 2001; Bates et al., 1995; Andonova et al., 2003; Bates, D'Amico et al., 2003) First, gender processing plays a role in every component of language, including phonology, grammar, lexical semantics, and discourse, hence the study of gender contributes to our understanding of interactions among various components of the language processor. Second, the relation between grammatical and semantic gender poses a particularly interesting example of arbitrary vs. semantically motivated sound-meaning mappings. The correlation between grammatical and semantic gender is weak in many languages, involving arbitrary or indirect relations (e.g., the word for 'bottle' is feminine in German, but the word for 'girl' is neuter). In contrast, there are often strong correlations between grammatical gender and the phonological shape of the word. The relative strength or weakness of these correlations varies across languages, which may lead to different profiles of sound-meaning interaction in the study of lexical access.

These aspects have been studied in three languages with structurally distinct gender systems: two genders only in Italian, masculine and feminine; three genders in Bulgarian and Russian, masculine, feminine, and neuter. Two different tasks were employed, varying in the degree to which they require conscious reflection on the property of gender. The first, repetition of spoken word targets ("cued shadowing"—Bates & Liu, 1996) requires very little metalinguistic reflection; the second task, classification of words according to gender (also known as gender monitoring or gender assignment) requires conscious attention to grammatical gender in order to reach a deliberate decision. Results show similarities and differences that may reflect interesting differences between languages, including language-specific principles of word formation and word structure, and the contrast between two- and three-gender systems. Reaction times were influenced by phonological factors, but grammatical gender only affected gender monitoring, suggesting that effects of surface gender marking may be restricted to a post-lexical stage in processing and/or to tasks in which conscious attention to the gender dimension is required. Syllabic structure affects Italians' performance. Semantic genders affect Bulgarian but not Italian in the gender monitoring task: specifically, words that refer to animate beings with recognizable semantic gender elicited faster and more accurate gender classifications. A possible interpretation is that it in two-gender languages like Italian, semantic gender is so arbitrary and indirect that it is ignored by native speakers even in a conscious gender-processing task; by contrast, the influence of semantic gender on processing a three-gender language system could be due to a higher correlation ("cue validity") between semantic and grammatical gender when the neuter category (with relatively few animate forms) is available.

Finally an interaction between sex of the participant and noun gender, reflecting a bias toward one's own grammatical gender (especially for females), was found in the Bulgarian data and in the reanalysis of Italian. In particular, women seem to be faster and (in Bulgarian) more accurate in classification of feminine nouns. The authors offer a tempting interpretation, suggesting that this result reflects a lifetime of experience in producing (in first person) and listening (in second and third person) to references about oneself—a kind of speech that is not only high in frequency, but also high in interest value for most listeners.

Studies that focus on verb morphology included inflectional complexity and regularity in Italian and Spanish (Devescovi et al.). A large parametric study of the effects of person, number, tense, conjugation class, and regularity/irregularity on recognition and processing of inflected verbs was conducted Spanish and Italian. Fifty common verbs were presented auditorily, in all person and number combinations, in four tenses (present indicative, future, remote past, imperfect past). These combinations do not exhaust the inflectional paradigms for verbs in either language (e.g. most Italian verbs can take more than 80 different forms), but this subset alone produces an experiment with close to 1000 items in each language, similar to psychophysical studies in size and purpose. Two versions of the experiment were conducted: a cued shadowing task (in which the auditorily presented verbs are simply repeated, in quasi-random lists) and a task in which participants generate a subject pronoun that agrees with the verb. Results are still preliminary, but the following trends have emerged. (1) To learn about the point at which decisions are made within richly inflected verbs, reaction times are measured and compared from various points (word onset, onset of sonorance [fundamental frequency], root onset, stem onset, word ending). These yield markedly different results, changing the order of difficulty among verb types as well as the factors that predict accuracy and RT. (2) In both languages, both tasks, and all verb conditions, acoustic-phonetic factors have a massive effect on verb recognition, in striking contrast to the ease and speed with which conjugated verbs are comprehended and produced in everyday life. These findings will be important for studies in which the same conjugated verbs are placed in a grammatically constraining context. (3) Effects of regularity seem to be an emergent property of other factors, including length, frequency, and similarity—a result that favors connectionist accounts over Dual Mechanism explanations for regularity effects; meanwhile, the traditional conjugational categories like tense, person, and number had a significant impact on response time in both tasks even after a large number confounded characteristics were controlled. Hence some abstract categories do appear to have psychological reality while others do not.

EFFECTS OF GRAMMATICAL CONTEXT
AND SENTENCE MEANING ON LEXICAL ACCESS

In recent years, several studies within the Competition Model have investigated effects of context priming on lexical access, exploring the interaction between grammatical structure and sentence meaning. These grammatical and sentence-level priming effects are controversial. In modular theories, grammatical and sentential priming is attributed to a controlled/post-lexical stage in which the products of a modular lexicon are integrated into the context. In interactive-activation theories (including the Competition Model), these effects can be automatic and predictive, affecting activation of an upcoming word within the lexicon.

Neely and colleagues (Neely, 1991; Neely, Keef & Ross, 1989) proposed empirical criteria to distinguish between automatic effects (which involve the internal workings of the lexicon) and strategic effects (which is how postlexical integration is usually viewed): Automatic priming effects are prelexical and bottom-up, characterized by faster reaction times, short time windows between prime and target (e.g. SOA < 250 ms), facilitation of lexical access, no metalinguistic operation implied, and a low proportion of related items. On the contrary, strategic/top-down controlled effects are postlexical, produce slower reaction times and inhibition, require long time windows between prime and target (e.g. SOA > 250 ms), metalinguistic operations, and a high proportion of related items.

These criteria were derived from the word-word priming literature; however, Bates and her colleagues thought that there was one criterion that sentential priming cannot meet: low proportion of semantic related trials, to discourage listeners from attempting integration. In word-word priming, integration has been regarded as a "bad thing," eliciting experiment-specific strategies that are unrelated to spreading activation in natural language use. But in connected discourse, normal listeners always expect the upcoming word to fit the context. Hence tasks that encourage integration may be a "good thing" that generalizes well to sentence-word interactions in real-life language use. For this reason, Bates and co-workers have opted for tasks in which the target is a potential continuation of the sentence.

To learn more about differences between word-word priming and sentence priming under these conditions, Hernandez, Fennema-Notestime,

Udel, and Bates (2001) compared the two directly in a single orthogonal design, with very short time windows, using two traditional priming tasks (cross-modal naming and visual lexical decision). Auditory sentences were occasionally interrupted by visual word pairs (e.g. "The man was walking down the [ROAD-STREET], when he . . ."), with instructions to judge or read the second word in each pair. Results were as follows. (1) Word-word and sentence-word priming occurred together in the earliest time windows (i.e. there was no window in which word-word priming was present but sentential effects had not yet occurred, as a modular two-stage theory would predict). (2) Sentential effects were larger and/or more robust than word-word effects across conditions. (3) Word-word priming effects observed out of context changed significantly when placed in context. (4) Word-word and sentence-word priming were additive in lexical decision, but they interacted in cross-modal naming (the fastest task, with no metalinguistic component). (5) Results were not affected by the presence or absence of lexical associates in the sentence context. These findings suggest that sentential effects are at least as early and robust as word-word priming, and meet most criteria for automatic priming.

On the basis of this finding, Bates inspired a series of seminal studies that have demonstrated robust and automatic grammatical priming across tasks and languages, applying similar designs and criteria to phrases and sentences with auditory word targets (see Table 6.2). These studies were designed to meet most criteria for automatic activation: tasks with rapid timing parameters, neutral baselines to differentiate between facilitation and inhibition, and no metalinguistic component, compared with others that asked subjects to focus explicitly and consciously on the grammatical dimensions.

Several studies have explored priming effects of grammatical gender on noun access in Italian (Bates, Devescovi, Hernandez & Pizzamiglio 1996), German (Hillert & Bates 1996; Jacobsen, 1999) and Russian (Akhutina, Kurgansky, Polinsky and Bates, 1999), using a word-word priming paradigm and different tasks: cued shadowing (e.g. subjects were asked to repeat the second word in a series of word pairs spoken by a female voice, where the first word was an adjective serving as grammatical pair), gender monitoring (e.g. subjects were asked to listen to a series of adjective-noun pairs and press one of two buttons indicating whether the noun target had feminine or masculine gender), grammaticality judgment (e.g. subjects were asked to decide whether adjective-noun pairs were grammatical or ungrammatical). These studies indicated that prenominal modifiers matched on grammatical gender can facilitate lexical access (decreasing reaction time relative to a neutral baseline) while mismatching gender can inhibit, suppress, or interfere with lexical access (increasing reaction times relative to the same baseline). Moreover, the reaction times monitored in the in the cued-

TABLE 6.2

Language	Tasks	Subject groups	References
Italian	CS, GM, GJ, Competition ModelV	Normal Adult, Aphasics	Bates, Devescovi, Hernandez, Pizzamiglio 1996; Bates, Pizzamiglio, Devescovi, Marangolo, Ciurli, Razzano 1996; Bates, Marangolo, Pizzamiglio, Dick 2001; Bentrovato, Devescovi, D'Amico, Bates 1999; Bentrovato, Devescovi, D'Amico, Wicha, Bates 2003.
English	PN, CS, Competition ModelV	Normal Children, Adult, Aged	Bates & Liu 1996; Herron and Bates, 1997; Ferdmeier, Bates 1997; Liu 1996; Liu, Bates, Powell & Wulfeck, 1997; Roe, Jahn-Samilo, Juarez, Mickel, Royer, Bates, 2000.
Spanish	PN, PJ, Competition ModelV	Normal Adult	Wicha, Bates, Hernandez, Reyes, Galvadon de Berreto (2000)
Chinese	CS, PN, GJ	Normal Adult	Lu, Bates, Hung, Tzeng, Hsu, Tsai, Roe (2001)
German	PN, Competition ModelV	Normal Adult	Hillert, Bates, 1996; Jakobsen 1999
Kswaili	PN	Normal Adult	Alcock, Ngorosho (2000)
Russian	CS, GJ	Normal Adult, Aphasics	Akhutina, T., Kurgansky, A., Polinsky, M., & Bates, E. (1999); Akhutina, T., Kurgansky, A., Kurganskaya, M., Polinsky, M., Polonskaya, N., Larina, O., Bates, E., & Appelbaum, M. (2000); Akhutina, T., Kurgansky, A., Kurganskaya, M., & Polinsky, M. (2000).

shadowing task were very fast (< 200 ms). These results for gender were replicated with other form of syntactic paradigms, including effects of nominal classifiers (a much larger class that is historically related to gender) on noun access in Chinese and Kiswahili, and effects of form-class context ("I like the_____" vs. "I like to_____") on processing of nouns and verbs in English and Chinese (Ferdmaier & Bates 1997; Liu 1996).

Some studies have also explored gender priming in fluent and non-fluent aphasic patients in Italian, using gender monitoring (Bates et al., in press) and in Russian, using cued shadowing (Akhutina et al., 1999, 2000). In Italian there was no evidence for gender priming in either patient group, though both performed above chance in judgment tasks (indicating preserved knowledge of noun gender and gender agreement). In Russian there was significant gender priming in both patient groups, but aphasics (independent of group or symptom profiles) did not show the normal gender markedness effect. The difference between these two aphasia studies underscores the importance of taking language, task, and modality into account in the interpretation of grammatical deficits.

Another line of research explored the contribution of sentence level context to word recognition and word production across the life-span (from 3 to 87 years). This effort forced the researchers to use methods that permit a comparison of subjects across the age range from preschool to late adulthood. Thus they avoided reading-based procedures (e.g. visual lexical decision, cross-modal naming; see Balota 1944 for review) and/or auditory techniques requiring metalinguistic judgments that are difficult for young children and older adults (e.g., auditory lexical decision, phoneme monitoring, word monitoring; see Grosjean & Frauenfelder for review). In studies of word recognition, the *cued shadowing* technique (Bates & Liu, 1996; Herron and Bates, 1997; Liu 1996; Liu et al. 1997) was adopted: subjects were instructed to listen to a sentence/story told by a man and then to repeat a target word in final position spoken by a woman, as fast as they could without making a mistake. For studying word production, subjects were asked to produce the name for a picture object (*picture naming*) embedded within an auditory sentence context (Roe et al. 2000). These studies show that these techniques yield lexical access effects (length, frequency, age of acquisition) and robust sentential priming effects, both facilitatory and inhibitory. In the recognition studies there were no differences in the magnitude of facilitation across the age range from 7–85 years, but there was a significant and monotonic increase with age in the size of inhibition scores.

In the production study as well, facilitation—established by at least 4 years of age—did not change markedly after that point. Inhibitory effects of sentence context on word production changed over time, but this change was not monotonic at all: inhibitory effects decrease between 3–5 years of age, remain stable from middle childhood through the adult years, and increase once again after 70 years of age.

Finally, some studies explored the interaction between grammatical cues and sentence context on word production in Italian and Spanish (Bentrovato, Devescovi, D'Amico, & Bates 1999, Bentrovato, Devescovi, D'Amico, Wicha, & Bates 2003; Wicha, Bates, Hernandez, Reyes, & Galvadon de Berreto 2000). In these studies, subjects were asked to name a picture/read a word presented at an unpredictable point within two-sentence auditory context. The factorial gender-by-semantic experimental design included all the four possible combinations of congruent/incongruent conditions in which the grammatical cues (an article indefinite/definitive), the target (picture/written word), and the context could take place: both gender and semantic congruent, both incongruent, semantic congruent/gender incongruent, semantic congruent/gender incongruent. Two neutral control baseline were used: in one of them each target word/picture was presented out of context, in the other it occurred inside control sentences containing no semantic or gender constrains.

In both Spanish and Italian, the picture naming paradigm yielded comparable results, despite differences in language, stimulus materials, and some methodological variation: large and significant interaction between sentence context and grammatical gender, due primarily to response facilitation when both sources of information converge. When both dimension were violated, a small but significant degree of response inhibition was observed. When only one dimension was incongruent, reaction times did not differ from the sentential baseline. Finally, faster response times in naming pictures than in any of the five experimental sentence conditions were observed, compared with latencies of naming the same picture out of context. These findings suggest that some linguistic context is better than none at all, even if that context contains misleading cues, due to some combination of prosodic and grammatical information that facilitates noun retrieval in the picture naming task.

Following the diagnostic empirical criteria proposed by Neely (1991) and Hernandez et al. (1996), all these studies support an automatic and prelexical interpretation of the grammatical and sentential priming effects: response times were relatively fast, and massive facilitative effects were found in tasks, with minimal SOA and that do not require a metalinguistic decision (word reading, cued shadowing, and picture naming). Moreover inhibitory effects play a role in tasks requiring both automatic/nonautomatic processing. This last finding suggests that inhibition may be not a useful guide to the locus of priming effects, even though such effects have been used to argue for controlled processing in large set of studies (see Dagenbach & Carr 1994). Its useful to point out that the results of life span studies (Roe et al., 2000, and Liu et al., 1997) show an interesting nonmonotonical developmental trend of the inhibitory effects, a decreasing trend in preschool children and an increasing trend in older adults. Following Roe et al. (2000), a possible interpretation is that this trend reflects the speaker's ability to suppress competitor words activated during processing in favor of more adequate candidates. In real life, a fluent speaker finds himself in situations in which the word he is looking for is activated together with one or more competitor words that may not be appropriate for the context. For several reasons (i.e. frequencies, recency, semantic/phonetic similarities, etc.) the competitor may be more accessible than the appropriate word, becoming difficult to be suppressed. From this point of view, this processing ability, that is efficient in adulthood, requires time to be mastered by children and could break down in older adults.

PROCESSING AT THE SENTENCE LEVEL

The largest body of work within the Competition Model comes from studies of comprehension and production at the sentence level, in normal adults and children and aphasics, including sentence interpretation (with both simple and complex sentences) and grammaticality judgment.

Interpretation of Simple Sentences (SI). The cue validity predictions of the Competition Model have been tested using a sentence interpretation paradigm that assesses "winners" and "losers" when cues compete and/or converge to indicate the agent role (MacWhinney & Bates 1989). In the off-line version, listeners were asked to indicate the agent (*Who did the action?*) by acting out sentences with small toys. In the online "mugshot" version of this task, subjects were asked to indicate the sentence agent by pushing a button under one of two pictures representing the two nouns in the sentence (side by side, counterbalanced with sentence order). Stimuli were transitive sentences with factorial combinations (competing and/or converging) of word order, subject-verb agreement, semantic reversibility (animate vs. inanimate nouns), and other factors specific to the languages in questions (e.g., casemarking, contrastive stress, topic-marking). Table 6.3 gives examples of the kinds of sentences (which are sometimes ungrammatical) that result from this factorial design. Adult subjects have been tested in such versions of the sentence interpretation procedure in English (Hernandez, Bates & Avila., 1994; Von Berger, Wulfeck, Bates & Fink., 1996), French (Kail, 1989), Italian (Devescovi, D'Amico, Gentile 1999), Spanish (Kail, 1989; Hernandez et al., 1994), Serbo-Croatian (Mimica, Sullivan & Smith, 1994), Chinese (Li, 1998) as well as bilingual populations (English-Chinese: Li 1996b. English-Spanish: Hernandez, Sierra, Bates, 2000). Results for assignment of sentence roles replicated most of the results obtained in off-line studies of sentence interpretation: strong quantitative differences between languages when cues compete, converge, or conspire against each other were observed. For example, given *The rock is kissing the rabbit,* English adult speakers usually choose the rock as the agent (a victory for Subject-Verb-Object (SVO) word order) but Italians and Chinese more often

TABLE 6.3

Example Sentence	Cues to Agency
The rock is kissing the rabbit.	SVO vs. animacy
The horse are kicking the cows	SVO vs. S-V agreement
The tiger the lions are chasing	OSV & S-V agreement
Is patting the rock the cat	VOS & animacy
The pencils is pushing the dog	SVO vs. animacy & agreement

choose the rabbit (a victory of semantics over word order, which is variable in both languages (Li, P 1994; Li, Bates & MacWhinney, 1993; Liu, Bates & Li 1992). Given *The horses are kicking the cows*, English adult speakers usually choose the horse as agent (another victory for SVO) while speakers of richly inflected languages choose the cow (basing choice on morphology more than on word order). The online crosslinguistic studies confirmed the different profiles or hierarchies of cues found in the previous study, in accordance with crosslinguistic differences in cue validity (e.g., word order > SV agreement > semantics > stress > topic in English; SV agreement > clitic agreement > animacy > word order > stress, topic in Italian; passive marking > semantics > word order > topic marking in Chinese; case marking > SV agreement > semantics > word order in Croatian;). Moreover, for any given language, these studies show that the most valid cues tend to be the most prone to transfer during second-language learning (Hernandez, Bates & Avila, 1994; Liu, 1996).

These studies also confirmed explicit predictions concerning response time, including: cue strength (decisions will be faster and more consistent in the presence of the most valid and reliable cues in the language), convergence (converging information leads to faster and more consistent decisions), competition (competing information leads to slower and less consistent decisions), and the "enough is enough" principle (cue strength can grow to the point where it overwhelms the effects of competition and convergence)

Only few online studies with children were conducted (Kail & Bassano 1994; Von Berger et al., 1996; Devescovi, D'Amico, Gentile 1999), also obtaining evidence for the cue strength, competition, and convergence predictions described above, providing further support for the Competition Model. The most valid cue tend to be the first ones used by children, but cue cost factors intervene to affect the size and shape of these effect. For example, subject-verb agreement is the cue that has highest cue validity for Italian listeners, and it is by far the strongest determinant of agent choice for adults, but this grammatical device may place heavy demands on memory before it can be used: very young children approach the problem of sentence interpretation with limited processing resources, a situation that improves over time. Hence, early in development these limitations raise the costs associated with this otherwise valid cue, to the point where children cannot use the cue, prefer not to use it, or use it only in conjunction with other sources of information that make the whole problem easier to handle. In the course of development, there is a transition point where children "give up" their immature avoidance of this valid but very costly cue, and opt for the best sources of information. Actually, choice data showed that agreement effects were in fact evident at every age level in Italian children as well. However, the use of agreement increased markedly across age groups. For children under 9 years of age, animacy was actually stronger than agreement, suggesting that younger children postpone the use of highly valid agreement information, due to the memory costs that such cues exact.

Response time data provided new information about reorganization and consolidation of sentence processing in children: overall, reaction times were slower in children than adults, but the increasing changes were not monotonic at all, simply becoming more efficient over time. For example, Von Berger et al. (1996) have observed that RT in English-speaking children actually increased between 7 and 9 years of age, coinciding with the emergence and consolidation of the adult-like word order strategy. Devescovi et al. (1999) observed a long plateau from 7;8 to 9;6 years of age in Italian-speaking children. This plateau appeared to be related to the integration of subject-verb agreement with other sources of information, reflected in the crossover from animacy dominance to agreement dominance that takes place in the same period.

Also, data coming from atypical child populations supported the cue cost effect in development. An online study has been conducted by Feldman, MacWhinney, and Sacco (2002) to study comprehension in 141 normal controls from 5–12 years of age, and 15 children with congenital unilateral brain injuries (12 to the left hemisphere, 3 to the right). As a group, the focal lesion population fell behind normal controls, showing later emergence of second-noun strategies and more persistent reliance on animacy in both agent choice and reaction times.

Interpretation of Complex Sentences.   Some studies focused on comprehension of complex syntax. One study (Bates, Devescovi & D'Amico, 1999) addressed the question as to whether the cue hierarchies found for simple sentences are also observed for sentences with relative clauses in English and Italian. The answer was "yes": Italians used agreement over word order in both the main clause and the relative; English speakers used word order at the expense of agreement in both the main and the relative. Response times yielded important information about the differential costs of complexity in these two languages: the English word order strategy was associated with more severe costs of center embedding; the Italian agreement strategy was less affected by embedding, but latencies were much longer for morphologically ambiguous items.

The "mugshot" technique was also used to investigate comprehension of actives, passives, subject clefts, and object clefts. A profile of above-chance performance on actives and subject clefts, but chance performance on passives and object clefts, has been considered "the core deficit of agrammatism" (Grodzinsky 2000). The study was interested in determining whether this profile occurs across languages, and is specific to agrammatic

Broca's aphasics. In the experimental sentences, there were no cue competitions (and no ungrammatical stimuli), but a contrast between converging agreement *(It's the horse that the cows are chasing)* and ambiguous agreement *(It's the horse that the cow is chasing)* were included. The English study (Dick et al. 2000) involved 58 patients and more than 300 controls. Work including normals and patients in Italian, and German normals, is still underway (Dick et al. 1999). We did find the expected agrammatic profile, but it occurred in all patient groups (Broca's, Wernicke's, anomics). All groups (including normals) showed lower accuracy and slower RTs on items with noncanonical word order (passives, object clefts). However, relative difficulty of noncanonical word order varied across these three languages, and (as predicted by the Competition Model) extra information from morphology was more helpful in Italian and German (Bates, Friederici & Wulfeck, 1987).

Two online study of children's comprehension of complex sentences in English and Italian (Devescovi & D'Amico, 1998; Dick, Wulfeck, Bates, Saltzman, Naucler, & Dronkers, 1999; Dick, Wulfeck, & Bates, 2003) confirmed the finding that language comprehension skills increase in speed and accuracy across childhood, and that this is especially true for sentence types that are low in frequency and word-order regularity. In both languages, sentences with canonical word order (actives, subject clefts) were interpreted more accurately and quickly than sentences with noncanonical word order (passives, object clefts). Correct response data showed a profile of accuracy such that CRs for Actives=Subject Clefts>Passives>Object Clefts; the same hierarchy of difficulty was seen in reaction times, where RTs for Actives=Subject Clefts<Passives<Object Clefts.

Dick et al. (2003) suggest that the sentence type effects observed are compatible with models in which whole sentence types like clefts and passives are represented in a distributed fashion, so that variations in frequency and validity apply in the "microstructure" of these sentence types. Subject clefts are actually quite low in frequency, but they bear a strong similarity to the highly frequent active sentence frame, in that the two structures share the same word order (Agent-Verb-Object) and similar morphology. Object clefts are not only low in frequency, but they also carry low-frequency word order within their microstructure (Object-Agent-Verb). Passives also have low frequency word order (Object-Verb-Agent), and atypical morphology (verbs in the participial form; presence of a by phrase), and yet they fare better than object clefts in our experiment. In the view of Dick et al., this is the case because passive morphology is both perceptually salient and high in cue validity, compensating partially for low frequency. The development of sentence comprehension skills appears to mirror these distributional facts, suggesting that representations are strengthened over development—not just at the level of the whole sentence type, but at the level of sentential microstructure, where principles of frequency and regularity, cue validity, and cue cost apply.

Grammaticality Judgment. Two online studies investigated the time course of grammaticality judgment in English (Blackwell & Bates 1995; Blackwell, Fisher & Bates 1995). Both studies yielded the same order of difficulty in error in aphasic patients (both fluent and nonfluent): sensitivity to agreement errors < omission errors < word order errors. However, the time course of error detection varied markedly for the three error types: agreement errors are detected immediately (if they are detected at all), movement errors are detected over a 2–3-word window, while detection of omission errors was a protracted process that often spans the entire sentence. This kind of information about the time course of "error monitoring" in receptive processing may help to explain why some error types are more common than others in the expressive language of aphasic patients (i.e. agreement and omission errors slip by the internal monitor), and enrich the notion of cue cost.

A grammaticality judgment study with Italian aphasics (Broca's, Wernicke's, anomics) and controls (Devescovi et al. 1997), focused only on subject-verb and adjective-noun agreement, varying the size of the violation (number of dimensions violated, e.g. number only vs. number + gender) and amount of contextual build-up (number of agreement cues leading up to the error). All groups showed greater sensitivity to errors with more than one violation (number + gender > number-only), which may help to explain why such errors are rare in aphasic speech (Bate & Wulfeck 1989). Effects of contextual build-up differed over patient groups: performance was *better* for controls and *even better* for anomics with multiple contextual cues ("more is better"), but it was *worse* with multiple contextual cues for both Broca's and Wernicke's aphasics ("more is worse"). Hence grammatical context can have a U-shaped effect: redundancy helps up to a point, beyond which more information can make things worse. Again, this increases our understanding of cue cost.

These findings for English and Italian indicate that detailed grammatical knowledge is preserved in aphasics (including agrammatics), in line with representational assumptions of the Competition Model. It was difficult to create stimuli for this purpose in Chinese, which has no inflectional morphology and permits extensive omission and word order variation. Nevertheless, the first study of grammaticality judgment in Chinese—using Broca's aphasics, Wernicke's aphasics, and controls (Lu et al. 2003)—did demonstrate above-chance sensitivity to grammatical violations in all groups. Profiles of relative sparing and impairment were the same for Broca's and Wernicke's, suggesting once again that receptive agrammatism is not specific to any single aphasic group.

NEW DIRECTIONS: STRESS CONTROL
AND BREAKPOINT STUDIES

Most of the studies within Competition Model framework have found common profiles of difficulty across different types of aphasia, within a given language. Furthermore, variants of these profiles in normal controls, especially elderly normals and/or nonaphasic patients, have been observed (Bates et al. 1994, 1999; Blackwell & Bates 1995; Dick et al. 2000). Within the Competition Model, such profiles reflect the response of a distributed knowledge system (organized around cue validity) to generic forms of stress (cue cost). Thus Bates and other researchers hypothesized that it should be possible to simulate profiles of receptive and expressive aphasia in normal controls, by testing them under adverse processing conditions that resemble the internal deficits proposed to explain aphasic symptoms. This would include temporal compression to approximate deficits in rate of processing, perceptual degradation (white noise, multitalker babble, low-pass filtering) to simulate deficits in the spectral quality of information, and cognitive overload or dual-task paradigms to simulate deficits in working memory and attentional resources. In the first study using stress controls (Kilborn 1991), German college students processing under a partial white noise mask showed precisely the same profile of sentence interpretation previously shown in German Broca's and Wernicke's aphasics. A later study (Bates et al. 1994) showed language-specific aphasia profiles in young Italian and English normals in the mugshot task with a concurrent digit load. Agrammatic profiles in English normals in the grammaticality judgment task were also elicited with a concurrent digit load (Blackwell & Bates 1995): detection of agreement errors slipped significantly with only two digits, omission errors fell with two digits, movement errors were robust to digit load at all levels and only slipped significantly at six digits. The largest stress control study involved the four sentence types described above (actives, passives, subject clefts, object clefts, Dick et al. 2000), with English normals tested under temporal compression, low-pass filtering, and digit load, alone and in combination. Results were as follows: (1) Mild but significant variants of the agrammatic profile occurred with compression or filtering alone. (2) With compression and filtering combined, results were superadditive, a quantitative and qualitative match to performance by aphasic patients. (3) In contrast with our results for morphology, digit load had no effect whatsoever on these syntactic contrasts, alone or in combination with the other stressors. Hence it was the first evidence for a dissociation between the stressors that affect morphology and those that affect syntax. Stress control studies of German and Italian are also underway, confirming these results but with language-specific variations in the magnitude of effects (Dick et al. 1999). In particular, the phonologically salient morphological system of Italian (and, to a lesser extent, German) is more resistant to all three stress controls, requiring a much higher "dose" of stress before an aphasia-like "breakpoint" is reached (further evidence for cross-language differences in both cue validity and cue cost).

Recently the stress controls have been extended to study lexical access. Several studies have shown differential lexical priming in Broca's aphasics (underactivation) and Wernicke's aphasics (underinhibition) (Milberg et al. 1995). They have also shown underactivation profiles in normals by using acoustically altered (degraded) prime words in a word-word semantic priming task. Bates and Utman looked at sentential priming of auditory lexical decision under temporal compression and low-pass filtering, alone and in combination (Utman & Bates 2000). The same stimuli were also administered to Broca's and Wernicke's aphasics (Utman & Bates 1998, Utman et al. 1999). Briefly summarized: (1) low-pass filtering of the context results in a Broca-like profile of reduced facilitation (but relatively little effect on sentential inhibition); (2) compression of the context results in a Wernicke-like profile of reduced inhibition (with little effect on sentential facilitation). A follow-up study using cued shadowing with the same sentence stimuli is underway; so far, results are a near-perfect replication of findings with auditory lexical decision.

Encouraged by these results, Bates and her collaborators have started to apply stress controls more broadly within all of our experimental paradigms. This includes a new study of picture-word verification in Spanish-English bilinguals (Moineau 2000) that testifies to the importance of crosslinguistic differences in the phonological properties of words. In the unaltered condition, these bilinguals (who have become English dominant) are faster and more accurate in recognizing English words. Under a combination of filtering and compression (the same in both languages), things reverse: Spanish words are now significantly easier to recognize (virtually unaffected by stress) but performance on English words drops markedly. It is possible to infer that specific structures in specific languages can vary in their "breakpoints," requiring a higher dose of compression or degradation before we see an aphasia-like profile.

The effects of acoustic degradation on lexical processing were investigated in children ranging from 12 to 31 month of age (Zangl, Klarman, Thal & Bates 2001). Using a visual fixation technique, familiar target words (infant-directed speech) were presented either acoustically unaltered, time compressed, or low-pass filtered. The children's ability to correctly identify the target was assessed by examining accuracy, response time, and visual engagement. All three measures were sensitive to the acoustic manipulation; the severity of the effect was dependent on the nature of the acoustic distortion, the child's age, and vocabulary level. Low-pass filtering, which had minimal effects on recognition in adults, had devastating effects on infants: accurate looking was observed only in the more sophisticated groups (vocabulary > 100 words). In contrast, infants had relatively little difficulty in recognizing temporally compressed stimuli. Moreover, reaction time data indicate a nonlinear increase in the efficiency of word recognition that coincides with the acceleration in expressive vocabulary observed in the literature on developmental studies of production.

CONCLUSION

The purpose of the Competition Model is to uncover universal processes that govern the development, use, and breakdown of language, assuming that psycholinguistic universals do exist. Languages such as English, Italian, and Chinese do not live in different parts of the brain, and children do no differ in the mechanisms required to learn each one. However, languages can differ (sometimes quite dramatically) in the way this mental substrate is taxed or configured, making differential use of the same basic mechanisms for perceptual processing, encoding and retrieval, working memory, and planning. It is known that languages can vary qualitatively, in the presence/absence of specific linguistic features (e.g. Chinese has lexical tone, Russian has nominal case markers, English has neither). The research summarized above shows that languages vary quantitatively in the challenges posed by equivalent structures (lexical, phonological, grammatical) for learning and/or real-time use. For example, relative clause constructions are more common in Italian than in English. To the extent that frequency and recency facilitate structural access, these differences should result in earlier acquisition and/or a processing advantage. As shown, this seem to be the case for relative clauses in Italian. That does not necessarily mean that some languages are inherently harder to learn, process, or retain under brain damage than others. All languages must have achieved a roughly comparable degree of learnability and processibility across the course of history, or they would not still be around. However, overall processibility is the product of cost-benefit tradeoffs, a constraint satisfaction problem that must be solved across multiple dimension of the language system. As result, powerful differences have been found between languages in the relative difficulty of specific linguistic structures, with differential effects on performance by children, aphasic patients, and healthy normal adults. In the perspective of the Competition Model this kind of cross-language variation in structural difficulty reflects universal facts of perception, learning, and processing that are not specific to language at all.

REFERENCES

Akhutina, T., Kurgansky, A., Kurganskaya, M., & Polinsky, M. (2000). Gender priming in Russian-speaking aphasics. (Abstract). *Brain and Language*, 74(3), 512–514.

Akhutina, T., Kurgansky, A., Kurganskaya, M., Polinsky, M., Polonskaya, N., Larina, O., Bates, E., & Appelbaum, M. (2000). *Gender priming in Russian-speaking aphasics* (submitted).

Akhutina, T., Kurgansky, A., Polinsky, M., & Bates, E. (1999). Processing of grammatical gender in a three-gender system: Experimental evidence from Russian. *Journal of Psycholinguistic Research*, 28(6), 695–713.

Andonova, E., Devescovi, D'Amico, & Bates (2003). Gender and lexical access in Bulgarian.

Bates, E., & MacWhinney, B. (1987). Competition, variation and language learning. In B. MacWhinney ed. *Mechanism of language acquisition*, Hillsdale, N.J., Erlbaum pp. 157–193.

Bates, E., & Liu, H. (1996). Cued shadowing. In F. Grosjean & U. Frauenfelder (Eds.), A guide to spoken word recognition paradigms. Special Issue of *Language and Cognitive Processes*, 11(6), 577–581. (also published as *A guide to spoken word recognition paradigms: Special issue of Language and Cognitive Processes*. Hove, England: Psychology Press, 577–581).

Bates, E., & Wulfeck, B. (1989b). Comparative aphasiology: A crosslinguistic approach to language breakdown. *Aphasiology*, 3, 111–142 and 161–168.

Bates, E., Chen, S., Li, P., Opie, M., & Tzeng, O. (1993). Where is the boundary between compounds and phrases in Chinese? A reply to Zhou et al. *Brain and Language*, 45, 94–107.

Bates, E., D'Amico, S., Jacobsen, T., Szekely, A., Andonova, E., Devescovi, A., Herron, D., Lu, C.-C., Pechmann, T., Pleh, C., Wicha, N., Federmeier, K., Gerdjikova, I., Gutierrez, G., Hung, D., Hsu, J., Iyer, G., Kohnert, K., Mehotcheva, T., Orozco-Figueroa, A., Tzeng, A., & Tzeng, O. (2003). Timed picture naming in seven languages. *Psychonomic Bulletin & Review*, 10(2), 344–380.

Bates, E., Devescovi, A., & D'Amico, S. (1999). Processing complex sentences: A crosslinguistic study. *Language and Cognitive Processes*, 14(1), 69–123.

Bates, E., Devescovi, A., Dronkers, N., Pizzamiglio, L., Wulfeck, B., Hernandez, A., Juarez, L., & Marangolo, P. (1994). Grammatical deficits in patients without agrammatism: Sentence interpretation under stress in English and Italian (Abstract). *Brain and Language*, 47(3), 400–402.

Bates, E., Devescovi, A., Hernandez, A., & Pizzamiglio, L. (1996). Gender priming in Italian. *Perception & Psychophysics*, 58(7), 992–1004.

Bates, E., Devescovi, A., Pizzamiglio, L., D'Amico, S., & Hernandez, A. (1995). Gender and lexical access in Italian. *Perception & Psychophysics*, 57(6), 847–862.

Bates, E., Devescovi, A., & Wulfeck, B. (in press). Psycholinguistics: A cross-language perspective. *Annual Review of Psychology*. Chippewa Falls, WI: Annual Reviews.

Bates, E., Dick, F., Martinez, A., Moses, P., Müller, R.-A., Saccuman, C., & Wulfeck, B. (2000). *In-progress pilot studies of fMRI language measures in English and Chinese* (Tech. Rep. CRL-0012). La Jolla: University of California, San Diego, Center for Research in Language.

Bates, E., Dick, F., & Wulfeck, B. (1999). Not so fast: Domain-general factors can account for selective deficits in grammatical processing. *Behavioral and Brain Sciences*, 22(1), 96–97.

Bates, E., Friederici, A., & Wulfeck, B. (1987). Comprehension in aphasia: A crosslinguistic study. *Brain and Language*, 32, 19–67.

Bentrovato, S., Devescovi, A., & Bates, E. (2000). Effects of grammatical gender and semantic context on word reading. *(Tech. Rep. CRL 0005)*. La Jolla: University of California, San Diego, Center for Research in Language.

Bentrovato, S., Devescovi, A., D'Amico, S., & Bates, E. (1999). The effect of grammatical gender and semantic context on lexical access in Italian. *Journal of Psycholinguistic Research*, 28(6), 677–693.

Blackwell, A., & Bates, E. (1995). Inducing agrammatic profiles in normals: Evidence for the selective vulnerability of morphology under cognitive resource limitation. *Journal of Cognitive Neuroscience, 7*(2), 228–257.

Blackwell, A., Fisher, D., & Bates, E. (1996). The time course of grammaticality judgment. *Language and Cognitive Processes, 11*(4), 337–406.

Chen, S., & Bates, E. (1998). The dissociation between nouns and verbs in Broca's and Wernicke's aphasia: Findings from Chinese. Special issue on Chinese Aphasia. *Aphasiology, 12*(1), 5–36.

Devescovi A., & D'Amico, S. *Effetti della focalizzazione sulla comprensione di frasi in bambini e adult.i* XII Congresso Nazionale A.I.P. Associazione Italiana di Psicologia. Sezione di Psicologia dello sviluppo. Bressanone 5–7 dicembre 1998

D'Amico, S., Devescovi, A., & Bates, E. (2001). Picture naming and lexical access in Italian children and adults. *Journal of Cognition and Development, 2*(1), 71–105.

D'Amico, S., Szekely, A., & Bates, E. (2003). Comparing modality in lexical access, *in preparation.*

Devescovi, A., D'Amico, S., Bentrovato, S, & Bates, E. (2003). Psychophysics of verbal conjugation. *In preparation.*

Devescovi, A., D'Amico, S., Smith, S., Mimica, I., & Bates, E. (1998). The development of sentence comprehension in Italian and Serbo-Croatian: Local versus distributed cues. In B. D. Joseph & C. Pollard (Series Eds.) & D. Hillert (Vol. Ed.), *Syntax and semantics: Vol. 31. Sentence processing: A crosslinguistic perspective.* San Diego: Academic Press, 345–377.

Dick, F., Bates, E., Ferstl, E., & Friederici, A. (1999). Receptive agrammatism in English- and German-speaking college students processing under stress (Abstract). *Journal of Cognitive Neuroscience, Supplement, 1,* 48.

Dick, F., Bates, E., Ferstl, E., (2003). Spectral and temporal degradation of speech as a simulation of morphosyntactic deficits in English and German *Brain and Language.*

Dick, F., Bates, E., Wulfeck, B., & Dronkers, N. (1998). Simulating deficits in the interpretation of complex sentences in normals under adverse processing conditions (Abstract). *Brain and Language, 65*(1), 57–59.

Dick, F., Bates, E., Wulfeck, B., Utman, J., & Dronkers, N. (2000). *Language deficits, localization and grammar:* Evidence for a distributive model of language breakdown in aphasics and normals. *Psychological Review, 108*(4), 759–788.

Federmeier, K. D., & Bates, E. (1997). Contexts that pack a punch: Lexical class priming of picture naming. *Center for Research in Language Newsletter, 11*(2). La Jolla: University of California, San Diego.

Gentner, D. (1982). Why nouns are learned before verbs: Linguistic relativity versus natural partitioning. In S. A. Kuczaj (Ed.), *Language development: Vol. 2. Language, thought and culture* (pp. 301–334). Hillsdale, NJ: Lawrence Erlbaum.

Grodzinsky Y. (2000) The neurology of syntax: language use without Broca's area. *Behavioral Brain Science, 23,* 1–71.

Hernandez, A. E., Bates, E., & Avila, L. X. (1994). Online sentence interpretation in Spanish-English bilinguals: What does it mean to be "in between"? *Applied Psycholinguistics, 15,* 417–446.

Hernandez, A. E., Bates, E., & Avila, L. X. (1996). Processing across the language boundary: A cross-modal priming study of Spanish-English bilinguals. *JEP: Learning, Memory and Cognition, 22*(4), 846–864.

Hernandez, A. E., Dapretto, M., Mazziotta, J., & Bookheimer, S. (submitted). *Language switching and language representation in Spanish-English bilinguals: An fMRI study.*

Hernandez, A. E., Martinez, A., & Kohnert, K. (2000). In search of the language switch: An fMRI study of picture naming in Spanish-English bilinguals. *Brain and Language, 73*(3), 421–431.

Hernandez, A. E., Sierra, I., & Bates, E. (in press). Sentence interpretation in bilingual and monolingual Spanish speakers: Grammatical processing in a monolingual mode. *Spanish Applied Linguistics.*

Hernandez, A. E., Fennema-Notestine, C., Udell, C., & Bates, E. (in press). Lexical and sentential priming in competition: Implications for two-stage theories of lexical access. *Applied Psycholinguistics.*

Herron, D., & Bates, E. (1997). Sentential and acoustic factors in the recognition of open- and closed-class words. *Journal of Memory and Language, 37*(2), 217–239.

Hillert, D., & Bates, E. (1996). *Morphological constraints on lexical access: Gender priming in German* (Tech. Rep. No. 9601). La Jolla: University of California, San Diego, Center for Research in Language.

Hung, D., & Tzeng, O. (1996). Neurolinguistics: A Chinese perspective. In C. T. James Huang & Y. H. Audrey Li (Eds.), *New horizons in Chinese linguistics* (pp. 357–380). Amsterdam: Kluwer Academic Publishers.

Iyer, G., Saccuman, C., Bates, E., & Wulfeck, B. (2000). A study of age-of-acquisition ratings in adults (Abstract). *Proceedings of the 22nd Annual Conference of the Cognitive Science Society*, 1033. New Jersey: Lawrence Erlbaum Associates.

Jacobsen, T. (1999). Effects of grammatical gender on picture and word naming: Evidence from German. *Journal of Psycholinguistic Research, 28*(5), 499–514.

Kail, M. (1989) Cue validity, cue cost and processing types in sentence comprehension in French and Spanish, in MacWhinney, B., & Bates, E. (Eds.). (1989). *The crosslinguistic study of sentence processing.* New York: Cambridge University Press.

Kilborn, K. (1987). *Sentence processing in a second language: Seeking a performance definition of fluency.* Doctoral dissertation, University of California, San Diego.

Kohnert, K. (2000). *Lexical skills in bilingual school-age children: Cross-sectional studies in Spanish and English.* Ph.D. Dissertation, University of California, San Diego and San Diego State University.

Kohnert, K., Bates, E., & Hernandez, A. (1999). Balancing bilinguals: Lexical-semantic production and cognitive processing in children learning Spanish and English. *Journal of Speech, Language, and Hearing Research, 42*, 1400–1413.

Li, P. (1998). Crosslinguistic variation and sentence processing: Evidence from Chinese. In D. Hillert (Ed.), *Sentence processing: A crosslinguistic perspective* (pp. 33–51). San Diego: Academic Press.

Liu, H. (1996). *Lexical access and differential processing in nouns and verbs in a second language.* Doctoral dissertation, University of California, San Diego.

Liu, H., Bates, E., Powell, T., & Wulfeck, B. (1997). Single-word shadowing and lexical access: A lifespan study. *Applied Psycholinguistics, 18*(2), 157–180.

Lu, C.-C., Bates, E., Li, P., Tzeng, O., Hung, D., Tsai, C.-H., Lee, S.-E., & Chung, Y.-M. (in press). Judgments of grammaticality in aphasia: The special case of Chinese. *Aphasiology, 14*(10), 1021–1054.

MacWhinney, B. (Ed.) (1999). *The emergence of language.* Mahwah, NJ: Lawrence Erlbaum.

MacWhinney, B., & Bates, E. (Eds.). (1989). *The crosslinguistic study of sentence processing.* New York: Cambridge University Press.

Marangolo, P. (1994). Grammatical deficits in patients without agrammatism: Sentence interpretation under stress in English and Italian (Abstract). *Brain and Language, 47*(3), 400–402.

Milberg, W., Blumstein, S. E., Katz, D., Gershberg, F., & Brown, T. (1995). Semantic facilitation in aphasia: Effects of time and expectancy. *J. of Cognitive Neuroscience, 7*(1), 33–50.

Moineau, S. (2000). *The effects of acoustic degradation on lexical processing in bilinguals* (Tech. Rep. CRL-0004). La Jolla: University of California, San Diego, Center for Research in Language.

Neely, J. H. (1991). Semantic priming effects in visual word recognition: A selective review of current findings and theories. In D. Besner & G. W. Humphreys (Eds.), *Basic processes in reading: Visual word recognition* (pp. 264–336). Hillsdale, NJ: Erlbaum.

Roe, K., Jahn-Samilo, J., & Bates, E. (2000). *The effect of stimulus repetition on contextual priming* (Tech. Rep. CRL-0002). La Jolla: University of California, San Diego, Center for Research in Language.

Roe, K., Jahn-Samilo, J., Juarez, L., Mickel, N., Royer, I., & Bates, E. (2000). Contextual effects on word production: A life-span study. *Memory & Cognition, 28,*(5), 756–765.

Szekely, A., & Bates, E. (2000). Objective visual complexity as a variable in studies of picture naming. *Center for Research in Language Newsletter, 12*(2). La Jolla: University of California, San Diego. http://crl.ucsd.edu/newsletter/12-2/article.html

Szekely, A., D'Amico, S., Devescovi, A., Federmeier, K., Herron, D., Iyer, G., Jacobsen, T., Arevalo, A., & Bates, E. (in press). *Timed action and object naming. Cortex.*

Utman, J., & Bates, E. (1998). Effects of acoustic degradation and semantic context on lexical access: Implications for aphasic deficits (Abstract). *Brain and Language, 65*(1), 217–218.

Utman, J., & Bates, E. (2000). *Effects of acoustic distortion and semantic context on lexical access.* (in press).

Utman, J., Dick, F., Prat, C., & Mills, D. (1999). Effects of acoustic distortion and semantic context on event-related potentials to spoken words (Abstract). Proceedings of the Cognitive Neuroscience Society, Washington, DC. *Supplement to Journal of Cognitive Neuroscience, 52.*

Von Berger, E., Wulfeck, B., Bates, E., & Fink, N. (1996). Developmental changes in real-time sentence processing. *First Language, 16,* 192–222.

Wicha, N., Bates, E., Moreno, E., & Kutas, M. (2000). Grammatical gender modulates semantic integration of a picture in a Spanish sentence (Abstract). *Journal of Cognitive Neuroscience, Supplement,* 126.

Wicha, N., Hernandez, A., Reyes, I., Gavaldón de Barreto, L., & Bates, E. (2000). *When zebras become painted donkeys: Interplay between gender and semantic priming in a Spanish sentence context.* (submitted).

Part IV

BIOLOGY AND LANGUAGE

Chapter 7

Rethinking Developmental Neurobiology

Barbara L. Finlay
Cornell University

Liz Bates gave a talk at ICIS, the International Conference on Infant Studies in 1996 and the conference organizers offered tapes of it, only $11. A bargain, as I have played it to my Developmental Neuroscience class ever since, and more than I bargained for, as the repetitions of this talk slowly restructured my thinking on developmental neurobiology. In my mind, the talk is titled "Unnecessary Entailments," though Liz probably titled it something pithier. I have since discovered it touches on virtually all of the major themes that weave through her imposing volume of work. In this talk, she dissected the unnecessary identities that have proliferated in the conceptual structure of cognitive neuroscience. How a complex problem, mapping the structure of the world onto a string of speech, may produce a unique and complicated neural structure but not entail a corresponding structure of complicated innate rules. How the fact that somewhere-localized, physical changes in the brain must accompany any new thought (in this case, her husband George's shoe size) neither entail biological determinism nor an impenetrable neural center for shoe size. How that the fact we can identify language as a unique human ability does not entail unique corresponding structure in the genome. And most important, this talk supplied the correct response to the "I can't imagine how . . ." argument—Liz correctly pointed out that this argument entails only incapacity in the speaker, but nothing about the structure of cognition, the brain, or the genome. Her own imagination has consistently outrun the opposition.

I have since applied this critical approach wholesale to the way people apply the information of developmental neurobiology to cognitive development and the reverse, and I hope here I can literally flesh out some of Liz Bates' deductions about the nature of the physical structure of the developing brain. Also, I will spend a little time tracing the tracks of entailments and assumptions back and forth between disciplines. One of my professional roles has come to be interdisciplinary translator, as my research and reading lies principally in developmental neurobiology and biology, while my departmental home and journal work are in psychology and cognitive science. I would hope to explain each group to the other, running the intermediary's perpetual risk of alienating both. Biologists and psychologists approach developmental questions in fundamentally different ways, but very often import each other's terminology without question, using words more often as metaphors than as items with particular definitions. In this paper, I will discuss theory-making in both disciplines first, and then discuss the concepts of modules and cortical areas which do service in both domains, both in their computational and developmental aspects.

THEORIES OF EVERYTHING

It's the rare neurobiologist who would make a wholesale claim like "Every neuron in the nervous system is capable of activity-dependent stabilization of its synapses" and then, as a research enterprise, set out to demonstrate the existence of one instance after another. Broad statements, such as, "Cognition is rule-based" are more typical of cognitive scientists. Neurobiologists more often address a prominent, and promising piece of organization. Hypothesis-generation comes second and concerns how the piece works, or how it got that way. For example, the curiously part-transient, first-generated neurons of the cortex, the subplate, were hypothesized to be a developmental scaffold for the cortex (Shatz, Chun et al. 1988), and the research race was on to confirm or deny the guess. In many cases, the piece of organization is often called a model system which is asked to stand for the actual system the researcher is interested in, but for reasons or complexity or inaccessibility, cannot. Thus we have the development of bird song motivated as a model system for human language, or long-term potentiation in the hippocampus as a model for learning, more generally. A suitably interesting model system soon takes on its own life and will apply to many more questions than initially motivated its choice, and will generate a set of researchers who will identify themselves with the system, "I work on LTP", "I'm a bird-song person."

Investigation of the striped arrangement of ocular dominance columns in primary visual cortex is an interesting case of a self-organizing neurobiological research system using this general approach. Hubel and Wiesel first noted that neurons in primary visual cortex were either sensitive to one eye, or the other, or both, in a columnar organization extending the depth of the cortex. Looking at the cortical surface, these columns were organized in a system of stripes (Hubel and Wiesel 1962, 1968). Further, if one eye were deprived of experience, the stripes belonging to the deprived eye all but disappeared (Wiesel and Hubel 1965; Hubel, Wiesel et al. 1977). The multifarious applications of these observations for understanding the nature of visual perception, activity-dependent learning, the nature of the visual cortex as a learning device, and for various ophthalmologic disorders were immediately apparent. Hundreds of papers have been written on various aspects of ocular dominance columns and stripes, with perhaps the most notable result (of a number of different results) a fairly complete mechanistic explication of how presynaptic axons whose activity are correlated take up and stabilize connections on the same neuron—the mechanism of the basic Hebbian synapse, "fire together, wire together" (for a reasonably recent exemplar, Kirkwood, Lee et al. 1995).

Whether ocular dominance columns themselves have any functional significance is not clear, curiously enough. To be sure, if a deprived eye claims no cortical territory at all, its acuity and capacities are meager (Wiesel 1982). Clearly, correlation and lack of correlation of input from the two eyes serves multiple functions. A difference of location of a single contour in the two eyes signifies depth relative to plane of focus (the use of binocular disparity for stereoscopic depth); a tag about the eye-of-origin of non-matching visual input can be used to segregate object boundaries; duplicate information from the two eyes in low light conditions can be used to confirm a guess about what's out there. It is the need to segregate eye-specific information into stripes, however, which is not clear. The separation of the two eyes into stripes in their cortical representation can apparently be eliminated with no obvious loss of visual function—old and recent reports of New World monkeys show animals in possession of good binocular vision with nonexistent or variable ocular dominance stripes (Livingstone, Nori et al. 1995; Livingstone, 1996; Adams and Horton, 2003). Just as any artificial neural net might recover correlated structure coming from two eyes without any corresponding spatial structure of stripes in its "hidden" layer, so can the visual system. So, after years of research, we have some clear answers to "How does it get that way?" and "How does it work?" (in the sense of how receptive fields organize their local input) in this eye-catching piece of morphology but can say little about the functional necessity of stripes per se. In fact, there is every reason to believe that the emergence of stripes is a non-essential epiphenomenon of the combined interaction of a set of neurons and their inputs whose activity-dependent sorting function is trying to satisfy two constraints simultaneously, eye-of-origin, and topographic position within the eye (for example, Swindale, 2000). Activity-dependent sorting parameters or initial conditions may predispose to the stripe solution, but in fact other perfectly functional configurations exist. I have extended this example in order to return to what I will claim is a similar evolution in the understanding of the significance of a "cortical area."

Cognitive scientists, both those with developmental interests and not, are more apt to begin from more principled, hypothetical stances about the structure of cognition, often as embodied in a particular intellectual leader—i.e. "Gibsonian," "Piagetian," "Vygotskian." The most salient stances in this context are those who try to understand language by the operation of general-purpose devices, connectionists, and those who in the Chomskian lineage who contend it is rule-based. I do not wish to caricature the members of either group, as various complex interactionist positions have evolved as the evidence evolves. I also acknowledge the cognitive scientists who behave like neurobiologists, those who latch onto juicy-looking phenomena whose explanations promise answers to interesting questions in a number of domains. In general, however, definitions are used quite differently depending what type of theoretical position you start from. A "module" in cognitive psychology has an accepted definition, due to Fodor (1992), history, and the requirements of deductive argumentation. A "module" to a neurobiologist has a fuzzier and inductively derived meaning, often referring to some sort of repeating functional unit, which carries with it no claims of impenetrability or special structure. "Rules" and "laws" have a different status in research areas that are phenomenon-driven versus concept-driven.

Scientists of all descriptions are very interested in importing confirmatory evidence of either the truth of their theory (cognitive scientists, principally) or the functional importance of the phenomenon they are investigating (neurobiologists). Neither group is likely to look quite as closely at the evidence supplied by another field as they are to their own, relying, as is quite reasonable, on a mapping of the principal terms used by one field into the other. In the case of the cortical area, cognitive scientists and neurobiologists have unwittingly colluded in their mutual interests in giving special prominence to the "cortical area." Cortical areas are reasonably prominent pieces of morphology that divide up an anatomical region that appears intractably large and uniform, and which promise a straightforward mechanistic answer to how they come to be; cognitive scientists, for quite some time, were looking for the physiological correlate of the boxes with arrows between them. Cortical areas have been given the status of an important unit in cognition, a location and a module (perhaps impenetrable) where a particular computation is done and shipped out to the next area/module. But increasingly, neither the definitions used nor the evidence evolving in either domain corresponds to reality, nor to each other. I will argue now that cortical areas may well be like the stripes formed by ocular dominance columns, easily-seen morphological divisions that carries information about the process of information segregation and dispersal in the nervous system, but that has little functional interest in its own right. Of course, Liz Bates has been arguing that searching for modules in the nervous system has been a poorly justified enterprise for years. Moreover, one of her very latest articles (Bates, Wilson et al. 2003 "Voxel-based lesion-symptom mapping") tells us what to do next when deprived of this fundamental piece of grammar/structure in theory-building as the identities of cognitive scientists and neurobiologist finally become entwined in functional brain imaging.

CORTICAL AREAS IN BRAIN SPACE
AND EVOLUTIONARY TIME

Brodmann's Enduring Influence. The obvious way to begin a talk in any number of areas of cognitive neuroscience or developmental neurobiology (and I do it myself) is to flash a picture of Brodmann's original delineation of substructure in cortical architecture, showing the divisions of the human cerebral cortex, ca. 1900. The whole cerebral cortex ("neocortex" or more properly "isocortex") has a consistent structure of layering of input and output, the reason it is given a single name. However, local differentiation exists. This local differentiation essentially comes down to thalamic input it attracts (or allows) and eventually receives (though the claim here is *not* that the cortex is entirely undifferentiated and receives its instructions through the thalamus, to be explained). First, a brief review of relevant cortical structure.

The key to understanding cortical structure, both in development and adulthood, is to understand that the "cortical column" (the fundamental, repeating unit of the cortex) does a stereotyped intake, transformation and distribution of information within a matrix of local and distant influences from the rest of the cortex. The functional contents of any particular column are wildly diverse, depending on their input. The defining input to the cortex (i.e. whether it is *called* "visual, motor, somatosensory") comes from the thalamus. The thalamus itself gets its input from 1) the senses including sight, sound, touch and body position 2) from other parts of the brain which give about the body's state of motion, emotion, homeostasis and arousal state and 3) from the cortex itself. The thalamus might be a kind of transduction device that takes these diverse inputs and transforms it to a common code appropriate to the uniform operations of the cortex, though this characterization remains a guess. The input from the thalamus goes to the middle layer, Layer IV, and to a lesser extent, to the upper part of Layer VI. This thalamic information in Layer IV is then relayed up and down, to Layers II and III, and to Layers V and VI. The majority of synaptic connections most input cells of the cortex will make are restricted to the column several cells wide that extends perpendicularly from Layer IV to the cortical surface, and down to Layer VI. All the cells in a particular column participate in similar contexts. For a few examples, taken from widely separated parts of the cortex, one column might fire to stimulation of a particular location and type of sensation on the body surface, another before a particular trajectory of arm movement, and another when the individual is anxious in a social context.

The activity in these columns is continually modified by the local, regional and distant context supplied from other cortical areas (Gilbert, Das et al. 1996; Albright and Stoner 2002; see also Merker (in press) for an interesting conceptualization of how to describe this context). Even in primary visual cortex, less than 5% of the excitatory input to a cortical column is estimated to be of thalamic origin, and the rest is intracortical and some external modulatory input (Peters and Payne 1993; Peters, Payne et al. 1994). Intracortical input comes from Layers II and III. Axons from these layers distribute to neighboring cortical areas (for example, from primary to secondary visual cortex); to distant cortical areas (for example, from secondary visual cortex to visuomotor fields in frontal cortex); and across the corpus callosum to the cortex on the other side of the brain. The principal output connection of Layer VI is a reciprocal connection back to the thalamus, which can be massive—even in the case of the lateral geniculate nucleus, the most primary of primary sensory areas in the thalamus, the vast majority of inputs to the nucleus itself are not from the retina, but rather are reciprocal inputs back from primary visual cortex and modulatory inputs from the brainstem (Erisir, Van Horn et al. 1997). The point of this description is to emphasize that while thalamic input brings new sensory information to the cortex, it might be better to think of the thalamus as installing new information in an immense current and historical context.

The next level of organization past the column, the "cortical area," has inputs, descending connections and relative specializations of layers that reflect its relative position in this intake and distribution of information. Primary visual cortex, which receives thalamic input of input relayed from the retina, has an unusually large number of cells in Layer IV. In motor cortex, Layer IV is almost absent, and the cells of Layer V, the output layer connecting to downstream motor centers and the spinal cord, are unusually large and prominent. Each cortical area typically contains a topographic representation of a sensory, motor or other computed dimension (any derived ordered array, for example, location in 3-D auditory space, which has no sensory surface like the retina). A large number of these represent egocentric space, in various modalities. The cortical topographic map is often a direct replication of the same topographic array already represented in the thalamus. Each area has unique input and output and a limited repertoire of physiological transformations of its thalamic input, such as the elongated, orientation-selective visual receptive fields of primary visual cortex that are constructed from the symmetrical center-surround visual fields of their visual input.

Making Areas. What is the source of the information that gives cortical areas their distinct input and output connections and other specialized local features? Only recently, the cortex has come to be understood in the same genomic terms that structures like the entire vertebrate body plan, or spinal cord segmentation are understood (Ragsdale and Grove 2001; Muzio and Mallamaci 2003). These schemes are rather counterintuitive to the amateur human architect, who typically imagines expression of Gene A corresponds to Segment A or Cortical Area A, and Gene B, Segment B and so on. Rather, adult "parts," like a spinal cord segment or cortical area, correspond to regions in overlapping and nested patterns of regulatory genes. The relative level of expression of these genes controls the expression of other regulatory genes, "transcription factors," and those in turn, direct the genes that direct the construction of particular molecules like structural proteins of cell bodies and axons, axon-dendrite recognition molecules and all the transmitter production and uptake systems that are the physical components of the cortex (and possibly still more transcription factors). Very rarely would the domain of expression of an early regulatory gene be identical with a recognizable chunk of adult morphology. With the exception of a few genes and other markers that are partially localized to the primary sensory cortices, particularly visual and somatosensory, there is no mosaic organization of gene expression that in any way mirrors the adult mosaic of cortical areas.

A "polarizer" has been discovered at the front of the growing cortical plate that appears to control the orientation of the areas of the cortex with respect to the whole cortical surface—if this region is transplanted to the back, the topographic organization of cortical areas turns around from the normal arrangement such that somatosensory cortex is at the back and visual cortex in the front (Fukuchi-Shimogori and Grove 2001). This polarizer controls the expression of transcription factors, genes that regulate the expression of other genes in the proliferative zone for the cortex and in the developing cortex itself. So far, predominating types of gene expression recognized to be under control of transcription factors are those that produce different kinds of cell recognition molecules that control axon pathway selection—the mileposts and signals that direct particular thalamic input to particular regions of the cortex (Leingartner, Richards et al. 2003). One of the first things that the developing cortex does, therefore, is specify which input it is to receive.

One clear outcome of this specification is that thalamic input to the cortex is very topographically precise in early development in those primary sensory regions where it has been studied (Crandall and Caviness 1984; Miller, Chou et al. 1993; Molnar, Adams et al. 1998). For example, in the adult, the lateral geniculate nucleus in the thalamus gets a point-to-point projection from the retina and confers this representation directly on the visual cortex. In the embryo, even on first contact, the topology of the projection from the retina to the cortex is nearly as specific as it is in adulthood. Once thalamic input is in place, it can be a source of information for further differentiation. The early arrival and precise placement of thalamic input is well suited to further specify many of the local features of cortical areas. Thalamus-controlled differentiation steps include differences in numbers of cells in the various layers, expression of particular transmitters, and perhaps most important, the effects of the nature and pattern of activity relayed through the thalamus on how cortical neurons wire up (Miller, Windrem et al. 1991; Windrem and Finlay 1991; Kingsbury and Finlay, 2001).

In marked contrast to the thalamic connections, which at least of the primary sensory zones, could be conceptualized as a list independent of who neighbors whom, that is, Nucleus A should connect to Cortical Area Z, Nucleus B to Cortical Area Y, and so on, the early connections of the cortex with itself are dominated by nearest-neighbor spatial relations. In a study of the development of intracortical connections in the hamster, Barbara Clancy and Marcy Kingsbury described initial projections that covered from one third to one half of the entire cortical area normally distributed from point of origin, quite distinct from an idiosyncratic list of particular projections from one cortical area to various other cortical areas (Prasad, Graf et al. 1999; Kingsbury and Finlay 2001). A similar observation has been made for much larger brains—the colleagues of Scannell and Young (Scannell, Blakemore et al. 1995; Hilgetag, Burns et al. 2000), analyzing the dataset of connectivity compiled for the monkey (Felleman and Van Essen 1991) and the cat, find that 85% of connections within the cortex fall under the rule "nearest neighbor plus one." Thus, in larger brains, the connections do not normally reach so far when expressed as percent of total area, but are well described by relatively simple rules about connecting to nearest neighbors.

Intracortical connections are also rather easy to rearrange, quite distinct from thalamocortical connections. Intracortical connections are the principal substrate of cortical plasticity of all types that involve reallocation of the cortex to new functions, from gross to fine functional readjustments. Demonstrations of this range from local plasticity that might be caused by producing a gap in the sensory information coming in from the periphery within a particular sensory modality, to experimental "rewiring" of cortex done by inducing retinal axons to innervate auditory centers, which causes the auditory cortex to take on visual properties (Pallas 1990; Pallas 2001).

Recent demonstration of multimodal activation of the visual cortex in the early blind, including activation during Braille reading, almost certainly uses intracortical pathways to produce the observed reorganization (Sadato, Pascualleone et al. 1996; Burton 2003).

The Significance of Embryology for Modularity and Plasticity. Understanding the cortex in terms of general vertebrate (and invertebrate!) mechanisms that produce the basic body plan opens a wealth of analogies and models. Segmentation of a uniform field into a number of repeating units, and then subsequent differentiation of each unit is the central strategy for creation of the body in embryos, from the segments of an insect body or a worm, to the segments of the vertebrate spinal cord. This "theme and variation" strategy maps in a fairly direct way onto an "easy" evolutionary alteration of the genome that preserves basic function while allowing adaptations (Gerhart and Kirschner 1997; Wilkins 2001). Individual gene or groups of genes are duplicated, followed by modification of the duplicate gene while the functions of the original one are conserved. A typical modification would allow new constellations of genes to come under the control of the regulatory genes in evolving segments of a segmented structure. Consider the spinal cord of a fish, which has a repeating segmental structure that maps onto the relatively uniform (front to back) musculature of the fish trunk for the propagation of the wavelike contraction and relaxation of body-wall musculature in swimming. In animals with limbs, those segments that innervate the limbs must have evolved to acquire new instructions, including some very specific new wiring for complicated limb musculature. Yet, if these limb segments are transplanted into the body trunk region, they are capable of expressing the old trunk pattern and wire up in general accord with their new environment (Lance-Jones and Landmesser 1981). To conscript a Batesian turn of phrase for this phenomenon, old regions may be adapted to new functions, but they don't give up their day jobs.

The question of whether particular cortical areas, like a "face area" or a "motion area" could have specializations for particular functions or are generic has a very likely answer in this developmental context: all of the above. Because a particular location in cortex is predictable in what information it will receive, that is, it has a very high likelihood of receiving particular thalamic input and standing in predictable neighboring relations to other cortical areas, regions of cortex could take on novel functions under genetic control. To hypothesize some possibilities, none of which have been demonstrated, coarse pattern generating genes like those that produce eye spots in butterfly wings could be sited in a likely spot in the temporal cortex, the patterns producing factors that induce mutual connectivity between spots rather than pigments for wings, this producing a crude face template (Beldade, Brakefield et al. 2002). Regions could express certain neurotransmitters or change the vigor of axon outgrowth, to name just a few possibilities. Were the expected thalamic input not available, or perhaps even in the normal case, the same area of cortex still possesses its generic functions.

The Proliferation of Cortical Areas in Evolution. Finding the right conceptual framework for understanding cortical evolution is important, since the large area of cortex of the human brain is its signature feature. As we also know that that number of cortical areas increases with brain size, it is reasonable to hypothesize that the cortical area might be the "unit" of cortical evolution—for example, that genes might exist that could simply duplicate an advantageous cortical region (Kaas 1989). The assumption that a cortical area has a particular function and is the same as a committed processing module makes this type of hypothesis particularly attractive. Many alternative possibilities have been stated—one, for example, Rakic's "radial unit hypothesis," that the developmental unit of a radial glial cells and the neurons that migrate on it that gives rise to a cortical column is the selectable unit, which can be made more numerous by increase in the numbers of cell cycles in cortical neurogenesis (Rakic, 1990). For the moment, however, we will concentrate on the hypothesis that it is the cortical area that is the important unit of cortical information processing, and of cortical evolution.

If the cortical area is the important feature of cortical evolution, and animals are selected on the functions that reside in cortical areas, we could make two predictions. First, that the number of cortical areas animals might have should be variable, as they are under different selection pressures, and there should be some kind of relationship between the size or number of cortical areas and the sensory or motor capacities on which an animal most depends. How do the numbers, sizes and arrangements of cortical areas vary in evolution?

At the most general level of allometric scaling, first, it is important to know that the volume of area of the cortex is a highly predictable from brain size (Hofman 1989; Finlay, Darlington et al. 2001). Primates as a group have a high volume of cerebral cortex compared to other mammals (a "grade shift") and also, the cortex in primates has "positive allometry"—its volume increases more rapidly than the volume of the whole brain as brain size increases. Yet, the volumetric change is totally predictable—humans have exactly the amount of cortex we should have for an animal of our brain size. So while it is certainly possible that we were selected for behaviors dependent upon the volume of cortex, it is not dissociable from total brain size. Further, cortical regions, like frontal cortex or visual cortex also scale in a predictable manner. Humans do not have an "overdeveloped" frontal lobe, but one that would be expected from scaling relationships with other great apes (Jerison 1997; Semendeferi, Lu et al. 2002).

Within this scaling context, Desmond Cheung in my laboratory undertook an analysis of how the number of cortical areas scale with cortex size (Cheung, Darlington et al. 2002), using the corpus of observations accumulated principally by Kaas, Krubitzer and their associates (see general reviews in Krubitzer 1995; Kaas 1996). He found a very predictable relationship, with R^2 ranging from .7's to .89's, depending upon the subsets of data considered and the method of analysis. The nature of the logarithmic relationship was such that the number of cortical areas increased very rapidly from the smallest cortices (in shrews) up until about a ferret-sized brain, and thereafter increased slowly. It is at the size of brain that includes ferrets, cats and monkeys where visible substructure of cortical areas becomes prominent, including ocular dominance stripes, cytochrome oxidase blobs and patches of interleaved axonal projections (to give this scaling relationship a physical referent, the entire cortex of a mouse would fit comfortably in the primary visual cortex of a cat).

In a separate study, Peter Kaskan looked at the scaling of the size of cortical areas, with respect to brain size and niche (Kaskan et al., submitted). He found that very reliable allometric scaling of cortical areas, including the primary sensory and motor areas, as others have shown—V1, S1 and so forth have a predictable relationship to brain size, or cortex area. Most interesting, though, was when the data were divided into primarily nocturnal or primarily diurnal animals, there was no difference whatsoever in the relative sizes of visual, somatosensory and auditory cortices—the data points lay directly on top of each other. Nor was there a difference whether the primary sensory cortices alone were considered, or the primary and secondary sensory regions were added together.

These and other observations suggest a cortical sheet that generates subdivisions in a rather mechanical way with increasing size, rather than by generating novel areas by specifying new connections and new circuitry to produce new and unique regions by adaptation and evolutionary selection. The lack of relationship of niche to cortex area size finds a complement in studies of plasticity, from Lashley to the present. Consider the example already cited, that in individuals blind from birth, the visual cortex becomes activated during Braille reading and other haptic functions (Sadato, Pascualleone et al. 1996; Burton, 2003). So, while the area defined anatomically by input from the lateral geniculate nucleus of the thalamus remains morphologically identifiable, it acquires new functions. Somewhat less dramatic, but significant remappings were also shown in other individuals with other sensory losses, or those using atypical means of communication (Bavalier, Brozinsky et al., 2001; Elbert, Storr et al, 2002, Newman, Balvalier et al., 2002). This ability of cortical areas to acquire new functions, or at least functions different from the name we have given it (primary "visual" cortex) suggest why the size of anatomically-defined cortical areas is not particularly sensitive to niche—there appears to be a robust mechanism already in place, working epigenetically, that assigns cortical regions to new functions on the basis of activity or importance, particularly if the thalamic input is relatively inactive.

Intracortical connections, both their distribution and their plasticity, suggest a different interpretation of the significance of the cortical area. While thalamic input to the cortex is entirely discrete from nucleus to nucleus, topographically ordered in detail, intracortical connections integrate across those areas, in an overlapping tiling pattern. There is an aspect of hierarchy in the laminar distribution of projections as one goes out from primary sensory areas, termed "feedforward" and "feedback" (Felleman and Van Essen 1991; Barone, Batardiere et al. 2000). Projections from primary to secondary areas target preferentially the "input" cortical lamina, Layer IV, while projections in the opposite direction distribute to intracortically-projecting zones, Layers II III and VI. The significance of this pattern of providing cortical context to the operations of individual cortical column is discussed at length Merker in "Cortex, countercurrent context, and the logistics of personal history." One piece of the anatomical puzzle is missing—while much is known about subcortical projections, area by area, little is know about whether subcortical projections have an obvious pattern with respect to the whole cortical sheet.

What I will suggest briefly now, and elaborate more after I have also discussed some issues in development of the cortex, is that much like the stripes made by ocular dominance columns in some brains, cortical areas are not particularly important features of cortical organization, and most certainly do not correspond to "modules"—localized regions that do a distinct input-output computation and are functionally isolated. Rather, they are epiphenomena of a particular way of maximally specifying and fanning out information from thalamus to cortex, while allowing intracortical projections to recombine this distributed input quite widely and use prior activity (memory) and other current activity to recognize emerging patterns across this matrix.

DEVELOPMENTAL STAGES IN CORTEX AND STAGES IN COGNITIVE ABILITIES: DEVELOPMENTAL MODULES?

The most common question asked by developmental psychologists of developmental neurobiologists is if there is a morphological or physiological marker of any sort that accompanies developmental transitions—for example, the development of stereoscopic vision and coordinated visual pursuit in the two eyes at about three months of age; the burst in vocabulary acquisition; the change from the A-not-B area in spatial memory; the emergence of autobiographical memory. Neurobiological candidates for such markers were events like marked synaptogenesis or synaptic loss, establishment or myelination of a connecting pathway, or the "switching on" of an entire cortical area/module. For years, when I was the developmental neurobiologist queried, I had to confess that I did not know of any but hadn't investigated the matter closely. In 1998, Liz Bates and her colleague Donna Thal asked me and my postdoctoral associate Barbara Clancy if we would be interested in making an update of the article "Early language development and its neural correlates" (Bates, Thal et al. 1992) to investigate specifically the question of the relationship of events in the developing biological system, the cortex, to language development. While the challenge given was more or less the traditional one—find biological markers that accompany behavioral events, Liz Bates and colleagues had already written a great deal about the fact that sharp behavioral accelerations and discontinuities can often be the results of underlying processes that are essentially continuous (Elman, Bates et al. 1996). That paper contains the data we surveyed, written out in detail, and here I will excerpt our principal conclusions that relate to modules, areas, and the general issue of brain/behavior mappings (Bates, Thal et al. 2002).

To my knowledge, there is no one place where the following is written out specifically, but I believe the following beliefs were (and are) commonly held about the relationship of cortical and behavioral maturation. Humans are quite neurally immature at birth, with many important functions awaiting simple maturation. Subcortical functions develop first, the cortex later, and functions carried out subcortically are often subsumed by the cortex as development proceeds. Within domains, primary sensory functions appear first, correlated with the coming on line of primary sensory areas, and then new functions are added as subsequent regions mature. Across the cortex, sensory functions develop first, then language and other integrative functions, and finally the executive and organizing functions dependent on the frontal cortex.

It was astonishing to find out how little actual evidence could be found for any single one of those statements, not to mention a rather wide range of contradictory empirical results. First, by precisely and quantitatively comparing the schedule of events in maturation from the nervous system of the monkey to human maturation, we found that contrary to our expectations, humans are born later in development with respect to neural milestones than are macaque monkeys—humans would be born at seven months postconception, not nine, if we followed the macaque schedule, and lag *in utero* an extra couple months (Clancy, Darlington et al. 1999; Clancy, Darlington et al. 2001). As anthropologists have known, the last couple months in utero for humans is characterized by the acquisition of much body fat

(Pawlowski 1998). Relatively little goes on at this time in the way of significant neural events. In fact, virtually all of the neurons and most of the main connectional architecture of the brain are generated and laid down very early in development, in the first three months of life (Clancy, Darlington et al. 1999).

The cortex itself presents a complicated picture. First, there is no evidence that any part of the cortex "switches on" postnatally—in fact, the cortex is electrophysiologically active even at the time it is under basic construction, in the first three months of life (for example, voltage- and ligand-related activity affects even cell migration—Rakic and Komuro, 1995). There is no single dimension of "maturational state" that any area of the isocortex can be retarded or advanced on (which makes it even less likely there could be a moment when a region "turns on"). Rather, each isocortical area is best viewed as an assembly of different features, including neurogenesis, the maturation of its input, and the maturation of its output, all of those in the context of the maturation of the entire organism (reviewed in Bates et al. 2002; see also Dannemiller, 2001 for a detailed examination of cortical layer, area and regional maturation and their relation to visual function). Because different areas of the brain follow maturational gradients that don't match in order, interesting mismatches occur—in some areas, intracortical connections will be relatively more mature than thalamic connections (the frontal cortex), and in others, the reverse will hold (primary visual cortex).

The cortical sheet has an intrinsic gradient of maturation. Neurogenesis begins at the front edge of the cortex and proceeds back to primary visual cortex; the limbic cortices on the midline also get an early start. Paradoxically, the frontal cortex, viewed in hierarchical models as the last maturing cortical area, is in fact one of the first to be produced and thus quite "mature" in some features. The order of thalamic development is quite different. In general, the primary sensory nuclei in the thalamus are generated first and establish their axonal connections to the cortex first. Of the various other nuclei, motor and cingulate are intermediate in their timing, and the last to be produced are the thalamic nuclei that innervate the frontal, parietal and part of the inferotemporal cortex (reviewed in Finlay, Darlington et al. 2001; Bates, Thal et al. 2002). The thalamic order of neurogenesis suggested a hierarchical notion of cortical development (primary sensory areas mature early, "association" areas late), but it's not the whole story. So what might the dual gradients mean for frontal cortex, the area so often described as "maturing late"? The fact that frontal cortex is generated early but receives its input from the thalamus relatively late could predispose it for intracortical processing. In other words, this difference in developmental gradients might mean that frontal cortex is primed for higher-order associative function by the nature of its position and connections, but not because any essential retardation in maturation of its neurons prevents its early function.

Synapses begin to be formed in the cortex from the time that the first neurons move into place and a fair number are in evidence at six months post-conception (Bourgeois and Rakic 1993). The first synapses must account for the many demonstrations of early activity-dependent organization in the cortex, and perhaps for several types of *in utero* learning, for example, preferences for the language rhythms of the mother (Jusczyk, Friederici et al. 1993). A few months later, though, anticipating birth and all over the cortex, the density and number of excitatory synapses surges ten to a hundredfold (Bourgeois 2001). This observation is quite species-general—synapse numbers surge when the maturing animal *anticipates* exit from the womb (or burrow) into the environment of real-world experience. It is not caused by the experience of the world (Bourgeois, Jastreboff et al. 1989). Many effects on types and distributions of synapses are caused by experience, but not the time nor amount of the burst of synaptogenesis.

Laying down great numbers of synapses on neurons prior to most experience and learning makes computational sense. The immediate postnatal phase of development is distinguished by axon retraction and synapse elimination, "regressive events," as well as growth and addition. In the mature nervous systems, synapses are both added and subtracted during learning. Perhaps the developing nervous system is both allowing activity (though initially disorganized) to be easily propagated through itself, and also allowing itself the possibility of subtraction of synapses, as well as additive ones (Quartz and Sejnowski, 1997), by the installation of large numbers of synapses just prior to experience. This initial "overproduction" of synapses may be a way of producing continuity in mechanisms of synaptic stabilization from initial development to adulthood. The impressive statistical learning capabilities of infants in their first year may require this highly elaborated substrate (Saffran, Aslin et al. 1996).

Experience-Induced Maturation. One of the longest- and best-studied features of perinatal development from both behavioral and neural perspectives is the development of binocular vision, and its relationship to binocular interactions in the visual cortex, both anatomically and physiologically defined (Movshon and Van Sluyters 1981; Teller and Movshon 1986; Dannemiller 2001). Several observations of interest about structure-function links arise from this work. First, in normally developing individuals with normal experience and reasonable optics, there is a critical period for the establishment of a balance of influence from the two eyes on perceptual decisions, for sorting information by eye-of-origin, and for the development of stereoscopic depth perception which happens in the first several years of life. Absence of activity in either eye or incoordination of the eyes can permanently derail the development of normal visual function during this period. If *all* visual experience is denied, however, and both eyes are closed, what occurs is delay of the critical period—the representation of the two eyes does not begin its segregation that results in the physical marker of ocular dominance column in those animals that possess them. The special neurotransmitters and receptors that are responsible for this structural change are held at their initial state (Kirkwood, Lee et al. 1995). When experience is reinstated, anatomical, pharmacological and physiological events then progress, as they would have independent of the animal's age (to a point). A similar phenomenon has been observed in birds that learn their songs from tutors—for the unfortunate nestlings born too late in the season to hear any of the spring songs that establish territories, the "critical period" is held over until the next spring, when singing begins again (Doupe and Kuhl 1999).

Presumably this allocation of neurons to particular functions on the basis of activity occurs everywhere in the cortex. Assignment of initial function to structure is often called "maturation" and the property of "maturity" is ascribed to the tissue, but the example above shows this need not be so. Returning to the frontal cortex, the "immaturity" of frontal cortex on which many executive and self-monitoring skills depend could reflect an absence of events likely to activate frontal cortex in early childhood, not a maturational deficit of the tissue itself.

Continuous Brain, Discontinuous Behavior. One instructive structure-function relationship that appeared in the binocular interaction research was a mismatch between the gradual spatial segregation of the neurons responsive to either the right or left eye in the cortex and a stepwise change in an aspect of visual behavior likely to be dependent on it, the development of binocular rivalry. Infants presented with horizontal stripes to one eye and vertical stripes to the other indicate by their pattern of habituation that their experience is a checkerboard, and not the alternating rivalry between the horizontal and vertical stripes that an adult experiences. In longitudinal studies, the infants switched in a matter of days from the immature checkerboard to the mature rivalrous state, at about 3 months of age, while no such instant of sharp segregation has ever been observed in the presumably corresponding anatomy—from single neurons to stripes, ocular dominance columns in the cortex move slowly to their mature organization (Held 1991; Movshon and Van Sluyters 1981). A different discontinuity with a similar lesson was described in the development of infant walking by Esther Thelen. At birth, all infants will show an alternating stepping movement when supported over a surface, which disappears around 2–3 months, with "real" walking appearing at about a year. This progression was first described as a "spinal reflex" becoming supplanted by cortical control as the cortex matured. In fact, the spinal reflex never disappears, is the basis of adult walking, and can be elicited at any time if the infant is appropriately weighted and balanced (Thelen, Fisher et al. 1984). In this case, spinal circuitry can produce many different rhythmic patterns at any age, dependent on the particular pattern of peripheral load, and "maturation" lies in the changing periphery.

Mapping Complex Changing Functions Onto Complex, Changing Tissue. The point of the prior section on maturation is to discount as much as possible the notion of cortical areas maturing as single functional modules blossoming one at a time, but rather to emphasize the continuous activity of the cortex from the time of its generation, with a single point of punctuation in the surge of synapse production at the time of birth. What then is known about the postnatal maturation of the cortex and its relationship to behavior? Until quite recently, very little. Attempts had been made to locate discontinuities or inflections in graphs of changes in the volume or structure of brain tissue, synapses and process and correlate them with discontinuities in behavior (for example, the period of very rapid vocabulary addition in learning), although, as we have discussed, the assumption that anatomical and physiological discontinuities should correspond in any case is questionable. Myelination, the growth of the insulating glial sheaths that increase the speed of axon conduction of impulses, is something that occurs postnatally and can be correlated with behavioral abnormalities, but has never produced any great insight unto the physical correlate of normal behavioral stages (Sampaio and Truwit 2001). Measurements of spontaneous electrical activity in the cortex and evoked activity (ERP's) could be compared from infant to adolescent to adult, with the typical result showing that the frontal cortex, and sometimes the parietal cortex showed the mature pattern later than sensory cortices, but the anatomical correlate of these physiological changes remained obscure.

With new structural and functional imaging techniques including new versions of ERP's, some striking results have already emerged that integrate well with the picture of the developing brain presented here, consistent across both brain damage and imaging studies (Nelson and Monk 2001; Casey, Thomas et al. 2001; Stiles, Bates et al. 1998). What is presented here are a few examples, with no attempt at review. Although the cortical areas involved in early and adult performance of the same tasks are rarely disjunct, they are never identical. The structures important for learning language are quite different to those required for mature language performance, both in laterality and in anterior-posterior position, as determined in longitudinal studies of children with early brain damage (Bates and Roe 2001). A different constellation of areas is activated for facial and spatial judgments in children, though general adult divisions are employed. Overall, there is an interesting tendency for the right hemisphere to be preferentially involved in initial stages of learning (both in children and adults). The frontal cortex was found to be more active in children engaged in response inhibition tasks than adults, though its activity was not related to success in the task (Casey, Thomas et al. 2001). Identification and understanding of neural structures that are preferentially engaged in the acquisition of new knowledge, rather than the performance of practiced abilities will probably be one of the first outcomes of this research enterprise.

DISTRIBUTION OF FUNCTIONS IN SPACE AND TIME

Following any of a number of interviews with the media, Liz Bates has bemoaned the lack of a simple, graspable result to convey the interest and the nature of the emergence of complicated distributed system. It seems to be news to say that the emergence of past tense in language depends on a spurt of synaptogenesis in Brodmann's area 41-b, the syntax module/area, which in turn reflects the activation of the FOX-PX gene on chromosome 18. To fully elaborate the interactionist position that production of the same ability requires virtually all the cortical areas, most of the genes, and a highly elaborated language experience does not make much of a sound bite, and there won't be one here. Yet, the picture that the cortex gives us about how information is deployed in both in development and in the mature functioning of the cortex does converge on a single story.

Brodmann pointed out discontinuities in the cortex, modules were proposed for behavior, cortical areas were proposed to be the biological analogue of those modules, and a list of those cortical areas is for the most part is what is produced in any current imaging study of the cortex when individuals are engaged in any cognitive task. Increasingly, however, it is clear that any particular cortical area makes a very poor one-to-one map with any perceptual or cognitive skill, even in those domains where perceptual decisions can be reasonably precisely defined, as in color or aspects of form-from-motion in vision. Rather, the thalamus lays out dimensions of sensory and motor experience on the cortical surface, losing little hard-won topographic detail in the projection. At least in primary visual cortex, and perhaps more generally, redundancy in this topographic projection is reduced within the processing class known as "sparse coding" (Field 1994). Information is relayed forward and back, recombining new information with processed information, or with other modalities (Shimojo and Shams, 2001). The scope of intracortical projections exceeds that of a cortical area, and we could view the concert of thalamocortical and intracortical projections as permuting and recombining relationships between the structure of new and incoming information, information recently perceived, remembered structure, and action. In this view, while presumably useful assemblies could arise in any one cortical area, it seems likely that perceptual or motor decisions of any complexity would involve many.

Cortical areas within general processing domains have had a disconcerting tendency to be just slightly different from each other, and rarely reflect what we would imagine to be processing "stages." I will take a few examples from visual processing. In posterior parietal cortex, there are several areas that participate in the coordinate transformation of visual space from a retinally-based code, to a eye-in-head based one, to a body-centered one, and perhaps, in concert with information about self-motion, to a body-independent allocentric code. Conceptually, this would appear to be successive additions of information to the retinal signal, but the neurons representing these coordinate additions do not appear in a stage-like manner in successive areas, but are distributed among the areas (Andersen 1997). Single neurons responsive to faces can be found in numerous locations over the ventral aspect of the orbitofrontal cortex, not confined to a single area, and responses to objects and faces can be discriminated even if the maximally-responsive area is eliminated from the analysis (Haxby, Gobbini et al. 2001). An area in visual cortex was described as "unusually responsive" to motion, particularly area MT, (but this is a statistical statement, as most of the visual cortex areas will respond to image motion), or unusually responsive to color (Area V4), and these two areas were perhaps the best candidates for special modules (Zeki, Watson et al. 1991). Complete ablation of either or both of these areas in macaque produces only mild and transient deficits in abilities in motion, color detection and stereopsis that these areas might be expected to be entirely responsible for, were the brain modular (Schiller 1993).

No claim is being made here that cortical areas do not differ from each other, or that they might not be genetically different, perhaps containing some area-specific computations, or that the process they represent is not critical to cognitive function. The claim is rather that the cortical areas we can see morphologically are the basic foundations of an information dispersal and recombination system, and as such, are extremely unlikely to correspond to any higher-order perceptual and cognitive functions, or even lower-order ones, if color and motion decisions should be construed that way.

The story of cortical development amplifies these same themes. In terms of maturation of its elements, each cortical area arises in time in a different place in converging maturational streams. There is no evidence that any part of cortex wholesale "switches on" as a module might be expected to, but rather, can be seen to be active from the very beginning of development, and changes function, contributing to different capacities and no doubt changing its own capacities as development proceeds.

NAVIGATING THE FUNCTIONING CORTEX

> He had bought a large map representing the sea
> Without the least vestige of land
> And the crew were much pleased when they found it to be
> A map they could all understand
>
> Lewis Carroll (1876)

Without cortical areas as an anchor to a functional description of the cortex, how are we to proceed? While it is certainly the case that the distribution of information that characterizes the thalamocortical projection may be of help discriminating cognitive operations from each other, it may also mislead, much like word-frequency counts might discriminate various writers from each other, but miss the most important components of meaning and message that writers optimally should be contrasted on. It was hard to imagine how to understand the cortex without the fundamental unit of the "cortical area," but as we know, this statement entails only incapacity in the speaker, not impossibility of the task.

Fortunately, Liz Bates and her team of colleagues have imagined it for us. The spatial layout of the cortex persists, whether or not we assign areas to it. A taxonomy of cortex wholly based on function, either function lost by the loss of cortical tissue, as in (Bates, Wilson et al. 2003) or by activation of cortex can replace an outmoded modular view of cortical function. The challenge then is to get the description of behavior right, and it is appreciating this necessity in future studies that makes yet another aspect of Liz Bates' work fall in place. She has laid out for us the complex and generative theoretical position minimally sketched at the outset of this chapter, perhaps best described in *Rethinking Innateness*. Consistent with this theoretical perspective, she outlines a better way to see the information that the cortex presents us in "voxel-based mapping." Finally, she tells us how to get the cortex to give us information we can use, producing the fundamental, basic descriptive, and grindingly difficult studies of language operations—the "MacArthur Communicative Development Inventories," cross-language picture-naming norming studies and gigantic longitudinal studies of the changing deficit patterns in language and cognition after early brain damage. These encyclopedic studies seem almost out of place in what would otherwise appear to be a very theory driven-corpus. But if we understand that our understanding of cortical function must arise from a good taxonomy of real-world cognition, and not from misapplied anatomy, this is the critical and essential step. She has given us latitude, longitude, a ship to sail with, and firm ground to sail from.

REFERENCES

Adams, D. L. and J. C. Horton (2003) Capricious expression of cortical columns in the primate brain. *Nature Neuroscience* **6**: 113–114.

Albright, T. D. and G. R. Stoner (2002) Contextual influences on visual processing. *Ann Rev Neurosci* **25**: 339–379.

Andersen, R. A. (1997). Multimodal integration for the representation of space in the posterior parietal cortex. *Philos Trans R Soc Lond [Biol]* **352**: 1421–1428.

Barone, P., A. Batardiere, K. Knoblauch and H. Kennedy (2000). Laminar distribution of neurons in extrastriate areas projecting to visual areas V1 and V4 correlates with the hierarchical rank and indicates the operation of a distance rule. *J Neurosci* **20**: 3263–3281.

Bates, E. and K. Roe (2001). Language development in children with unilateral brain injury. *Handbook of Developmental Cognitive Neuroscience*. C. A. Nelson and M. Luciana. Cambridge, MA, MIT Press: 281–307.

Bates, E., D. Thal, B. L. Finlay and B. Clancy (2002). Early language development and its neural correlates. *Child Neurology*. S. J. Segalowitz and I. Rapin. Amsterdam, Elsevier Science B.V. **8**: 109–1076.

Bates, E., D. Thal, and J. Janowsky (1992). Early language development and its neural correlates. *Child Neuropsychology*. S. J. Segalowitz and I. Rapin. New York, Elsevier. **7**: 69–110.

Bates, E., S. M. Wilson, A. P. Saygin, F. Dick, M. I. Sereno, R. T. Knight and N. F. Dronkers (2003). Voxel-based lesion-symptom mapping. *Nature Neuroscience* **6**: 448–450.

Bavelier, D., C. Brozinsky, A. Tomann, T, Mitchell, H. Neville and G. Y. Liu. (2001). Impact of early deafness and early exposure to sign language on the cerebral organization for motion processing. *J Neurosci* **21**: 8931–8942.

Beldade, P., P. M. Brakefield and A. D. Long. (2002). Contribution of Distal-less to quantitative variation in butterfly eyespots. *Nature* **415**: 315–318.

Bourgeois, J.-P. (2001). Synaptogenesis in the neocortex of the newborn: the ultimate frontier for individuation. *Handbook of Developmental Cognitive Neuroscience*. C. A. Nelson and M. Luciana. Cambridge, MA, MIT Press: 23–34.

Bourgeois, J. P., P. J. Jastreboff and P. Rakic. (1989). Synaptogenesis in visual cortex of normal and preterm monkey: evidence for intrinsic regulation of synaptic overproduction. *Proc Natl Acad Sci (USA)* **86**: 4297–4301.

Bourgeois, J. P. and P. Rakic (1993). Changes of synaptic density in the primary visual cortex of the macaque monkey from fetal to adult stage. *J Neurosci* **13**: 2801–2820.

Burton, H. (2003). Visual cortex activity in early and late blind people. *J Neurosci* **23**: 4005–4011.

Carroll, L. (1876). *The Hunting of the Snark.*

Casey, B. J., K. M. Thomas, and B. McCandless (2001). Applications of magnetic resonance imaging to the study of cognitive development. *Handbook of Developmental Cognitive Neuroscience*. C. A. Nelson and M. Luciana. Cambridge, MA, MIT Press: 137–148.

Cheung, D. T., R. B. Darlington, and B. L. Finlay (2002). Scalable structure in cortical cartography: Rules for the proliferation of cortical areas. *Soc. Neurosci Abs* **27**: 877.

Clancy, B., R. B. Darlington, and B. L. Finlay (1999). The course of human events: predicting the timing of primate neural development. *Devel Sci* **3**: 57–66.

Clancy, B., R. B. Darlington, and B. L. Finlay (2001). Translating developmental time across mammalian species. *Neuroscience* **105**: 7–17.

Crandall, J. E. and V. S. Caviness (1984). Thalamocortical connections in newborn mice. *J Comp Neurol* **228**: 542–556.

Dannemiller, J. M. (2001). Brain-behavior relationships in early visual development. *Handbook of Developmental Cognitive Neuroscience.* C. A. Nelson and M. Luciana. Cambridge, MA, MIT Press: 221–236.

Doupe, A. J. and P. K. Kuhl (1999). Birdsong and human speech: Common themes and mechanisms. *Annu Rev Neurosci* **22**: 567–631.

Elbert, T., A. Sterr, B. Rockstroh, C. Pantev, M. M. Muller and E. Taub. (2002). Expansion of the tonotopic area in the auditory cortex of the blind. *J Neurosci* **22**: 9941–9944.

Elman, J. L., E. A. Bates, M. H. Johnson, A. Karmiloff-Smith, D. Parisi and K. Plunkett (1996). *Rethinking innateness: A connectionist perspective on development.* Cambridge, MA, MIT Press.

Erisir, A., S. C. Van Horn, et al. (1997). Relative numbers of cortical and brainstem inputs to the lateral geniculate nucleus. *Proc Natl Acad Sci USA* **94**: 1517–1520.

Felleman, D. J. and D. C. Van Essen (1991). Distributed hierarchical processing in the primate cerebral cortex. *Cerebral Cortex* **1**: 1–47.

Field, D. J. (1994). What is the goal of sensory coding? *Neural Comput* **6**(4): 559–601.

Finlay, B. L., R. B. Darlington, et al. (2001). Developmental structure in brain evolution. *Behav Brain Sci* **24**: 263–307.

Fodor, J. A. (1992). Precis of the modularity of mind. *Behav Brain Sci* **8**: 1–42.

Fukuchi-Shimogori, T. and E. A. Grove (2001). Neocortex patterning by the secreted signaling molecule FGF8. *Science* **294**: 1071–1074.

Gerhart, J. and M. Kirschner (1997). *Cells, Embryos and Evolution.* Malden, Massachusetts, Blackwell Science.

Gilbert, C. D., A. Das, et al. (1996). Spatial integration and cortical dynamics. *Proc Natl Acad Sci USA* **93**: 615–622.

Haxby, J. V., M. I. Gobbini, et al. (2001). Distributed and overlapping representations of faces and objects in ventral temporal cortex. *Science* **293**: 2425–2430.

Held, R. (1991). Development of binocular vision and stereopsis. *Vision and visual dysfunction.* D. Regan. Hillsdale, NJ, Erlbaum: 170–178.

Hilgetag, C. C., G. Burns, M. A. O'Neill, J. W. Scannell and M. P. Young. (2000). Anatomical connectivity defines the organization of clusters of cortical areas in the macaque monkey and the cat. *Phil Trans Roy Soc London B* **355** : 91–110.

Hofman, M. A. (1989). On the evolution and geometry of the brain in mammals. *Prog Neurobiol* **32**: 137–158.

Hubel, D. H. and T. N. Wiesel (1962). Receptive fields, binocular interaction and functional architecture in the cat's visual cortex. *J Physiol* **160**: 106–154.

Hubel, D. H. and T. N. Wiesel (1968). Receptive fields and functional architecture of monkey striate cortex *J Physiol* **195**: 215–243.

Hubel, D. H., T. S. Wiesel and S. LeVay. (1977). Plasticity of ocular dominance columns in monkey striate cortex. *Phil Trans Roy Soc Lond (B)* **278**: 377–409.

Jerison, H. J. (1997). Evolution of prefrontal cortex. *Development of the Prefrontal Cortex: Evolution, Neurobiology and Behavior.* N. A. Krasnegor, G. R. Lyon and P. S. Goldman-Rakic. Baltimore, Pall H. Brooks Publishing Co: 9–26.

Jusczyk, P. W., A. D. Friederici, J. M. I. Wessels, V. Svenkerud and A. M. Juscyk (1993). Infants' sensitivity to the sound pattern of native-language words. *J. Memory and Language,* **32**: 402–420.

Kaas, J. H. (1989). The evolution of complex sensory systems in mammals. *Principles of Sensory Coding and Processing.* S. B. Laughlin. Cambridge, UK, the Company of Biologists, LTD. **146**: 165–176.

Kaas, J. H. (1996). What comparative studies of neocortex tell us about the human brain. *Rev. Brasil. Biol.* **56**: 315–322.

Kingsbury, M. A. and B. L. Finlay (2001). The cortex in multidimensional space: where do cortical areas come from? *Developmental Science* 4: 125–156.

Kirkwood, A., H. K. Lee, et al. (1995). Co-regulation of long-term potentiation and experience- dependent synaptic plasticity in visual cortex by age and experience. *Nature* 375 : 328–331.

Krubitzer, L. (1995). The organization of neocortex in mammals: are species differences really so different? *Trends Neurosci* 18 : 408–417.

Lance-Jones, C. and L. Landmesser (1981). Pathway selection by embryonic chick motoneurons in an experimentally altered environment. *Proc. R. Soc. Lond. B* 214: 19–52.

Leingartner, A., L. J. Richards, R. H. Dyck, C. Akazawa and D. D. M. O'Leary (2003). Cloning and cortical expression of rat Emx2 and adenovirus-mediated overexpression to assess its regulation of area-specific targeting of thalamocortical axons. *Cerebral Cortex* 13: 648–660.

Livingstone, M. S. (1996). Ocular dominance columns in new world monkeys. *J Neurosci* 16(6): 2086–2096.

Livingstone, M. S., S. Nori, D. C. Freeman and D. H. Hubel. (1995). Stereopsis and binocularity in the squirrel monkey. *Vision Res* 35: 345–354.

Merker, B. (In press). Cortex, countercurrent context and the logistics of personal history. *Cortex.*

Miller, B., L. Chou and B. L. Finlay (1993). The early development of thalamocortical and corticothalamic projections. *J Comp Neurol* 335(1): 16–41.

Miller, B., M. S. Windrem and B. L. Finlay. (1991). Thalamic ablations and neocortical development: alterations in thalamic and callosal connectivity. *Cerebral Cortex* 1: 1–24

Molnar, Z., R. Adams, and C. Blakemore. (1998). Mechanisms underlying the early establishment of thalamocortical connections in the rat. *J Neurosci* 18: 5723–5745.

Movshon, J. A. and R. C. Van Sluyters (1981). Visual neural development. *Ann Rev Psychol* 32: 477–522.

Muzio, L. and A. Mallamaci (2003). Emx1, Emx2 and Pax6 in specification, regionalization and arealization of the cerebral cortex. *Cerebral Cortex* 13: 641–647.

Nelson, C. A. and C. S. Monk (2001). The use of event-related potentials in the study of cognitive development. *Handbook of Developmental Cognitive Neuroscience*. C. A. Nelson and M. Luciana. Cambridge, MA, MIT Press: 125–136.

Newman, A. J., D. Bavelier, D. Corine, P. Jezzard and H. J. Neville (2002). A critical period for right hemisphere recruitment in American Sign Language processing. *Nature Neurosci* 5: 76–80.

Pallas, S. L. (1990). Cross-modal plasticity in sensory cortex: visual response properties in primary auditory cortex in ferrets with induced retinal projections to the medial geniculate nucleus. *The Neocortex: Ontogeny and Phylogeny*. B. L. Finlay, G. Innocenti and H. Scheich. New York, Plenum Press: 205–218.

Pallas, S. L. (2001). Intrinsic and extrinsic factors that shape neocortical specification. *Trends in Neurosciences* 24: 417–423.

Pawlowski, B. (1998). Why are human newborns so big and fat? *Human Evolution* 13: 65–72.

Peters, A. and B. Payne (1993). Numerical relationships between geniculocortical afferents and pyramidal cell modulaes in cat primary visual cortex. *Cerebral Cortex* 3: 69–78.

Peters, A., B. R. Payne, and J. Budd. (1994). A numerical analysis of the geniculocortical input to striate cortex in the monkey. *Cerebral Cortex* 4: 215–229.

Prasad, D., E. Graf, M. A. Kingsbury, B. Clancy and B. L. Finlay (1999). Development of callosal and corticocortical projections in neonatal hamster isocortex. *Soc. Neurosci. Abs.*(25): 504.

Quartz, S. R. and T. J. Sejnowski (1997). The neural basis of cognitive development: A constructivist manifesto. *Behav Brain Sci* 20: 537.

Ragsdale, C. W. and E. A. Grove (2001). Patterning the mammalian cerebral cortex. *Curr Op Neurobiol* 11: 50–58.

Rakic, P. (1990). Critical cellular events in cortical evolution: radial unit hypothesis. *The Neocortex: Ontogeny and Phylogeny.* B. L. Finlay, G. Innocenti and H. Scheich. New York, Plenum: 21–32.

Rakic, P. and H. Komuro (1995). The role of receptor/channel activity in neuronal cell migration. *J Neurobiol* **26**: 299–315.

Sadato, N., A. Pascualleone, J. Grafman, V. Ibanez, M. P. Deiber, G Dold and M. Hallett. (1996). Activation of the primary visual cortex by Braille reading in blind subjects. *Nature* **380** : 526–528.

Saffran, J. R., R. N. Aslin, and E. Newport (1996). Statistical learning by 8-month-old infants. *Science* **274** : 1926–1928.

Sampaio, R. C. and C. L. Truwit (2001). Myelination in the developing human brain. *Handbook of Developmental Cognitive Neuroscience.* C. A. Nelson and M. Luciana. Cambridge, MA, MIT Press: 35–44.

Scannell, J. W., C. Blakemore, and M. P. Young. (1995). Analysis of connectivity in the cat cerebral cortex. *J Neurosci* **15**: 1463–1483.

Schiller, P. H. (1993). The effects of V4 and middle temporal (MT) area lesions on visual performance in the rhesus monkey. *Visual Neurosci* **10**: 717–746.

Semendeferi, K., A. Lu, et al. (2002). Humans and great apes share a large frontal cortex. *Nature Neurosci* **5** : 272–276.

Shatz, C. J., J. J. M. Chun, and M. B. Luskin (1988). The role of the subplate in the development of the mammalian telencephalon. *The Cerebral Cortex.* A. Peters and E. G. Jones. New York, Plenum. **7**.

Shimojo, S. and L. Shams (2001). Sensory modalities are not separate modalities: plasticity and interactions. *Curr Opin Neurobiol* **11**: 505–509.

Stiles, J., E. Bates, D. Thal, D. Trauner and J. Reilly (1998). Linguistic, cognitive and affective development in children with pre- and perinatal focal brain injury: A ten-year overview from the San Diego longitudinal project. *Advances in Infancy Research.* C. Rovee-Collier, L. Lipsitt and H. Hayne. Norwood, NJ, Ablex: 131–163.

Swindale, N. V. (2000). How many maps are there in visual cortex? *Cerebral Cortex* **10**(7): 633–643.

Teller, D. Y. and J. A. Movshon (1986). Visual development. *Vision Research* **26**: 1483–1506.

Thelen, E., D. M. Fisher, and R. Ridley-Johnson. (1984). The relationship between physical growth and a newborn reflex. *Infant Behavior and Development* **7**: 479–493.

Wiesel, T. N. (1982). Postnatal development of the visual cortex and the influence of the environment. *Nature* **299**: 583–591.

Wiesel, T. N. and D. H. Hubel (1965). Comparison of the effects of unilateral and bilateral eye closure on cortical unit responses in kittens. *J Neurophysiol* **28**: 1029–1040.

Wilkins, A. S. (2001). *The Evolution of Developmental Pathways.* Sunderland, Massachusetts, Sinauer Associates.

Windrem, M. S. and B. L. Finlay (1991). Thalamic ablations and neocortical development: alterations of cortical cytoarchitecture and cell number. *Cerebral Cortex* **1**: 1–24.

Zeki, S., J. D. G. Watson, C. J. Lueck, K. J. Friston, C. Kennard and R. S. J. Frackowiack. (1991). A direct demonstration of functional specialization in the human visual cortex. *J Neurosci* **11**: 641–649.

Chapter 8

Bates's Emergentist Theory and Its Relevance to Understanding Genotype/Phenotype Relations

Annette Karmiloff-Smith
Neurocognitive Development Unit,
Institute of Child Health, London

INTRODUCTION

Elizabeth Bates (Liz, to us all) was a very dear friend and colleague, so I am sure that she would have forgiven me if I start the chapter that I have written in her honor with five quotations that would have given her goose pimples and raised her blood pressure momentarily! My purpose of course is rhetorical, and I will use Bates's Emergentist Theory to challenge the common theoretical thread that underlies each of these statements.

> We argue that human reasoning is guided by a collection of innate domain-specific systems of knowledge. (Carey & Spelke, 1994)

> The mind is likely to contain blueprints for grammatical rules . . . and a special set of genes that help wire it in place. (Pinker, 1994)

> The genes of one group of children [Specific Language Impairment] impair their grammar while sparing their intelligence; the genes of another group of children [Williams syndrome] impair their intelligence while sparing their grammar. (Pinker, 1999)

> It is uncontroversial that the development [of Universal Grammar] is essentially guided by a biological, genetically determined program . . . Experience-dependent variation in biological structures or processes . . . is an exception . . . and is called 'plasticity'. (Wexler, 1996)

The discovery of the [sic] gene implicated in speech and language is amongst the first fruits of the Human Genome Project for the cognitive sciences. (Pinker, 2001)

A naïve student reading the above literature would be forgiven if s/he were immediately to conclude that language and other domains of higher-level cognition are genetically determined, each ready to operate as soon as appropriate stimuli present themselves, with each functioning in isolation of the rest of the system, and that plasticity is not involved in normal development but merely acts as a response to injury. Our hypothetical student might well go on to infer that the main task for the scientist is to search for single genes that somehow map directly onto specific higher-level cognitive outcomes like grammar, face processing, number and the like. How has this position become so attractive to many linguists, philosophers and psychologists? Why does the popular press welcome this approach and jump at concepts like "a gene for language" or "a gene for spatial cognition"? What is the attraction of the notion that single genes code specifically for higher-level cognitive outcomes? Why are mouse models of human cognition, which often involve single gene knockouts and their relationship to phenotypic outcomes, not examined more critically? In the rest of this chapter, I will attempt to address these questions and show how a very different and more interactive theoretical approach—the Emergentist Theory embraced by Bates—offers a far deeper insight into the mind and brain of the developing child.

MOUSE MODELS OF HUMAN COGNITION

Obviously, there can be no mouse models directly of human language. Apart from in cartoons, mice don't communicate through a linguistically structured system like spoken or sign language. But there are many other aspects of human cognition that have been modeled using knockout mice. Since later in the chapter I will discuss genetic syndromes and focus in particular on one neurodevelopmental disorder, Williams syndrome (WS), I will take as my examples in this section two mouse models of WS.

First, a word about the syndrome itself. This will be very brief since WS has now been extensively described in the philosophical, linguistic and psychological literature (see Donnai & Karmiloff-Smith, 2000, for full details). Suffice it to say that WS is a genetic disorder in which some 25 genes are deleted on one copy of chromosome 7, causing serious deficits in spatial cognition, number, planning and problem solving. Of particular interest to cognitive neuroscientists is the fact that two domains—language and face processing—show particular behavioral proficiency compared to the general levels of intelligence reached by this clinical group. Indeed, while IQ scores are in the 50s to 60s range, WS behavior on some language and face processing tasks gives rise to scores that fall in the normal range, whereas spatial cognition is always seriously impaired.

Twenty-five genes within the typical WS critical region have been identified, although the function of many of them is not yet known (Donnai & Karmiloff-Smith, 2000). In the middle of the deletion are the elastin (ELN) and Limkinase1 (LIMK1) genes that have been the focus of considerable research. ELN was initially hailed as the gene that caused the facial dysmorphology in WS (Frangaskakis et al., 1996), but our group subsequently demonstrated that patients with small deletions could lose one copy of ELN and yet have nothing of the WS elfin-like facial dysmorphology (Tassabehji et al., 1999). The only clear-cut genotype/phenotype correlation confirmed so far is between ELN and supravalvular aortic stenosis (a narrowing of the aorta in its trajectory to the heart), due to the role that ELN plays in connective tissue development. If ELN contributes in any way to the WS facial dysmorphology, it must be in interaction with other genes on chromosome 7 which are deleted in WS. More interesting, however, are genes that are expressed in the brain. Could having only one copy of any of these genes be insufficient for the normal development of certain aspects of cognition? Note that we all can have genetic mutations of various kinds without that seeming to affect outcome at all. Only some genes are dosage sensitive, necessitating two copies to function normally. Two of the WS deleted genes that are expressed in the brain have recently been singled out as being of potential interest to the cognitive outcome: LIMK1 which is contiguous with ELN, and CYLN2 which is at the telomeric end of the deletion. Let us look at each of these in turn.

LIMK1 is expressed in early embryonic brain development as well as postnatally. Its product is thought to contribute to synaptic regulation and the modification of dendritic spines. In an initial study (Frankaskakis et al., 1996), two families were identified in which some members had two genes deleted within the WS critical region on chromosome 7—ELN and LIMK1—whereas other members had no such deletion. The family members with the deletions were shown to have spatial impairments on tasks involving pattern construction and block building, whereas the others were unimpaired on these tasks. The authors concluded that they had "discovered that hemizygosity of LIMK1, a protein kinase gene expressed in the brain ... leads to impaired visuospatial constructive cognition in WS" (Frangiskakis et al. 1996). However, a subsequent study by Tassabehji and collaborators (Tassabehji et al., 1999) examined four patients from three unrelated families who had deletions within the WS critical region, including ELN and LIMK1. They displayed no such spatial impairments. Indeed, unlike studies of patients with WS that consistently reveal a marked disparity between verbal and spatial scores, the patients tested in the Tassabehji et al. study displayed similar levels for both domains, with scores within the normal range. In fact, one of these patients, CS, was well above normal levels in all domains, despite in her case a very large deletion of some 20 of the genes in the WS critical region.

A mouse model created subsequently seems at first blush to challenge these findings. Meng and colleagues produced a LIMK1-knockout and showed that in the water maze the mouse had poor spatial learning, especially with respect to the flexibility required for reversal learning (Meng et al., 2002). This was hailed once again as showing that the deletion of LIMK1 in WS is the gene responsible for spatial learning. Note, though, that the knockout mouse was not only impaired spatially but also developed spinal cord deficits and a number of other problems. I will return to this point later.

A second mouse model of WS was created by Hoogenraad and collaborators, knocking out one copy of CYLN2 at the telomeric end of the WS critical region (Hoogenraad et al., 2002). CYLN2 is expressed in dendrites and cell bodies of the brain and its product is thought to contribute to the development of several areas such as the cerebellum, cerebrum, hippocampus and amygdala. The knockout mouse developed memory deficits, impairments of contextual fear conditioning and spatial deficits.

Our team subsequently identified a 3-year-old girl who has the largest deletion to date in the WS critical region without the full-blown WS phenotype. As well as deletions of one copy of ELN, LIMK1 and some 19 other genes, this patient also has CYLN2 deleted (one more gene than CS above) but not the final two telomeric genes in the WS critical region. The 3 year old has the typical short stature of children with WS, mild hypercalcaemia, mild stenoses, and a relatively mild dysmorphic face. However, her cognitive phenotype turns out to be different from the typical WS pattern, although this could of course change over developmental time. In this 3 year old, language scores were significantly worse than spatial scores. Indeed, unlike most children and adults with WS, she was in the normal range (lower end) on the pattern construction and block design sub-tests of the British Ability Scales–II. However, when we subsequently tested her in a human equivalent of the mouse maze (a pool filled with balls through which the child had to walk in order to locate a gift box hidden in two different positions and searching from different starting points), our preliminary results pointed to significant impairments in this child, compared to a group of 3-year-old healthy controls as well as to individual controls matched on each of the other spatial tasks. (We have yet to test WS toddlers with the full WS deletion on this new task, but are about to embark on the comparison.)

What can we derive from these two mouse models compared to the human tests done with various patients? First, there are particular advantages of mouse models of WS. All the genes involved in the WS critical deletion on chromosome 7 are present in the same albeit inverted order on mouse chromosome 5G. However, in my view, there remain a number of serious problems with mouse models in general, and with these two WS models in particular. First, identical genes in two species do not necessarily entail identical functions. This has to be demonstrated rather than simply assumed. Second, two species may not have identical timing of gene expression, even when particular genes are the same. Third, haploinsufficiency (one copy only) of genes can turn out to be lethal in one species, and give rise to no observable effects in the other, or one copy deleted in the human case may require both genes deleted in the mouse model to generate similar effects. Fourth, the models discussed above involve the deletion of a single gene in each case. Yet, WS involves a multiple gene deletion. It is highly likely that the deleted genes interact with one another and, of course, with genes on the rest of the genome in very complex ways. One-to-one mapping between each single gene and each phenotypic outcome is most unlikely. Fifth, as hinted above, single gene knockouts do not only give rise to a single impairment, like spatial learning. As is to be expected given the complexities of gene expression, single knockouts frequently result in multiple impairments to various aspects of the resulting phenotype. And, whereas reports comparing mouse and human stress spatial impairments, little is made of the fact that other impairments, such as spinal cord deficits in the LIKK1 mouse knockout, do not occur in the human WS case. Sixth, in general single gene knockouts of a variety of different genes on the mouse genome frequently give rise to spatial impairments. This is probably due in part to the fact that the mouse repertoire tested is fairly limited, with spatial memory in mazes being one of the preferred measures. This leads to my final, and seventh point, i.e., that we often encounter direct generalizations from mouse to human that involve behaviors at very different levels. The demonstration of the existence of a mouse deficit in the water maze and a human deficit in block design is not, I submit, the same thing. The former involves navigational skills, i.e., the animal's own body position and orientation needs to be represented in space. By contrast, in table-top tasks like block design, the position of the individual's own body in space is not relevant to the task; it is a given. Rather, the featural and configural relationships between objects themselves need to be represented. Large-scale navigational and small-scale spatial representations may well call on different abilities. Relevant to this point is the fact that the 3-year-old patient discussed above was significantly more impaired in our ball-pool version of the water maze in which she had to represent the position of her own body in space than on the tasks measuring table-top spatial construction.

In sum, mouse models of human genes, although often fascinating, must always be considered with caution when generalizing to the human phenotype. Although mouse models of human language are not directly possible, there are many other ways to investigate the genetic contribution to speech and language. Clearly genes do play *some* role in language development. The question is what that role might be.

GENES AND LANGUAGE

In 1998, and more specifically in 2001, the scientific world became very excited about the discovery of what came to be known as "the gene for speech and language" (Pinker, 2001). A British family, the now well-known KE family, had been identified, in whom an allelic variation in the FOXP2 gene in some family members gave rise to serious impairments in speech and language, whereas family members without this allele developed language normally (Vargha-Khadem et al., 1998; Pinker, 2001). Is the FOXP2 allele novel to the human genome, and could it explain the onset of language in the human species? Does such a gene have a unique and specific effect only on speech and language in humans? Some researchers have claimed that this might indeed be the case (Pinker, 2001; but see more cautious discussion from evolutionary biologists in Enard et al., 2002). However, a closer look at the phenotypic outcome in the affected KE family members highlights the need to consider a far more complex story. First, the deficits are neither specific to language, nor even to speech output. The dysfunctions in the affected family members not only involve serious problems with oral-facial movements which impact on the development of language, but also affect particular aspects of the perception of rhythm as well as the production of rhythmic movements of the hands (Alcock, 1995; Varga-Khadem et al., 1998). Moreover, this gene cannot alone explain human language for several reasons. First, we must not lose sight of the general point that when a genetic mutation is found to cause dysfunction of a particular behavior, this does *not* mean that intactness of that same gene causes the proper functioning of the behavior. The effects of a single gene may represent a very minuscule contribution to the total functioning and yet be sufficient to disrupt it. Numerous analogies make this point obvious. For example, if the carburetor of a car is not functioning properly, the car will not run. But it is not the carburetor that alone explains how the car runs in normal circumstances; it is just a small part of an extremely complex machinery of interactions. But a second point is as important. It is highly unlikely that a single gene or even specific set of genes will explain the development of human language. In the vast majority of cases, genes involve many-to-many mappings, not one-to-one mappings. Furthermore, effects are not only in the direction of genes to phenotypic outcomes; the outcomes themselves can affect subsequent gene expression in return. Even in the case of single gene disorders (e.g., Fragile X syndrome), the phenotypic outcome displays multiple impairments, because the gene in question is deeply involved in synaptogenesis across the developing system (Scerif et al., 2003).

Third is a point stressed frequently by Bates (e.g., Bates, 1984, 1997a), i.e., that there are many ways in which language can end up being impaired due to genetic mutations in numerous parts of the genome (and/ or, of course, to social and other non-genetic causes, Bates, Bretherton, Beeghly-Smith & McNew, 1982). So it is highly unlikely that a single gene will explain all such impairments. Moreover, the use of the shorthand of "the gene for language" is a particularly dangerous one (see discussion in Karmiloff-Smith, 1998) and likely to be wrong. Indeed, a recent paper from the field of behavioral genetics challenged the conclusions from the FOXP2 genetics studies (Meaburn, Dale, Craig & Plomin, 2002). The authors reported on the genotyping of the FOXP2 mutation for 270 four-year olds selected for low language scores from a representative sample of more than 18,000 children. Not a single one of the language-impaired children turned out to have the FOXP2 mutation (Meaburn, et al., 2002). Thus, although a disorder may of course at times be the result of a single gene mutation, language impairment is, as the authors claim, far more likely to be the quantitative extreme of the same multiple genetic factors responsible for heritability throughout the distribution. The notion that the evolution of human language involved a de nova single gene, or a specific set of genes, devoted to wiring language in place (Pinker, 1994), is most unlikely to turn out to be true.

Bates's subtle position on this debate is of particular interest (Bates, personal communication, September 2002). She of course agrees that genes play a crucial role in human development in general and in language in particular. But she argues that we need to consider the multiple functions that each gene may have, including genetic contributions to language over evolutionary time. Amongst these Bates points to the interaction of *all* of the following: (a) genetic alterations that gave us better fine motor control (like FOXP2), (b) genetic alterations that permitted a more direct mapping from perception to production (cross-modal perception which is essential for imitation, a major tool of cultural transmission), (c) genetic alterations that made us faster information processors, (d) genetic alterations that gave us better perceptual abilities, and (e) genetic alterations that led to the particular social makeup that makes us want to imitate each other, share eye gaze direction, and think about the mental states of others that motivate their behaviors rather than focusing merely on the behavior itself. In Bates's view, none of these genes will end up being specific to speech/language and yet, in conjunction, all of them will turn out to have been important for the emergence of speech, language, culture and technology in our species. Such an interactive, emergentist position is far removed from the notion of a specific gene for language (see the emergence of Bates's Emergentist Theory in Bates, 1978, 1979a, 1979b, 1992, 1994, 1997b, 1999a, 1999b, 2002; Bates, Dick & Wulfeck, 1999; Bates & Elman, 2000; Bates & Thal, 1990; Bates, Thal, & Marchman, 1991; Bates & Volterra, 1984; Dick, Saygin, Moineau, Aydelott & Bates, in press; Elman, Bates, Johnson, Karmiloff-Smith, Parisi & Plunkett, 1996).

Now, language is a relatively recent development within the human species. So, some might argue that this recency explains why genes don't *yet* directly code for language. Behind such reasoning is the notion that evolution is always aimed at creating genetically-determined, specialized modules for higher-level cognitive domains. So let's momentarily leave the topic of language and examine another possible candidate for genetic specification and direct genotype/phenotype relations.

FACE PROCESSING

One of the most fundamental abilities across the animal kingdom is the capacity for species recognition. One might therefore expect this to be a strong candidate for an innate ability in the case of the human infant. Yet the past couple of decades have revealed, at both the behavioral and brain levels, that the recognition of faces is a very gradual developmental process in both humans and other species such as the chick (Johnson & Morton, 1991). Indeed, brain localization and specialization in the processing of human faces, i.e., the gradual modularization over developmental time of face processing (Karmiloff-Smith, 1992), extends very progressively across the first 12 months of life and beyond (Johnson & de Haan, 2001). If infants start with anything resembling an innately specified template, it is not face specific but likely to be in the form of a T-shape in which more information at the top of a stimulus parsed as an object is particularly attractive to the young infant's visual system (Simion, Cassia, Turati & Valenza, 2001). With developmental time, however, the human face itself becomes increasingly the preferred stimulus (Johnson & Morton, 1991), enhanced not only by the massive input of faces but also by the fact that faces form a crucial site of attention for the social interactional patterns that develop over the first months of life.

Brain imaging experiments have shown that young infants initially process upright human faces, inverted human faces, monkey faces and objects, all in a relatively similar way across both hemispheres (Johnson & de Hann, 2001; de Hann, 2001). However, with development, infant processing of human upright faces becomes increasingly localized to the fusiform gyrus in the right hemisphere. It also becomes increasingly specialized, in that an electrophysiological marker emerges specifically for upright faces, differentiating it henceforth from the processing of inverted faces and objects. This is in the form of the activation of a predominantly right-lateralized equivalent of the adult N170 waveform whenever the older infant is presented with an upright human face (Halit, de Haan & Johnson, 2003). By 12 months of age, then, the electrophysiology of the infant brain when processing faces begins to look relatively similar to that of adults, although development of the N170 continues throughout childhood to adolescence (Taylor, Edmonds, McCarthy, Saliba, & Degiovanni, 1999).

In the light of the above findings, it seems very unlikely that the human genome contains a blueprint for face processing, resulting in a neonate face processing module, ready to operate once appropriate face stimuli are presented, a module that is intact or damaged in certain disorders. Yet this is exactly the kind of reasoning that underlies the assumptions of many researchers who invoke data from both adult neuropsychological patients and from children with developmental disorders to make claims about the existence of an innately specified face-processing module. Indeed, the fact that adult patients can present with prosopagnosia, i.e., the inability to recognize familiar faces, despite showing no obvious impairments elsewhere, has led theorists to claim that the human brain is equipped with an independently-functioning face-processing module (Buyer, Laterre, Seron, Feyereisen, Strypstein, Pierrad & Rectem, 1983; De Renzi, 1986; Farah & Levinston, 1995; Temple, 1997) and to go on to claim that this is part of the hardwired, genetically specified functional architecture of the infant brain (Temple, 1997). However, it must always be recalled that such neuropsychological patients are adults whose brains had developed normally prior to their brain insult in adulthood. And, as argued elsewhere, if independently-functioning modules do exist in the adult brain, they are likely to be the end product of a developmental process of gradual modularization, not its starting point (Karmiloff-Smith, 1992, 1998), in which many low-level processes contribute together to the final phenotypic outcome. So, the existence of adult prosopagnosics cannot be used to bolster claims about the genetic encoding of a face processing module.

What about developmental disorders? If genetic disorders were to be identified that display either a single deficit in face processing alongside normal intelligence, or a single proficiency in face processing alongside low levels of general intelligence, would that provide evidence of innately-specified face-processing module and a gene or specific set of genes to wire it in place?

Williams syndrome seemed at first glance to present such a case. Indeed, the fact that people with WS scored in the normal range on some standardized face-processing tasks was immediately heralded as demonstrating that WS presents with a genetically-specified "intact/preserved" face-processing module (e.g. Bellugi, Sabo & Vaid, 1988a; Bellugi, Wang & Jernigan, 1994;

Udwin & Yule, 1991; Wang, Doherty, Rourke & Bellugi, 1995) and that people with the syndrome process faces in exactly the same way as healthy controls (e.g., Tager-Flusberg, Plesa-Skwerer, Faja, & Joseph, 2003).

One of the problems with many of the WS face processing studies is that sets of terms like featural/piecemeal/componential/local/analytical versus configural/holistic/global/gestalt have been used as if they were synonymous, and have therefore not been adequately specified. The term "featural" refers to the ability to identify individual features (eyes, nose, mouth, chin) separately from one another, and the term "configural" to the ability to differentiate faces based on a sensitivity to the spatial distances amongst internal features, i.e., second order relational information. By contrast, the term "holistic" means the gluing together of facial features (and hairline) into a gestalt, without necessarily conserving the spatial distances between features (Tanaka & Farah, 1993; Maurer, Le Grand & Mondloch, 2002). In other words, the capacity to process information holistically does not involve the processing of second order relational information.

There are as yet no published experimental studies regarding infant face processing in Williams syndrome to compliment the now abundant studies of healthy infants mentioned above. However, some observational work, as well as experiments indirectly tapping face processing, revealed that infants with WS spend significantly more time focused on faces than on objects (Bellugi, Lichtenberger, Jones, Lai, St. George, 2000; Laing, Ansari, Gsodl, Longhi, Panagiotaki, Paterson & Karmiloff-Smith, 2002; Mervis & Bertrand, 1997). This inordinate attention to faces was argued to be due to a genetic predisposition and has led many authors to assume that it explains why individuals with WS end up achieving good behavioral scores on some faces processing tasks. But does such early attention to faces necessarily lead to configural processing? Our ongoing work on face processing in WS infants and toddlers (Karmiloff-Smith et al., in press) suggests that it may turn out that the longer infants look at a stimulus, the more likely they are to focus on features rather than overall configuration. So, there are initial indications from early development in WS that face processing may not proceed in the same way as in healthy controls. Thus, even if at the behavioral level adults have face-processing scores in the normal range on some tasks, they may not process faces in the same way as normal controls. If this were the case, then it cannot be claimed the WS presents with an intact gene or set of genes for setting up pre-determined, specialized circuits for face processing.

As mentioned above, in the early work on adolescents and adults with WS, many researches claimed that face recognition in the syndrome was 'intact'/'spared' (i.e., developed normally), based on findings that performance on the standardized face processing tasks like the Benton Facial Recognition Test and the Rivermead Face Memory Task was at normal or near normal levels (e.g., Bellugi, Sabo & Vaid, 1988a; Bellugi, Wang & Jernigan, 1994; Udwin & Yule, 1991; Wang, Doherty, Rourke & Bellugi, 1995). However, several recent studies have challenged the notion of an 'intact' face-processing module and suggest that people with WS achieve their normal scores by using different strategies from controls (Deruelle, Mancini, Livet, Cassé-Perrot, & de Schonen, 1999; Karmiloff-Smith, 1997).

Deruelle and her collaborators tested children and adults with WS, as well as two control groups, one matched on chronological age and the other on mental age (Deruelle et al., 1999). In one of their experiments, children were shown a series of pictures of faces and of houses. Their task was to decide whether the two face or two house pictures were same or different when presented in upright or inverted conditions. In the face condition, the clinical group performed differently from the controls and was less subject to an inversion effect. The authors explained these results by a greater reliance of the WS children on featural analysis in both the upright and inverted conditions, whereas the controls used predominantly featural processing for the inverted faces and configural processing for upright faces. Another experiment by Deruelle and colleagues had participants make a decision as to whether a model house/face was the same or different from one that had been modified either configurally or featurally. The WS group performed more poorly than the controls on the configurally-modified stimuli, but did not differ from controls on the featurally-modified ones. Moreover, again unlike the controls, performance in the clinical population correlated with neither chronological nor mental age. This led the authors to speculate that WS face processing is not merely delayed but follows a different developmental pathway. However, in a recent paper, Tager-Flusberg and her collaborators challenged this now rather widely accepted conclusion and claimed that people with WS process faces in exactly the same way as controls (Tager-Flusberg et al., 2003). While this study had the merit of using a considerably larger sample than previous work, several problems emerge.

First, it is not without interest that in their report, Tager-Flugberg and colleagues avoid the term "configural" in favor of "holistic." But the debate is not about whether individuals with WS can process stimuli holistically. Most authors accept that they can. Rather, the question is whether or not individuals with WS make use of *second-order configural relations* when processing faces, a capacity which emerges over time developmentally in healthy controls. But several studies have now shown that the inversion effect, considered to be the hallmark of configural processing of faces in normal controls (Yin, 1969), is significantly smaller in WS (Deruelle, et al., 1999; Rossen, Jones, Wang & Klima, 1995), again suggesting that this clinical population is impaired in configural processing.

A further challenge to Tager-Flusberg's claims about the normality of WS face processing comes from a number of brain imaging studies which have identified atypical processing of faces in adolescents and adults with WS (Grice, de Haan, Halit, Johnson, Csibra & Karmiloff-Smith, 2001; Mills, Alvarez, St. George, Appelbaum, Bellugi & Neville, 2000), as well as atypical brain processes for the binding of features (Grice, de Haan, Halit, Johnson, Csibra, Grant & Karmiloff-Smith, 2003). For example, Grice et al. (2001) investigated the neural basis of face processing in adolescents and adults with WS, as well as participants with autism, by examining EEG binding-related gamma-band activity in response to upright and inverted faces. We found that, unlike the controls, the brains of both clinical groups failed to show differences in gamma activity between upright and inverted faces. However, important differences also emerged between the clinical populations in the types of gamma burst identified. The brains of the group with autism yielded gamma bursts that were qualitatively similar to controls, but were not as well tied to stimulus onset. By contrast, the gamma-band activity in the WS adolescents and adults was flattened and resembled that of typically-developing 2-month-old infants. This raises the possibility that the brains of adolescents and adults with WS fail or at best are much slower to bind isolated features into an integrated whole. Moreover, in a further analysis of ERP data, adolescents and adults with WS were shown to have problems even in the very first 200 milliseconds that involve the brain's structural encoding of a face. Their N170—which, as we saw above, is almost adult-like by 12 months in normal infants—was very atypical and resembled that of young infants, despite the massive experience of the WS group with faces by the time they had already reached adulthood (Grice et al., 2001; 2003).

So, what seemed at first sight to be a nice example of an independently functioning, intact face processing module, determined by evolution and the genes, turns out to be a much more complex story in Williams syndrome. Almost all authors agree that individuals with WS are delayed in their face processing. But delay cannot simply be dismissed as theoretically irrelevant (Karmiloff-Smith, Scerif & Ansari, 2003). Delay in one domain or one aspect of a domain will interact over developmental time with other parts of the system. Timing is of essence in ontogenetic development (Karmiloff-Smith, 1998). And, even in the case of normal development, it has become clear that face processing develops very gradually in the infant brain across the first year of life and beyond. Some might argue that this could be viewed simply as the late onset of a maturationally-constrained, genetically determined specialized circuit. However, research shows that it is not a new additional circuit (not new gene expression) that comes on line as the child reaches the end of the first year of life. Rather, the change is characterized by *less* but increasingly specialized and localized activity in the way in which the brain processes faces. This body of infant literature is unfortunately largely ignored by those who use data from adult neuropsychology and genetic disorders to bolster their nativist, evolutionary claims

(Barkow, Cosmides & Tooby, 1992; Duchaine, Cosmides, & Tooby, 2001; Pinker, 1997). Yet, to understand how human development proceeds, one should not simply look to the contribution of genes, but rather also focus on the gradual process of ontogenetic development over time as opposed to the notion of impaired and intact modules.

Finally, we might ask how the study of developmental disorders helps us to examine the independence or interactions between domains. For two decades, the literature has claimed that face processing and visuo-spatial processing are independent of one another in WS and thus involve different genes. But this is unlikely to be the case. It could well be that spatial cognition is simply more vulnerable to the early impairments in WS development than is the case for overt behavior in face processing. In other words, while the behavior in one domain (face processing) may in some cases vastly outstrip scores in the other domain (visuo-spatial cognition), they may *both* be affected by similar deficient, low-level processes, but one domain may reveal this impairment more overtly and the other more subtly, simply because of their different problem spaces.

We are left with the puzzle of where the configural deficit in WS might stem from if it is not from a faulty gene that codes for configural processing. A study by Johnson, Mareschal and Csibra (2001) offers an interesting clue. These authors argued that a delay in the development of the magnocellular system would bias bottom-up processes from parvocellular pathways leading to an increased focus on detail. Likewise, atypical development of the dorsal stream may give rise to problems controlling disengagement of attention from central stimuli. Both of these problems have been identified in WS. A study by Atkinson and collaborators revealed a dorsal deficit in WS (Atkinson et al., 1997). In our own lab we studied visual saccade planning in toddlers with WS and with Down syndrome (DS) and found that those with WS, but not those with DS, were seriously impaired compared to MA and CA controls. The pattern of errors in the WS toddlers suggested sticky fixation on initial stimuli and a difficulty disengaging therefrom to plan subsequent eye movements (Brown, Johnson, Paterson, Gilmore, Longhi & Karmiloff-Smith, 2003). These two sources of data point to early problems in the general domain of visual processing that would have cascading but differential effects on the developing system over time, with more obvious impairments showing up for spatial cognition, and more subtle deficits underlying proficient behavior in face processing.

CONCLUDING THOUGHTS

So, why are processes as crucial to interacting with conspecifics as language and face processing not genetically specified and cordoned off to function independently from all other processes? The reason may well lie in two dif-

of control, and the fact that some higher-level cognitive out-
not be possible without the gradual ontogenetic process of
learning (Elman, Bates, et al., 1996).

It is generally accepted that there are two forms of biological control:
mosaic control and regulatory control. Mosaic control involves deterministic epigenesis: the genes tightly control timing and outcome, the process is
fast and operates independently of other processes. This form of control
works well under optimal conditions. However, it places serious limits on
complexity and on the flexibility of the developmental process. Yet, some
parts of human development do involve mosaic control. However, the
other type of control, regulatory control, is much more common in human
development, particularly in higher-level cognitive outcomes. It involves
probabilistic epigenesis. It is under broad rather than tight genetic control,
is slow and progressive, with limited pre-specification. In this type of control, different parts of a system develop *interdependently*. And, unlike mosaic
control, there are fewer constraints on complexity and plasticity. This does
not mean, of course, that there are no biological constraints, as the empiricist position would claim, but it is far less constrained than mosaic control.
This means that plasticity is the *rule* for all development, not merely a response to injury. Genes and their products are unlikely to code for anything
like higher-level cognitive outcomes like language and face processing, but
rather for differences in developmental timing, neuronal density, neuronal
migration, neuronal type, firing thresholds, and neurotransmitter differences, that impact on the developing system in interaction with the inputs
being processed.

The neuroconstructivist, emergentist approach embodies that of regulatory control, not mosaic control, with ontogeny seen as the prime force for
turning a number of domain-relevant processes progressively into domain-specific outcomes in the adult. This does not imply that the infant brain is a
single, homogeneous learning device. On the contrary. There is, no doubt,
much heterogeneity in the initial gross wiring of the brain. But, contrary to
what is often claimed, this heterogeneity bears little resemblance to the ultimate functional structures that can only emerge through interaction with a
structured environment. The question we must all ask is not whether human development is due to evolution *or* ontogeny. Clearly both play a vital
role, but the gradual process of ontogeny, rather than solely the genes, does
a lot of the work in establishing higher-level cognitive specializations like
language and face processing. Evolution may have heeded the need for the
adult cognitive system to be specialized. But it seems to have abdicated
quite a lot of the responsibility for achieving this specialization to the process of ontogenetic development. So, if we are to understand what it is to be
human, to have language and recognize our conspecifics, our continuing
emphasis must be on the process of development itself. In other words,

rather than the mosaic form of tight genetic control which some evolutionary psychology theories invoke, evolution's solution for the human brain may well have been to avoid too much pre-specification in favor of gradual development and neuroconstructivist plasticity: the essence of Bates's emergentist approach.

REFERENCES

Alcock, K. J. (1995). *Motor aphasia—A comparative study.* Unpublished doctoral thesis, University of Oxford.

Atkinson, J., King, J., Braddick, O., Nokes, L., Anker, S., & Braddick, F. (1997). A specific deficit of dorsal stream function in Williams Syndrome. *Neuroreport: An International Journal for the Rapid Communication of Research in Neuroscience, 8,* 1912–1922.

Barkow, J. H., Leda Cosmides, & John Tooby (eds). (1992). *The Adapted Mind: Evolutionary Psychology and the Generation of Culture.* New York, NY: Oxford University Press.

Bates, E. (1978). Functionalism and the biology of language. *Papers & Reports in Child Language.* Stanford University, Department of Linguistics.

Bates, E. (1979a). In the beginning, before the word: Review of S. Harnad, H. Steklis, & T. Lancaster, "Origins of Language and Speech." In *Contemporary Psychology, 24*(3), 169–171.

Bates, E. (1979b). On the emergence of symbols: Ontogeny and phylogeny. In A. Collins (Ed.), *Children's language and communication: The Minnesota Symposium on Child Psychology, Vol. 12.* Hillsdale, NJ: Erlbaum Associates, 121–157.

Bates, E. (1984). Bioprograms and the innateness hypothesis: Response to D. Bickerton. *Behavioral and Brain Sciences, 7*(2), 188–190.

Bates, E. (1992). Language development. In E. Kandel & L. Squire (Eds.), Special Issue on Cognitive Neuroscience. *Current Opinion in Neurobiology, 2,* 180–185.

Bates, E. (1994). Modularity, domain specificity and the development of language. In D. C. Gajdusek, G. M. McKhann, & C. L. Bolis (Eds.), Evolution and neurology of language. *Discussions in Neuroscience, 10*(1–2), 136–149. [Reprinted in W. Bechtel, P. Mandik, J. Mundale, & R. Stufflebeam (Eds.). *Philosophy and the neurosciences: a reader.* Oxford: Blackwell, 134–151].

Bates, E. (1997a). Origins of language disorders: A comparative approach. In D. Thal & J. Reilly (Eds.), Special issue on Origins of Communication Disorders, *Developmental Neuropsychology, 13*(3), 275–343.

Bates, E. (1997b). On language savants and the structure of the mind: a review of Neil Smith and Ianthi-Maria Tsimpli, "The mind of a savant: language learning and modularity." *International Journal of Bilingualism, 1*(2), 163–186.

Bates, E. (1999a). Nativism vs. development: Comments on Baillargeon & Smith. *Developmental Science, 2*(2), 148–149.

Bates, E. (1999b). Plasticity, localization and language development. In S. H. Broman & J. M. Fletcher (Eds.), *The changing nervous system: Neurobehavioral consequences of early brain disorders.* New York: Oxford University Press, 214–253.

Bates, E. (1999c). On the nature and nurture of language. In R. Levi-Montalcini, D. Baltimore, R. Dulbecco, & F. Jacob (Series Eds.) & E. Bizzi, P. Calissano, & V. Volterra (Vol. Eds.), *Frontiere della biologia* [Frontiers of biology]. The brain of homo sapiens Rome: Giovanni Trecanni.

Bates, E. (2002). Specific language impairment: why it is NOT specific. *Developmental Medicine and Child Neurology, 44,* 4. (Supplement No. 92).

Bates, E., Bretherton, I., Beeghly-Smith, M., & McNew, S. (1982). Social factors in language acquisition: A reassessment. In H. Reese & L. Lipsett (Eds.), *Advances in child development & behavior: Volume 16.* New York: Academic Press, 8–68.

Bates, E., Dick, F., & Wulfeck, B. (1999). Not so fast: domain-general factors can account for domain-specific deficits in grammatical processing. *Behavioral & Brain Sciences, 22*(1), 96–97.

Bates, E., & Elman, J. L. (2000). The ontogeny and phylogeny of language: A neural network perspective. In S. Parker, J. Langer & M. McKinney (Eds.), *Biology, brains, and behavior: The evolution of human development.* Santa Fe: School of American Research Press, 89–130.

Bates, E., & Thal, D. (1990). Associations and dissociations in language development. In J. Miller (Ed.), *Research on child language disorders: A decade of progress.* Austin, Texas: Pro-Ed, 147–168.

Bates, E., Thal, D., & Marchman, V. (1991). Symbols and syntax: A Darwinian approach to language development. In N. Krasnegor, D. Rumbaugh, R. Schiefelbush & M. Studdert-Kennedy (Eds.), *Biological and behavioral determinants of language development.* Hillsdale, NJ: Erlbaum, 29–65.

Bates, E., & Volterra, V. (1984). On the invention of language: An alternative view. Response to S. Goldin-Meadow & C. Mylander, Gestural communication in deaf children: the effects and noneffects of parental input on early language development. *Monographs of the Society for Research in Child Development, Serial No. 207, Vol. 49,* Nos. 3–4.

Bellugi, U., Lichtenberger, L., Jones, W., Lai, Z., & St. George, M. (2000). The neurocognitive profile of Williams syndrome: A complex pattern of strengths and weaknesses. *Journal of Cognitive Neuroscience, 1*(12), pp. 1–29.

Bellugi, U., Sabo, H., & Vaid, J. (1988). Spatial deficits in children with Williams syndrome. In J. Stiles-Davis, M. Kritchevsky & U. Bellugi (Eds.), *Spatial Cognition: Brain Bases and Development.* Hillsdale, NJ: Lawrence Erlbaum.

Bellugi, U., Wang, P. P., & Jernigan, T. L. (1994). Williams syndrome: An unusual neuropsychological profile. In S. H. Broman & J. Grafman (Eds.), *Atypical cognitive deficits in developmental disorders: implications for brain function.* Hillsdale, NJ: Lawrence Erlbaum Associates, pp. 23–56.

Brown, J., Johnson, M. H., Paterson, S., Gilmore, R. O., Gsödl, M., Longhi, E., & Karmiloff-Smith, A. (2003). Spatial representation and attention in toddlers with Williams syndrome and Down syndrome. *Neuropsychologia, 41*(8), 1037–1046.

Bruyer, R., Laterre, C., Seron, X., Feyereisen, P., Strypstein, E., Pierrand, E., Rectem, D. (1983). A case of prosopagnosia with some preserved covert remembrance of familiar faces. *Brain Cognition, 2,* 257–284.

Carey, S., & Spelke, E. S. (1994). Domain-specific knowledge and conceptual change. In L. Hirschfeld & S. Gelman (Eds.), *Mapping the mind: Domain specificity in cognition and culture,* pp. 169–200. Cambridge, UK: Cambridge University Press.

De Haan, M. (2001). The neuropsychology of face processing during infancy and childhood. In C. A. Nelson & M. Luciana (Eds.), *Handbook of Developmental Cognitive Neuroscience,* 381–398, Cambridge, Mass: MIT Press.

De Renzi, E. (1986). Current issues on prosopagnosia. In H. D. Ellis, M. A. Jeeves, F. Newcombe & A. Young (Eds.), *Aspects of Face Processing.* Dordrecht: Martinus Nijhoff Publ., 243–252.

Deruelle, C., Mancini, J., Livet, M. O., Casse-Perrot, C., & de Schonen, S. (1999). Configural and local processing of faces in children with Williams syndrome. *Brain & Cognition, 41*(3), 276–98.

Dick, F., Saygin, A. P., Moineau, S., Aydelott, J., & Bates, E. (in press). Language in an embodied brain: The role of animal models. *Cortex.*

Donnai, D., & Karmiloff-Smith, A. (2002). Williams syndrome: from genotype through to the cognitive phenotype. *American Journal of Medical Genetics, 97,* 164–171.

Duchaine, B., Cosmides, L., & Tooby, J. (2001). Evolutionary psychology and the brain. *Current Opinion in Neurobiology, 11*, 225–230.

Elliott, C. D. (1997). *British Abilities Scale—2nd Edition.* Windsor, UK: NFER-Nelson.

Elman, J. L., Bates, E., Johnson, M. H., Karmiloff-Smith, A., Parisi, D., & Plunkett, K. (1996). *Rethinking innateness: A connectionist perspective on development.* Cambridge, MA: MIT Press.

Enart, W., Przeworski, M., Fisher, S. E., Lai, C. S. L., Wiebe, V., Kitano, T., Monaco, A. P., & Pääbo, S. (2002). Molecular evolution of FOXP2, a gene involved in speech and language. *Nature,* Advanced on-line copy.

Farah, M. J., Levinson, K. L., Klein, K. L. (1995). Face perception and within-category discrimination in prosopagnosia. *Neuropsychologia, 33*, 661–671.

Frangiskakis, M. J., Ewart A. K., Morris C. A., Mervis C. B., Bertrand, J., Robinson, B. F., Klien B. P., Ensing G. J. Everette, L. A., Green, E. D., Proschel, C., Gutowski N. J., Noble, M., Atkinson, D. L., Odelberg S. J., & Keating M. T. (1996). LIM-kinase1 hemizygosity implicated in impaired visuospatial constructive cognition. *Cell, 86*, 59–67.

Grice, S. J., de Haan, M., Halit, H., Johnson, M. H., Csibra, G., Grant, J., & Karmiloff-Smith, A. (2003). ERP abnormalities of visual perception in Williams syndrome. *NeuroReport, 14*, 1773–1777.

Grice, S. J., Spratling, M. W., Karmiloff-Smith, A., Halit, H., Csibra, G., de Haan, M., & Johnson, M. H. (2001). Disordered visual processing and oscillatory brain activity in autism and Williams Syndrome. *NeuroReport, 12*, 2697–2700.

Halit, H., de Haan, M., & Johnson, M. H. (2003). Cortical Specialization for Face Processing: Face-sensitive Event Related Potential components in 3 and 12 month old infants. *NeuroImage, 1*(9), 1180–1193.

Hoogenraad, C. C., Koekkoek, B., Akhmanova, A., Krugers, H., Dortland, B., Miedema, M., van Alphen, A., Kistler, W. M., Jaegle, M., Koutsourakis, M., Van Camp, N., Verhoye, M., van der Linden, A., Kaverina, I., Grosveld, F., De Zeeuw, C. I., Galjart, N. (2002). Targeted mutation of Cyln2 in the Williams syndrome critical region links CLIP-115 haploinsufficiency to neurodevelopmental abnormalities in mice. *Nature Genetics, 32*, 116–27.

Johnson, M. J., Halit, H., Grice, S. J., & Karmiloff-Smith, A. (2002). Neuroimaging and Developmental Disorders: A perspective from multiple levels of analysis. *Development and Psychopathology, 14*(3), 521–536.

Johnson, M. H., & Haan, M. D. (2001). Developing cortical specialization for visual-cognitive function: The case of face recognition. In J. L. McClelland & R. S. Siegler (Eds.), *Mechanisms of cognitive development: Behavioral and neural perspectives* (pp. 253–270). Mahwah, NJ, US: Lawrence Erlbaum Associates, Inc., Publishers.

Johnson, M. H., Mareschal, D., & Csibra, G. (2001). The development and integration of the dorsal and ventral visual pathways: A neurocomputational approach. In C. A. Nelson & M. Luciana (Eds.), *Handbook of Developmental Cognitive Neuroscience* (pp. 139–151). Cambridge: MIT Press.

Johnson, M. H., & Morton, J. (1991). *Biology and cognitive development: The case of face recognition.* Oxford, England: Blackwell.

Karmiloff-Smith, A. (1992). *Beyond Modularity: A Developmental Perspective on Cognitive Science.* Cambridge, Mass.: MIT Press/Bradford Books.

Karmiloff-Smith, A. (1997). Crucial differences between developmental cognitive neuroscience and adult neuropsychology. *Developmental Neuropsychology, 13*, 513–524.

Karmiloff-Smith, A. (1998). Development itself is the key to understanding developmental disorders. *Trends in Cognitive Sciences, 2*, 10, 389–398.

Karmiloff-Smith, A., Scerif, G., & Thomas, M. (2002). Different approaches to relating genotype to phenotype in developmental disorders. *Developmental Psychobiology, 40*, 311–322.

Karmiloff-Smith, A., Scerif, G., & Ansari, D. (2003). Double dissociations in developmental disorders? Theoretically misconceived, empirically dubious. *Cortex, 39*, 161–163.

Karmiloff-Smith, A., Thomas, M. S. C., Annaz, D., Humphreys, K., Ewing, S., Grice, S., Brace, N., Van Duuren, M., Pike, G., & Campbell, R. (in press). Exploring the Williams syndrome face processing debate: The importance of building developmental trajectories. *Journal of Child Psychology and Psychiatry.*

Laing, E., Butterworth, G., Ansari, D., Gsödl, M., Longhi, E. Panagiotaki, G., Paterson, S., & Karmiloff-Smith, A. (2002). Atypical development of language and social communication in toddlers with Williams syndrome. *Developmental Science, 5,* 233–246.

Maurer, D., Le Grand, R., & Mondloch, C. J. (2002). The many faces of configural processing. *Trends in Cognitive Sciences, 6,* 255–260.

Meaburn, E., Dale, P. S., Craig, I. W., & Plomin R. (2002). Language-impaired children: No sign of the FOXP2 mutation. *NeuroReport,* 13, 8, 1075–1077.

Meng, Y., Zhang, Y., Tregoubov, V., Janus, C., Cruz, L., Jackson, M., Lu, W.-Y., MacDonald, J. F., Wang, J. Y., Falls, D. L., Jia, Z. (2002). Abnormal spine morphology and enhanced LTP in LIMK-1 knockout mice. *Neuron, 35,* 121–133.

Mervis, C. B., & Bertrand, J. (1997). Developmental relations between cognition and language: evidence from Williams syndrome. In L. B. Adamson & M. A. Romski (Eds.), *Research on communication and language disorders: Contributions to theories of language development* (pp. 75–106). New York: Brookes.

Mills, D. L., Alvarez, T. D., St. George, M., Appelbaum, L. G., Bellugi, U., & Neville, H. (2000). Electrophysiological studies of face processing in Williams syndrome. *Journal of Cognitive Neuroscience, 12,* 47–64.

Pinker, S. (1994). *The Language Instinct.* Penguin Books.

Pinker, S. (1997). *How the Mind Works.* New York: Norton; London: Penguin.

Pinker, S. (2001). Talk of genetics and vice-versa. *Nature, 413,* 465–466.

Rossen, M. L., Jones, W., Wang, P. P., & Klima, E. S. (1995). Face processing: Remarkable sparing in Williams syndrome. Special Issue, *Genetic Counseling, 6*(1), 138–140.

Scerif, G., Cornish, K., Wilding, J., Driver, J., & Karmiloff-Smith, A. (2004). Visual search in typically developing toddlers and toddlers with fragile X and Williams syndrome. *Developmental Science, 7,* 116–130.

Tager-Flusberg, H., Plesa-Skwerer, D., Faja, S., & Joseph, R. M. (2003). People with Williams syndrome process faces holistically. *Cognition, 89*(1), 11–24.

Tanaka, J. W., & Farah, M. J. (1993). Parts and wholes in face recognition. *Quarterly Journal of Experimental Psychology, 46A,* 225–245.

Tassabehji, M., Metcalfe, K., Karmiloff-Smith, A., Carette, M. J., Grant, J., Dennis, N., Reardon, W., Splitt, M., Read, A. P., Donnai, D. (1999). Williams syndrome: use of chromosomal microdeletions as a tool to dissect cognitive and physical phenotypes. *American Journal of Human Genetics, 64*(1), 118–25.

Taylor, M. J., McCarthy, G., Saliba, E., Degiovanni, E. (1999). ERP evidence of developmental changes in processing of faces. *Clinical Neurophysiology, 110*(5), 910–5.

Temple, C. M. (1997a). Cognitive neuropsychology and its application to children. *Journal of Child Psychology and Psychiatry, 38,* 27–52.

Temple, C. M. (1997b). *Developmental Cognitive Neuropsychology.* Erlbaum/Psychology Press.

Udwin, O., & Yule, W. (1991). A cognitive and behavioral phenotype in Williams syndrome. *Journal of Clinical and Experimental Neuropsychology, 13,* 232–244.

Vargha-Khadem, F., Watkins, K. E., Price, C. J., Ashburner, J., Alcock, K. J., Connelly, A., Frackowiak, R. S. J., Friston, K. J., Pembrey, M. E., Mishkin, M., Gadian, D. G., & Passingham, R. E. (1998). Neural basis of an inherited speech and language disorder. *Proceedings of the National Academy of Sciences of the USA* (95), 12695–12700.

Wang, P. P., Doherty, S., Rourke, S. B., & Bellugi, U. (1995). Unique Profile of visual-spatial skills in a genetic syndrome. *Brain and Cognition, 29,* 64–65.

Wexler, K. (1996). The development of inflection in a biologically based theory of language acquisition. In M. L. Rice (Ed.), *Toward a Genetics of Language.* Mahwah, NJ: Lawrence Erlbaum Associates, Inc.

Yin, R. (1969). Looking at upside down faces. *Journal of Experimental Psychology, 81*(1), 141–145.

Chapter 9

Language and the Brain

Frederic Dick
Center for Research in Language, University of California, San Diego
Birkbeck College, University of London

Nina F. Dronkers
Center for Research in Language, University of California, San Diego
VA Northern California Health Care System
University of California, Davis

Luigi Pizzamiglio
Università La Sapienza, Rome, Italy

Ayse Pinar Saygin
Center for Research in Language, University of California, San Diego

Steven L. Small
Brain Research Imaging Center, University of Chicago

Stephen Wilson
Center for Research in Language, University of California, San Diego
Neuroscience Interdepartmental Program, UCLA

For centuries, opinions regarding the fundamental character of neural organization have swung between two often caricatured poles: a phrenological view (Fodor, 1983; Gall, 1810), where each sensorimotor and cognitive function is subserved by a single region of neural tissue, and an equipotential view (Goldstein, 1948; Lashley, 1950), where the functions of particular brain regions are not sharply defined, and contribute to multiple mental processes. Over the last 40 years, the field of language research has been particularly polarized by an analogous debate regarding mental organization, with both generative linguistics and psycholinguistics often taking an explicitly modular and often phrenological position (Grodzinsky, 2000; Mauner, Fromkin, & Cornell, 1993), in which mental processes are subserved in specific "loci" of information processing systems and/or specific brain regions. By contrast, some psycholinguistic and neuropsychological research has moved away from this extreme position, but without resorting to a theory of equipotentiality. This alternative is consistent both with neurobiological notions of regional specialization as well as observed overlap in the regional responsibilities for high-level computations. This major revision, known as "embodied cognition," reflects a change in the functional primitives used to characterize the mental processes produced by the brain.

Embodied cognition is an approach originally charted by early researchers in affect (James, 1994), perception (Gibson, 1951) and cognitive development (Piaget, 1928). Here, the (primate) brain is acknowledged to have significant functional and anatomical divisions of labor; however, the brain's parcellation is driven not by abstract psychological constructs (such as those proposed by Gall and Fodor), but by the body that inhabits it. In this view, language (as well as other abstract or higher-order skills) emerges from, and is intimately linked to, the more evolutionarily entrenched sensorimotor substrates that allow us to comprehend (auditory/visual) and produce (motor) it.

Indeed, results from a half-century of research strongly suggest that the ability to comprehend and produce language is based upon an interwoven constellation of skills that emerges from everyday human behavior: social, physical, and linguistic interactions with the environment (exogenous) combined with the consequent interactions among neural systems (endogenous). Studies of language development and breakdown suggest that sensorimotor and language processes develop with similar trajectories (i.e., the ability to manipulate an object in a certain way emerges at the same time in development as does production of a certain language structure); conversely, lesions causing language deficits often cause problems with other sensorimotor skills (i.e., patients with aphasia are very likely to have problems producing gestures or interacting with objects—see Bates & Dick, 2002, for review and discussion).

Such an "emergentist" (MacWhinney, 1999) view of language evolution, development, and processing is often paired with a commitment to a distributive or connectionist account of language processing and its neural instantiation (Elman et al., 1996; Small, 1997; cf. Ullman, 1999, for a more modular 'embodied' account). In connectionist accounts, complex skills like language (or even simple ones) are subserved by a 'vast neuronal conspiracy' of locally and distally connected computational units that also contribute to processing of other domains having similar underlying perceptuo-motor demands (see Todorov, 2000, for an example of higher-level properties emerging from purely physical constraints in the motor domain). A key tenet of this approach is that the pattern of connections underlying knowledge and/or skill representations is *dynamic* or *plastic*, continually adjusting to new contingencies in the internal and external milieu.

In this chapter, we summarize findings from a variety of studies that support this new perspective. First we review recent findings from studies of adult aphasia, suggesting that the relationship between the character of language breakdown and the locus of brain damage is much less straightforward than had previously been believed; indeed, the divisions that are revealed seem to have more to do with language's conceptual or sensorimotor processing demands than with abstract linguistic distinctions such as syntax vs. semantics. We then move to results from studies of children with early-occurring focal lesions that shed new light on issues of plasticity and neural reorganization, and on developmental processes more generally. We then examine the processing and neural resources that language does—and doesn't—share with other domains, and review findings from both lesion and functional magnetic resonance imaging (fMRI) studies that illustrate the tight links between language and its sensorimotor substrate. We close by presenting some methodological advances that may allow us to better understand the relationship between brain and language.

BRAIN AND LANGUAGE: EVIDENCE FROM APHASIA

Systematic studies of the language breakdown that can occur after neurological injury are the bedrock supporting our understanding of the relationship between brain and language. By investigating the linguistic changes that result from injuries such as stroke, head trauma, tumor, or dementia, we are better equipped both to treat people with aphasia and to understand better the language system itself. The wide variation in the manifestations of aphasia can inform us about the individual components of the language system that may be differentially affected. Further, the relationship between the observed deficits and the areas of the brain that are affected can inform us about how the brain supports language functions. Investigations of aphasia have grown exponentially over the last several decades. These studies have begun to change the 19th century view that language consisted of two simple parts, production and comprehension, localized in Broca's and Wernicke's areas of the brain, respectively. After a period of abandonment, this localizationist perspective returned years later with the idea that it was functional modules defined by linguistic theory (such as syntax and semantics) that were supported by these brain regions. Broca's area was believed to subserve syntactic processing because patients with perceived deficits in processing grammatical information had damage to Broca's area. Similarly, Wernicke's area was believed to be a center for semantic processing, as patients with Wernicke's aphasia had lexical processing deficits and many had damage to Wernicke's area. It was assumed that these patterns would be observed worldwide, in all aphasic patients, regardless of the language(s) they spoke, and that these functions were therefore hard-wired into the brains of humans.

There is now a significant body of evidence suggesting that the relationship between function—be it clinically or linguistically defined—and specific brain region is considerably more complicated, and more variable, than was previously believed. For instance, lesions confined entirely to Broca's area do *not* lead to a persisting Broca's aphasia, nor do lesions affecting only Wernicke's area lead to a persisting Wernicke's aphasia (Mohr et al., 1978; Dronkers, Redfern, & Knight, 2000). Furthermore, the classical theory that production and comprehension are subserved by Broca's and Wernicke's areas, respectively, cannot be supported. For example, Bates et al. (2003b) utilized a new system of lesion-symptom mapping to demonstrate the effects of lesions to the brain on general performance in fluency and auditory comprehension in 101 chronic aphasic patients (see below for further details). The authors showed that when involvement in other brain regions was covaried out (the anterior insula and middle temporal gyrus, respectively), damage to Broca's area was not strongly associated with reduced fluency, and damage to Wernicke's area likewise did not correlate robustly with impairments in auditory comprehension.

Indeed, the original speech articulation deficit described by Broca—*aphemia*, roughly, a severe disruption in the patient's voluntary speech production ability, associated with "recurring utterances" such as "tan tan tan"—is associated not with injury to a specific cortical area, but with damage to the left superior arcuate fasciculus, a major fiber tract passing from the temporal lobe over the lateral ventricle to anterior cortical regions (Dronkers, Redfern, & Shapiro, 1993). A related deficit typically seen in patients with Broca's aphasia—namely a loss of articulatory agility, or apraxia of speech—also appears not to be associated with the third frontal convolution as previously thought, but rather with damage to the superior portion of the left precentral (short) gyrus of the insula. In a study of 44 aphasic patients with left hemisphere damage, Dronkers (1996) showed that all 25 patients with speech apraxia suffered from a lesion extending into this portion of the anterior insula, while the remaining 19 aphasic patients without speech apraxia had approximately equivalently-sized lesions, but ones that spared exactly this region of cortex.

We should emphasize that mapping symptoms to lesions does *not* presume that the associated brain area is solely responsible for the function in question. Metter, Kempler, and colleagues have elegantly demonstrated this fact in a series of PET studies, showing that the locus and extent of structural lesions (as detected by CT scans) often vastly underestimate the functional impact of seemingly focal damage, and that functional changes (as demonstrated by the presence of brain hypometabolism) are often more tightly yoked to the resulting behavioral deficits than are the lesions themselves. As an example, Kempler, Metter, Curtiss, Jackson, and Hanson (1991) showed that structural damage to the classical "language areas"—

the left inferior frontal gyrus ("Broca's") and left superior and middle temporal gyri ("Wernicke's")—correlated only weakly with the degree of syntactic deficit observed in the 43 aphasic patients they studied. However, examination of the same patients' PET data showed that comprehension deficits in morphology and syntax were highly correlated with hypometabolism in left occipital and temporal regions; syntactic deficits were further correlated with hypometabolism in the parietal lobe. Such findings suggest not only that the effect of "focal" brain lesions is considerably less circumscribed than is generally believed, but also that language may rely upon a much broader confederacy of cortical and subcortical regions than those classically associated with language function.

Not surprisingly, claims regarding the specificity of mapping between discrete linguistically-defined abilities and particular (if loosely defined) brain regions and/or aphasia syndromes have been difficult to uphold. For instance, Grodzinsky (1995, 2000) has claimed that Broca's area ". . . is neural home to mechanisms involved in the computation of transformational relations between moved phrasal constituents and their extraction sites" (Grodzinsky, 2000, p. 2), a computation posited by some linguists to be crucial for comprehension of sentence types such as passives and object relatives, but not for comprehension of "canonical" sentence types such as simple transitives. However, the results of several large studies of aphasic patients' syntactic comprehension have in fact found no systematic relationship between damage to *any* single brain region and the presence of syntactic comprehension deficits (Caplan, Baker, & Dehaut, 1985; Caplan, Hildebrandt, & Makris, 1996; Dick, Bates, Wulfeck, Utman, Dronkers, & Gernsbacher, 2001; Dronkers et al., 1994). What is more, the signature profile of syntactic deficits cited by Grodzinsky (2000) as evidence for the modularity and localizability of syntactic operations can be reproduced both qualitatively and quantitatively in *neurologically intact* college students operating under "stressful" or degraded conditions—a finding that holds for both speakers of English (Dick et al., 2001) and German (Dick, Bates, & Ferstl, 2003—see chapter by Aydelott, Kutas, & Federmeier, this volume, for details of the "stress" techniques used). Similarly, Wilson & Saygin (2004) reexamined Grodzinsky & Finkel's (1998) claim that agrammatic aphasics were selectively impaired in their ability to process syntactic structures involving "traces of maximal projections" in grammaticality judgment tasks. Wilson & Saygin found no evidence that agrammatic aphasics (or any other aphasic subgroup) were selectively impaired on structures involving traces. In fact, groups of patients had remarkably similar profiles of performance across sentence types, regardless of whether the grouping was made by aphasia type, screening for agrammatic comprehension, or lesion site. Furthermore, Wilson, Saygin, Schleicher, Dick & Bates (2003) examned grammaticality judgment on sentences with and without traces of max -

imal projections when healthy young controls performed the task under "stressful" conditions and found that the breakdown of performance under non-optimal processing conditions closely resembled the breakdown observed in aphasic patients.

In summary, the lesion correlates of "specific" linguistic deficits in adult aphasic patients are much more variable and complicated than was previously thought, supporting the contention that higher-level language skills are dynamic, and distributed throughout the brain. On the other hand, there are obviously quite dramatic global differences in the character of linguistic deficits depending on lesion site, e.g., left hemisphere injury in adults is much more apt to cause severe and lasting language problems, and damage to frontal regions tends to correlate with production and articulation difficulties, while posterior damage correlates with comprehension difficulties. Moreover, these coarse mappings tend to be quite consistent over individuals (indeed, ~95% of neurologically intact right-handed adults appear to be "left-dominant" for language, based on the results of WADA tests—Rasmussen and Milner, 1977). Does this quasi-inevitability of left-hemisphere-dominated processing of language imply not only that the left hemisphere is "purpose-built" for processing language, but in addition, that a special mechanism or mechanisms are needed for successful language acquisition and processing? Or is the typical adult profile of language organization a result of softer constraints or regional biological predispositions to perform certain types of computations? Perhaps the emerging processing biases of the constituent regions of the left hemisphere are more suited to the demands of language (e.g., rapid coordination of effectors, analyses of fast formant transitions), but given enough time and learning, alternate organizations for language production and comprehension could arise. Such plasticity might be anticipated *a priori* given the significant individual variability in language organization found in typically developing children and adults (Dick et al., 2001b). We address these issues in the next section.

LEARNING LANGUAGE AFTER EARLY BRAIN INJURY

Results from 30 years of studies of children with early-onset brain injury (for example, due to congenital arterovenous malformation, pre- or perinatal stroke, chronic seizures, or hemispherectomy) suggest that the intrinsic biases needed to get language off and running are very soft indeed. As reviewed by Bates & Roe (2001), the overall picture from the literature on children with early focal lesions and hemispherectomy tends *not* to show consistent differences between early left and right hemisphere injury in terms of language abilities. If differences are observed, they are much smaller than those observed in adults with commensurate injuries, and generally are noted for only a few language subscales. As Bates and Roe point out, these are particularly thorny studies to conduct, and to evaluate; the variability over patients and over studies in lesion onset time, seizure history, type and extent of injury, sample size, and statistical method tremendously complicate the interpretation of putative differences. Indeed, when samples sizes are large, and direct statistical comparisons between lesion groups are made, (e.g., right-hemisphere-damage (RHD) vs. left-hemisphere-damage (LHD), controlling for seizure history and lesion onset time), lesion side and site appears not to predict language proficiency (Bates and Roe, 2001—see also Brizzolara et al., 2002).

For instance, in a study of 43 English-speaking and 33 Italian-speaking children ages 5 and up with pre- and peri-natal-onset focal lesions, Bates, Vicari, and Trauner (1999) found that there was an *overall* delay in language acquisition associated with *any* lesion, with IQ scores in the low-to-normal range. In contrast to the expected adult profile (where LHD patients show more pronounced language deficits, and RHD patients show more pronounced spatial deficits), Bates et al. observed *no* difference between children with RHD and LHD on standard IQ measures (both verbal and non-verbal) or on any language comprehension/production measures (available for the Italian sample only). With regard to the latter result, the overall differences in language comprehension and production between Italian-speaking patient and control children disappeared after controlling for mental age.

Bates and her colleagues have also directly compared school-age children and adults with comparable focal lesions on a number of different measures. For instance, Kempler et al. (1999) tested adult and child (ages 6–12) patients' comprehension of familiar versus novel phrases. Results with adult patients revealed a classic double dissociation, with RHD patients showing impaired comprehension of familiar phrases and idioms with relatively preserved comprehension of novel phrases, while LHD patients showed the opposite pattern of deficits. In stark contrast, not only was there no difference between children with LHD and RHD on either measure, but both groups performed in the low-normal range relative to their age-matched controls, whereas their adult aphasic counterparts were massively impaired relative to healthy age-matched controls.

Dick et al. (1999, 2004) tested the online syntactic comprehension of 20 children ages 7–18 with RHD or LHD, comparing them to a large sample of typically developing children. Children with lesions to either hemisphere showed developmental delays in both accuracy and reaction time though their comprehension was similar to that of the youngest typically developing children. Again there was little evidence for a RHD/LHD difference in accuracy or response times. Similar results were found by Feldman, Mac-

Whinney, and Sacco, 2002, where children with focal lesions were delayed, and not deviant, in a standard competition model task—see chapter by MacWhinney in this volume. Direct comparisons between adults and children revealed a substantial quantitative but marginally significant interaction between lesion and age, where RH-damaged adults and RH- or LH-damaged children performed roughly equivalently, while LH-damaged adults aphasics fared considerably worse, with massive inter-subject variability.

The dramatic differences between language comprehension skills after early- and late-onset focal lesions are echoed in a recent study of language production (Bates, Reilly, Wulfeck, et al., 2001). Here, children and adults with right- or left-hemisphere focal brain damage were asked to narrate brief biographical sketches; these narratives were transcribed and further analyzed in terms of patterns of errors (omission versus commission), propositional content, sentence length, and so forth. As would be expected, adults with LHD were significantly more impaired than their RHD-counterparts, with each group showing a very different pattern of relative strengths and weaknesses. But comparisons between children with RHD and LHD revealed absolutely no differences on any production measures; moreover, this sample of children with early-onset lesions differed very little from age matched controls, where children with lesions used fewer words and made more omission errors than did their age-matched controls.

In short, the results of these studies of school-age children with early-onset focal lesions provide compelling evidence for the plasticity of the developing brain. Although these children do tend to show language processing delays relative to their age-matched peers, they show remarkably spared comprehension and production relative to adults with comparable focal lesions. What is more, these results suggest that the usual pattern of brain organization for language—e.g., left hemisphere dominance—is neither inevitable nor even necessary for successful language processing. In tandem with a bevy of behavioral results with neurologically intact subjects, these results further suggest that there is considerable change in children's neural underpinnings for language, even well into the school-age years (see chapters by Marchman & Thal, and Devescovi & D'Amico, this volume).

In this regard, the few functional MRI studies that have been directed at typical language development have shown interesting differences between activation patterns for adults and school-age children, even when very simple tasks are employed. Using a variety of word generation tasks (verb/ rhyme/opposites), Schlaggar et al. (2002) found that young adults showed activation in a left dorsal prefrontal region that was completely absent in children; conversely, children showed increased activation in a left fusiform region that was significantly greater than that evoked in adults. Saccuman et al. (2002) showed similar findings, where young adults in a covert picture naming task demonstrated significantly more activation in left lateral prefrontal and superior temporal regions than did children ages 10–12. These differences in activation could not easily be attributed to group differences in behavior, suggesting that as learning and development progress there are qualitative changes in the way that our brains structure themselves to process language, even after much of the "heavy lifting" in language acquisition has taken place.

It might be anticipated that significant neural circuit modifications take place early on, concomitant with the development of language skills. Unfortunately there are as of now no functional imaging studies of typically developing children under the age of 5 that bear on this issue (but see a recent study of young infants—Stanislas-Dehaene, Dehaene, & Hertz-Pannier, 2003). However, Bates and colleagues have conducted prospective cross-sectional studies of children with peri-natal focal lesions at the dawn of language comprehension and production, allowing a direct contrast between various "stages" of brain organization for language. In three similar studies of English- and Italian-speaking children with either LHD or RHD (Thal et al., 1991; Bates et al., 1997; and Vicari et al. 2000) data from several communicative inventories (MacArthur CDI, Fenson et al., 1993) and free speech samples were collected from children from 10–40 months, a period beginning with early language comprehension and word production (10–17 months) and continuing to multi-word utterances and grammatical development (18–40 months). The results of these studies serve as *prima facie* evidence against the theoretical notion that the developing brain is a conglomeration of inexorably maturing modules devoted to different processing needs.

For example, Thal et al. (1991), Bates et al. (1997), and Vicari et al. (2000) showed that early in the development of language skills (10–18 months), some children with peri-natal focal lesions show delays in language *comprehension* as well as gestural communication. However, these delays were observed only in children with *right* hemisphere injury; those with LHD (even with left temporal damage) were within the normal range on word comprehension. Not only is this the opposite of what one would expect from an adult model of language comprehension—where left temporal damage tends to correlate with comprehension disorders—but is also opposite the usual lesion correlate of deficits in gesture production and comprehension, which in adults are strongly associated with left hemisphere damage (see Bates and Dick, 2002 for extended discussion, as well as Wang and Goodglass, 1992). For early single word *production* in the same cohort of children (again 10–18 months), lesions to either hemisphere provoke delays in development, but are particularly severe in children with left *temporal* damage; this is again in contrast to the adult model, where language production deficits tend to correlate with left *frontal* damage.

Results from all three studies showed that left temporal damage continues to be a predictor of delayed language *production* somewhat later in development (e.g., 19–31 months). Here, toddlers with left temporal damage show impaired lexical *production*, with commensurate delays in grammatical development (as measured in free speech and the toddler version of the MacArthur CDI). With regard to this unexpected finding, Bates et al. (1997) suggest that whereas successful naturalistic auditory language comprehension relies on a wide range of partially redundant cues (such as temporal and spectral structure, prosody, gesture, and environmental cues) that allow for good comprehension in the face of incomplete or imperfect perception, language production requires a more fine-tuned and detailed set of acoustic representations, ones that would take longer to develop in the face of disrupted acoustic processing. In contrast to the left temporal findings, frontal damage to *either* hemisphere was also implicated in production delays—again unlike the adult model of left frontal damage leading to production difficulties.

Interestingly, these lesion-specific (left-temporal) deficits are observed in somewhat older and/or more advanced children (at the stage of multiword production in Vicari et al. (2000), and at age 5 in Reilly, Bates, & Marchman (1998)). At this point in development, children with focal lesions are on average slightly delayed relative to their age-matched peers, but still function in the low-to-normal range overall.

Clearly these children's brains are organizing themselves differently than they would in typical development. Does this indicate that the brain is equipotential for language, or—as might be expected from an embodied account—that are there early-forming connections and architectures that make some developing brain regions more hospitable to language than others? More concretely, if left frontal and temporal regions are damaged early in development, will the brain regions enabling language function emerge throughout the brain (as one might predict given strict equipotentiality) or will contralateral regions homologous to those characteristically associated with language be recruited for language tasks?

Axel Müller and colleagues (Müller et al., 1998; Müller et al., 1999; Müller et al., 1998b) have investigated this question using PET imaging on patients with early-onset lesions that resulted in intractable epilepsy. Using sentence listening and repetition tasks, Müller et al. (1998) compared activation profiles for children with perinatal left and right focal lesions (with the functional deficit confirmed by resting hypometabolism in the affected hemisphere). Here, children and adolescents with early LH lesions showed extensive right-lateralization of activation in both traditional perisylvian "language" areas, as well as much of the right temporal lobe (particularly the anterior temporal lobe), the angular gyrus, the precuneus, and the anterior cingulate. Roughly the opposite pattern was seen for the group with RH lesions—see Müller et al. (1998) for details. (A more recent fMRI study (Staudt et al., 2002) of 5 children with left periventricular lesions (causing hemiplegia but no epilepsy) showed a similar hemispheric mirroring of typical left lateralized activation in a covert verb generation task).

In an imaging analogue to the behavioral studies of Bates and colleagues discussed above, Müller et al. (1999) directly compared typical adult language-related activation to children and adults with early- and late-onset left hemisphere focal lesions, respectively, with the expectation that earlier injuries would allow greater potential for reorganization of function. Here, neurologically intact adults showed the usual left-lateralized perisylvian activation profile for sentence comprehension, while patients with early-onset focal lesions showed a mirrored, right-lateralized profile and late-onset patients showed highly symmetrical perisylvian activation. The dramatic lateralization difference between the early- and late-lesion group suggests that at least some of the remarkable capacity of the early-lesion group to acquire normal language may be due to development of these (or closely related) functions in the right hemisphere. These findings argue against the notion that language functions are inexorably hard-wired within specific left hemisphere regions.

Interestingly, this early-lesion-induced shift in interhemispheric activation is not seen in all domains, even in the face of early cerebral insult. In this regard, Müller et al. (1998b) directly compared left-right FDG PET activation asymmetries for sentence listening and repetition versus a basic motor task (finger tapping) in a sample of nine patients with relatively early-onset left hemisphere lesions. The difference in activation asymmetry was striking: for the language tasks, patients showed strong rightward activation asymmetries in the regions typically associated with these tasks (e.g., superior and middle temporal gyri, inferior frontal gyri)—again, a pattern opposite that of healthy control subjects. However, the same patients showed strong *leftward* activation asymmetries in the motor task, asymmetries very similar to controls. As with the behavioral studies discussed above, these results suggest that the development and commitment of neural resources for language is a protracted process, and one that might be more flexible than development of more developmentally and evolutionarily entrenched capacities such as the motor system. However, it is worth emphasizing that lesion-induced reorganization of language function appears to recruit roughly homologous regions in the right hemisphere rather than, for instance, co-opting left-hemisphere visual and somatosensory regions to accomplish language tasks. This suggests that regions with certain patterns of cortical and subcortical connections may be more amenable than others to cooption or "shared use" by language—a point we turn to in the next section (see also Small and Hoffman, 1994).

THE RELATIONSHIP OF LANGUAGE TO OTHER DOMAINS: EVIDENCE FROM APHASIA AND BRAIN IMAGING

As we noted in the introduction, the study of language as a special, independent system has been a dominant approach in the cognitive sciences and linguistics. But there is ever-increasing evidence that language maybe more profitably viewed as an "embodied" system, one tightly interwoven with sensory and motor faculties and other cognitive processes. There is ample historical precedent for this view: since the early days of neurology, there has been speculation—and empirical evidence—supporting a more intimate relationship between language processing and other cognitive and sensorimotor domains. To our knowledge, Finkelnburg (1870 lecture translated by Duffy & Liles, 1979) was the first to propose that an underlying factor was common to both the language impairments in aphasia and the deficits in nonverbal domains that these patients can exhibit. This idea received some support from subsequent pioneers in neurology (Goldstein, 1948; Head, 1926). More recently, aphasic patients' impairments in nonverbal domains have been demonstrated in experimental settings using such tasks as gesture (e.g., Duffy & Duffy, 1981), and environmental sound comprehension (e.g., Varney, 1980).

Despite such a long history of evidence to the contrary, aphasia is most commonly viewed as a deficit restricted to the linguistic domain. It is true that aphasic patients often have spared abilities in domains not clearly related to language. For instance, Italian aphasic patients with impaired grammatical gender priming do show intact color priming (Bates, Marangolo, Pizzamiglio, & Dick, 2001). Nevertheless, there is growing evidence that an "embodied" and distributive account of language function may be more viable, one that would predict tight links between linguistic and nonlinguistic tasks sharing similar processing demands.

In one neuropsychological study, our group assessed the relationship between verbal and nonverbal comprehension of complex, meaningful information in the auditory modality by examining aphasic patients' abilities to match environmental sounds (such as the sound of a cow mooing, or a car starting) and corresponding linguistic phrases to associated pictures, using a forced-choice task (Saygin, Dick, Wilson, Dronkers, & Bates, 2003). Task demands, stimulus characteristics, and semantic features were all carefully controlled in order to test the association between the linguistic and nonlinguistic processing without introducing additional confounds. Results from 30 LHD and 5 RHD patients (along with 21 neurologically intact age-matched control subjects) were consistent with the embodied view of language. Aphasic patients' deficits were *not* restricted to the linguistic domain; rather, patients were impaired to the same extent in comprehending language and environmental sounds, as measured by both accuracy and reaction time. In addition, there was a surprisingly high correlation between performance scores for language and environmental sounds, strongly suggesting that the two domains utilize common brain regions and/or processes. Furthermore, a lesion-symptom mapping analysis (Bates et al., 2003b) found that damage to posterior regions in the left middle and superior temporal gyri and to the inferior parietal lobe was a predictor of deficits for *both* speech and environmental sounds. Interestingly, these left-hemisphere regions are often considered to be language-specific areas. Indeed the posterior portion of Brodmann's area 22 (as roughly identified in stereotactic space) corresponds to the original Wernicke's area. Our results indicate that this area and the surrounding mid-temporal and parietal regions are also implicated in environmental sound processing. In fact, Wernicke's area itself, in the posterior superior temporal gyrus, while significantly associated with deficits in both domains, was more highly associated with performance in the nonverbal domain than the verbal domain.

In a related fMRI study on comprehension of environmental sounds and linguistic descriptions (Dick, Saygin, Pitzalis, Galati, Bentrovato, D'Amico, Wilson, Bates, & Pizzamiglio, 2003; submitted), we asked whether these left-hemisphere regions, shown in patients with brain injury to be *necessary* for the processing of environmental sounds are also the most *active* when studied with brain imaging of normal adults. This does appear to be the case: The more consistent the lesion-deficit mapping in a given region, the more that same region tended to be activated in the fMRI experiments. Consistent with the aphasia findings and with a "shared resources" view of language, the lesion maps (environmental sound- or language-based) were better predictors of environmental sound activation than language activation. And similar to the results of other studies of environmental sound and language comprehension (Adams & Janata, 2002; Humphries, Willard, Buchsbaum, & Hickok, 2001; Lewis, Wightman, Junion Dienger, & DeYoe, 2001; Thierry, Giraud, & Price, 2003), our fMRI subjects showed substantial overlap in activation for environmental sounds and language, particularly in the left hemisphere. ERP and fMRI studies by Koelsch, Friederici, and colleagues have revealed commensurate similarities between music- and language-related activation (Koelsch, Gunter, von Cramon, Zysset, Lohmann, & Friederici, 2002).

Note that such findings are not limited to the auditory modality. Saygin, Wilson, Dronkers & Bates (in press) carried out an analogous experiment in the visual modality, examining patients' processing of meaningful, transitive actions using corresponding linguistic and nonlinguistic stimuli. In another study, Saygin & Wilson (in press) tested point-light biological motion perception in the same patient group. In both of these studies aphasic patients showed significant deficits in nonverbal domains compared with control subjects. Lesion sites also overlapped significantly with anterior and posterior language processing areas described earlier.

We now turn from studies that directly compare lesion maps or activation profiles across linguistic and nonlinguistic domains to those that probe the interaction of language with its sensorimotor substrate. In line with more than a decade of behavioral findings regarding online interactions between sensorimotor and language processing (Gentilucci et al., 2000; Gentilucci & Gangitano, 1998; Glenberg, 1997, Glenberg, Schroeder, & Robertson, 1998), results from recent neuroimaging studies by Cappa, Perani, Rizzolatti, Saccuman, Tettamanti, and colleagues (Tettamanti et al., 2002; Saccuman et al., 2003) have shown that language processing is deeply entwined with its sensorimotor roots. For example, subjects asked to listen to a series of transitive sentences involving movements of the mouth, hand, or leg (versus similar but abstract transitive sentences), show somatotopic brain activation in premotor cortex along the precentral gyrus and in the parietal operculum but, most importantly, there was in addition a common activation in the inferior frontal gyrus (Broca's area). This suggests that at least some of the brain regions important for language comprehension are also involved in sensing and moving the body (Tettamanti et al., 2002). This hypothesis is supported by results from another study by the same group (Saccuman et al., 2003) showing that fMRI activation related to action and object naming is strongly modulated by whether or not the action or object involves manipulation by the hand. Here, naming of manipulable objects or associated actions (e.g., golfing, hammering) when compared to the naming of actions or objects that do not involve hand manipulation (such as diving), preferentially activates a neural system, including premotor, sensorimotor cortex, frontal operculum and parietal regions, all of them shown to be involved in action representations by other imaging studies. Moreover, this "manipulable/non-manipulable" activation contrast is much more dramatic than the contrast between activation for nouns and verbs in the same study. This suggests that a manipulation of the semantic content of nouns and verbs might have a stronger effect on activation than what can be attributable to the morpho-syntactic differences between the two lexical classes.

In a related vein, Small, Nusbaum, and Skipper have shown that activation in traditional "language" areas is contingent upon the sensorimotor demands of the experimental task used. Here subjects were imaged with fMRI while listening to interesting stories (audio only), listening to stories while seeing the storyteller (audiovisual), or just seeing the storyteller (visual). Analyses revealed far more activation in the inferior frontal cortex (stereotactically defined BA 44/45, often referred to as "Broca's area" in the imaging literature) in the audiovisual condition than in either of the other conditions (Skipper, Nusbaum, & Small, 2002a; Skipper, Nusbaum, & Small, 2002b; Skipper, Nusbaum, & Small, 2003). Moreover, the presence of the visuo-motor information both greatly increased and slightly left-lateralized activity in the superior temporal gyrus, demonstrating an interaction between face and speech processing in traditional receptive language regions—see also Wright et al. (2003), and Stephan et al. (2003) for similar findings in temporal and frontal regions, respectively.

In summary, we see that language has considerable—if complicated—behavioral and neural links with related nonlinguistic skills and with the sensorimotor substrate that allows language to be perceived and produced. In order to understand more fully how language colonizes, inhabits, and shares a brain that is truly ensnared by the demands of the body, we will need to develop new tools that will allow us to begin to untangle the changes in, and contributions of, different brain regions to language function over learning, development, and breakdown. In the final section of this chapter, we outline several new approaches to investigating brain-behavior mappings that attempt to characterize the continuous, complex, and multifaceted nature of brain-behavior mappings.

NEW TOOLS FOR EXPLORING BRAIN-LANGUAGE RELATIONSHIPS

In this section, we elaborate on three new techniques for analyzing links between brain and behavior. The first is a novel method of "quantifying dissociations" in samples of aphasic patients; the second is a method of characterizing lesion symptoms in a continuous, rather than discrete symptom space. The final method is a new way of analyzing and visualizing lesion-symptom mapping, a method that can also be used to quantitatively combine lesion and fMRI data.

A long-standing debate in neuropsychology concerns the relative merits and problems of group vs. single-case studies (see Bub & Bub, 1988; Caplan & Hildebrandt, 1988; Caramazza, 1986; Shallice, 1988). Critics of the single-case approach note the limits on generalizability of results to larger populations and the lack of statistical power, while critics of group studies point out the limited validity of syndromes and classic neuropsychological taxonomies, and the potentially important information about individual patients that is masked by such groupings.[1]

---

[1]Note that the use of double dissociations as a theoretical testing ground is increasingly criticized, based in part on the results of connectionist and/or statistical simulations (Juola & Plunkett, 1998; Van Orden, Pennington, & Stone, in press).

It is possible to approach neuropsychological data in a way that minimizes the problems associated with both single case and standard group studies? One method of addressing this question involves "quantifying dissociations". Double dissociations have played an immense role in neuropsychology, but surprisingly little work has been done on how these dissociations can be characterized statistically. In theory, neuropsychological dissociations are interesting because they represent unusual relationships between two measures, and in some cases they can reveal underlying functional "fault lines" in the intact brain. However, as Bates, Appelbaum, Salcedo, Saygin, & Pizzamiglio (2003a) argue, the degree to which these relationships are unusual is difficult to assess without reference to the correlation that is observed between the variables of interest. Bates et al. (2003a) demonstrated a new approach to quantifying dissociations, based both on illustrative examples and on large neuropsychological datasets (two measures from a language battery administered to a large sample of patients at risk for aphasia, and two from a nonverbal battery administered to a large sample of patients at risk for neglect). The same datasets were analyzed using different definitions of what constitutes a dissociated individual. Results showed that the probability of labeling an individual case as a single or double dissociation is strongly influenced by the distribution of scores in the population from which the patients are drawn. This includes not only the way that extreme scores are defined for each measure, but also the correlation between those measures. More specifically, not only is the number of dissociations detected related to the magnitude of the correlation between measures, but the set of patients identified as showing dissociations varies with the choice of statistical method. Bates et al. (2003a) point out that, by taking into account the correlation between measures, one can not only guard against false positives that may arise when the measures are not correlated, but also false negatives when the measures are strongly correlated.

In another study, Bates, Saygin, Moineau, Marangolo, & Pizzamiglio (in press) demonstrated that classical aphasia taxonomies based on symptom dimensions need not limit analysis methods in neuropsychological group studies. Here, nominal taxonomies based on arbitrary cut-offs and groupings are replaced by multivariate analyses in which individual patients are treated as vectors or points in a multidimensional symptom space. This approach preserves the continuous range of information available for all measures obtained from each patient, without drawing boundaries that lose or distort information about the individual patient's symptom profile. As a demonstration case, Bates et al. (in press) used a large archival data set of fluency, naming, comprehension, and repetition scores for 126 Italian-speaking patients. Here, standard aphasia taxonomies (e.g., Broca's vs. Wernicke's aphasia) or continuous WAB subscores (fluency, comprehension, repetition, naming) were used to predict behavior on a single external validation measure, the Token Test. Results showed that the continuous multivariate scores predicted significantly more variance in Token Test performance than did the standard aphasia subtypes. In short, the continuous approach is more efficient as all information inherently present in the data is used. In addition, and in contrast with studies where patients are grouped by aphasia type, these multivariate analyses do not discard or obscure any information about individuals, thus eliminating the conflict between group and individual approaches to neuropsychological data. Moreover, outliers and dissociations can be identified and further studied using the "quantifying dissociations" methods described above.

The principle of avoiding discrete classifications based on cutoff scores and the like has also led to the technique of voxel-based lesion-symptom mapping (VLSM—Bates et al., 2003b). Lesion-symptom mapping is a way of making inferences about brain-behavior relationships that combines information about lesion location and behavioral performance. Most previous lesion-symptom mapping work has employed one of two basic approaches, which will refer to as the "groups defined by behavior" and "groups defined by lesion" methods. Both methods have the disadvantage of having to discard potentially useful data.

In the "groups defined by behavior" method, a cutoff score is stipulated. Patients who score below the cutoff are designated as "impaired," whereas those who score above it are designated as "spared". An overlay of all the impaired patients' lesions is then constructed to determine whether there is some area which is consistently damaged in impaired patients. Likewise, a complimentary overlay can be made of the behaviorally spared patients' lesions to ensure that any such area is indeed intact in these patients. This method is ideal if the symptom of interest is relatively discrete—for instance Dronkers (1996) used this method in the study of apraxia of speech described above. However, when deficits are graded in nature, the method is not ideal because an arbitrary cutoff must be stipulated and information about the degree of impairment in both groups is discarded.

The other common method of lesion-mapping is the "groups defined by lesion" technique. Here, patients are grouped based on their lesions according to broad neuroanatomical criteria. For instance, patients might be divided into groups according to whether or not their lesions affected the temporal lobe. These anatomically-defined groups are then compared on one or more behavioral measures. This technique can also be useful, especially when there is an *a priori* brain region of interest, or when a relatively small number of patients are available (e.g. Chao & Knight, 1998). But by grouping patients on gross anatomical criteria, this method cannot use all available lesion information; furthermore, because it is based on regions of interest, it generally cannot identify multiple regions which contribute to a behavior.

Voxel-based lesion-symptom mapping goes beyond these methods by utilizing both continuous behavioral information and continuous lesion information (Bates et al., 2003b). The relative importance of brain regions for a behavior of interest is inferred on a voxel-by-voxel basis. At each voxel, patients are divided into two groups according to whether or not their lesion includes that particular voxel. The behavioral scores of these two groups are then compared statistically (e.g., using a t-test) with the results plotted as color or intensity maps, where the intensity value at each voxel indicates the severity of deficits associated with having a lesion in that location. An example is shown in Fig. 9.1, based on Figure 1 from Bates et al. (2003b). The behavioral measures used in this study were Western Aphasia Battery (Kertesz, 1979) fluency and comprehension subscores for 101 left-hemisphere-dam-

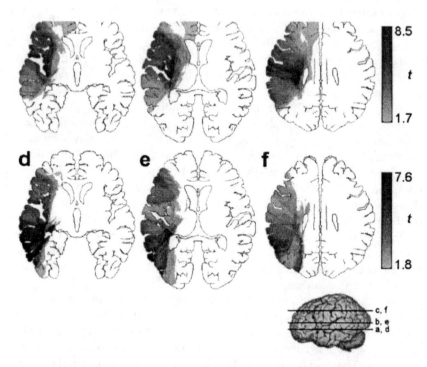

FIG. 9.1.   Representative slices from VLSM maps computed for fluency and auditory comprehension performance of 101 aphasic stroke patients. At each voxel, a t-test was carried out, comparing patients with lesions in that voxel to patients whose lesions spared that voxel. High t-scores (black and dark gray) indicate that lesions to these voxels had a highly significant effect on behavior, whereas lighter gray voxels indicate regions where the presence of a lesion had relatively little impact on the behavioral measure.

aged stroke patients. The top three panels show that damage to the anterior insula and the superior longitudinal fasciculus were most strongly associated with poor fluency scores. The bottom three panels show that for comprehension, the most severe deficits were associated with lesions to the middle temporal gyrus. The VLSM method thus replicates the basic idea that anterior areas are more important for production and posterior areas for comprehension, but differs somewhat from traditional accounts in terms of exactly which areas are most likely to cause severe deficits.

While the Bates et al. (2003b) study relies upon behavioral measures taken from a standard clinical battery, it is also interesting to examine behavioral measures which are more theoretically motivated. For instance, the comprehension subscore on the WAB conflates single word comprehension as well as sentence comprehension; thus, the resulting VLSM maps can be expected to reveal areas which are important for any aspect of the comprehension process. More constrained behavioral measures might allow for a more nuanced understanding of areas involved in language or other skills. Several studies have applied VLSM to more specific behavioral measures, although to date none have enjoyed the large sample size of the Bates et al. (2003b) study. Using VLSM, Saygin et al. (in press) found that deficits in pantomime comprehension are associated with lesions to frontal areas. Wilson & Saygin (2004) found that grammaticality judgment performance is most affected by posterior temporal lesions, regardless of the specific syntactic structure being judged. Finally, Dronkers et al. (in press) have used VLSM to uncover multiple brain areas involved in sentence comprehension.

CONCLUSIONS

The field of brain and language has veered back and forth between the Scylla of phrenological determinism and the Charybdis of tabula rasa empiricism, with neither account providing a sufficient explanatory framework for more than a century of data from behavioral, neuropsychological, and neuroimaging experiments. In this chapter we have tried to chart the progress of a fledgling "third way" of thinking about language in the brain—one that takes into consideration basic (phylo)genetic, developmental, and anatomical constraints on the brain while also acknowledging both the extraordinary plasticity of the mammalian nervous system (during development and throughout the lifespan) and the information-processing capacities afforded by a distributive processing system. This approach brings with it formidable theoretical and methodological challenges. It requires a commitment to new analytical techniques that can distill data from the massively multivariate, dynamic, and non-linear system that we believe the brain to be, ones that avoid imposing overly simplistic assumptions about mechanism or behavior. This approach will also require taking into account the "embodiment" of complex functions, both in terms of the constraints an organism's sensorimotor system might place on the brain, and the possibilities for distributed co-representation of sensorimotor and higher cognitive functions. Indeed, such an approach will force us to begin to see language on the brain's terms, rather than simply assuming a one-to-one correspondence between alluring linguistic taxonomies and underlying neural mechanisms.

AUTHOR NOTE

The authors would like to thank Dan Slobin, Mike Tomasello, and Erlbaum Publishing for having made this Festschrift possible.

REFERENCES

Adams, R., & Janata, P. (2002). A comparison of neural circuits underlying auditory and visual object categorization. *NeuroImage, 16*, 361–377.

Bates, E., & Dick, F. (2002). Language, gesture, and the developing brain. *Developmental Psychobiology, 40*(3), 293–310.

Bates, E., & Roe, K. (2001). Language development in children with unilateral brain injury. In C. A. Nelson & M. Luciana (Eds.), *Handbook of developmental cognitive neuroscience* (pp. 281–307). Cambridge, MA: MIT Press.

Bates, E., Appelbaum, M., Salcedo, J., Saygin, A. P., & Pizzamiglio, L. (2003a). Quantifying dissociations in neuropsychological research. *Journal of Clinical and Experimental Neuropsychology, 25*(8), 1128–1153.

Bates, E., Marangolo, P., Pizzamiglio, L., & Dick, F. (2001). Linguistic and nonlinguistic priming in aphasia. *Brain and Language, 75*(4), 1–8.

Bates, E., Reilly, J., Wulfeck, B., Dronkers, N., Opie, M., Fenson, J., Kriz, S., Jeffries, R., Miller, L., & Herbst, K. (2001). Differential effects of unilateral lesions on language production in children and adults. *Brain and Language, 79*, 223–265.

Bates, E., Saygin, A. P., Moineau, S., Marangolo, P., & Pizzamiglio, L. (in press). Analyzing aphasia data in a multidimensional symptom space. *Brain and Language.*

Bates, E., Thal, D., Trauner, D., Fenson, J., Aram, D., Eisele, J., & Nass, R. (1997). From first words to grammar in children with focal brain injury. *Developmental Neuropsychology, 13*, 447–476.

Bates, E., Vicari, S., & Trauner, D. (1999). Neural mediation of language development: Perspectives from lesion studies of infants and children. In H. Tager-Flusberg (Ed.), *Neurodevelopmental disorders* (pp. 533–581). Cambridge, MA: MIT Press.

Bates, E., Wilson, S. M., Saygin, A. P., Dick, F., Sereno, M. I., Knight, R. T., & Dronkers, N. F. (2003b). Voxel-based lesion-symptom mapping. *Nature Neuroscience, 6*(5), 448–450.

Brizzolara, D., Pecini, C., Brovedani, P., Ferretti, G., Cipriani, P., & Cioni, G. (2002). Timing and type of congenital brain lesion determine different patterns of language lateralization in hemiplegic children. *Neuropsychologia, 40*, 620–632.

Bub, J., & Bub, D. (1988). On the methodology of single-case studies in cognitive neuropsychology. *Cognitive Neuropsychology, 5*, 565–582.

Caplan, D., Baker, C., & Dehaut, F. (1985). Syntactic determinants of sentence comprehension in aphasia. *Cognition, 21,* 117–125.

Caplan, D., & Hildebrandt, N. (1988). *Disorders of syntactic comprehension.* Cambridge, MA: MIT Press.

Caplan, D., Hildebrandt, N., & Makris, N. (1996). Location of lesions in stroke patients with deficits in syntactic processing in sentence comprehension. *Brain, 119,* 933–949.

Caramazza, A. (1986). On drawing inferences about the structure of normal cognitive systems from the analysis of patterns of impaired performance: The case for single-patient studies. *Brain and Cognition, 5,* 41–66.

Chao, L. L., & Knight, R. T. (1998). Contribution of human prefrontal cortex to delay performance. *Journal of Cognitive Neuroscience, 10,* 167–177.

Dehaene-Lambertz, G., Dehaene, S., & Hertz-Pannier, L. (2002). Functional neuroimaging of speech perception in infants. *Science, 298,* 2013–2015.

Dick, F., Bates, E., & Ferstl, E. C. (2003). Spectral and temporal degradation of speech as a simulation of morphosyntactic deficits in English and German. *Brain and Language, 85*(3), 535–542.

Dick, F., Bates, E., Wulfeck, B., Utman, J., Dronkers, N., & Gernsbacher, M. A. (2001). Language deficits, localization and grammar: evidence for a distributive model of language breakdown in aphasics and normals. *Psychological Review, 108*(4), 759–788.

Dick, F., Saccuman, C., Sereno, M., Müller, R. A., Bates, E., & Wulfeck, B. (2001b). Language production and comprehension in fMRI: Consistency and variability over individuals and group averages. Poster presented at the Meeting of the Society for Cognitive Neuroscience, New York, NY, 2001.

Dick, F., Saygin, A. P., Pitzalis, S., Galati, G., Bentrovato, S., D'Amico, S., Wilson, S., Bates, E., & Pizzamiglio, L. (submitted). *What is involved and what is necessary for complex linguistic and nonlinguistic auditory processing.* Manuscript submitted for publication.

Dick, F., Wulfeck, B., Bates, E., Saltzman, D., Naucler, N., & Dronkers, N. (1999). Interpretation of complex syntax in aphasic adults and children with focal lesions or specific language impairment. *Brain and Language, 69,* 335–336.

Dick, F., Wulfeck, B., Krupa-Kwiatkowski, M., & Bates, E. (2004). The development of complex sentence interpretation in typically developing children compared with children with specific language impairments or early unilateral focal lesions. *Developmental Science, 7*(3), 360–377.

Dronkers, N. (1996) A new brain region for coordinating speech articulation. *Nature, 14;384(6605),* 159–61.

Dronkers, N. F., Redfern, B. B., & Knight, R. T. (2000). The neural architecture of language disorders. In M. S. Gazzaniga (Ed.), *The new cognitive neurosciences* (2nd ed.) (pp. 949–960). Cambridge, MA: MIT Press.

Dronkers, N., Redfern, B., & Shapiro, J. (1993). Neuroanatomic correlates of production deficits in severe Broca's aphasia. *Experimental Neuropsychology, 15*(1), 59–60.

Dronkers, N. F., Wilkins, D. P., Redfern, B. B., Van Valin, J. R., & Jaeger, J. J. (1994). A reconsideration of the brain areas involved in the disruption of morphosyntactic comprehension. *Brain and Language, 47*(3), 461–463.

Dronkers, N. F., Wilkins, D. P., Van Valin, R. D. Jr., Redfern, B. B., & Jaeger, J. J. (in press). Exploring brain areas involved in language comprehension using a new method of lesion analysis. *Cognition.*

Duffy, R., & Duffy, J. (1981). Three studies of deficits in pantomimic expression and pantomimic recognition in aphasia. *Journal of Speech and Hearing Research, 24,* 70–84.

Duffy, R., & Liles, B. (1979). A translation of Finkelnburg's (1870) lecture on aphasia as "asymbolia" with commentary. *Journal of Speech and Hearing Disorders, 44*(2), 156–168.

Elman, J. L., Bates, E. A., Johnson, M. H., & Karmiloff-Smith, A., Parisi, D., & Plunkett, K. (1996). *Rethinking innateness: A connectionist perspective on development.* Cambridge, MA: MIT Press.

Feldman, H., MacWhinney, B., & Sacco, K. (2002). Sentence processing in children with early unilateral brain injury. *Brain and Language, 83,* 335–352.

Fenson, L., Dale, P. S., Reznick, J., Thal, D., Bates, E., Hartung, J. P., Pethick, S., & Reilly, J. S. (1993). *The MacArthur Communicative Development Inventories: User's guide and technical manual.* San Diego, CA: Singular Publishing Group.

Fodor, J. A. (1983). *The modularity of mind : An essay on faculty psychology.* Cambridge, MA: MIT Press.

Gall, F. J. (1810). *Anatomie et physiologie du système nerveux* (Vol. 1). Paris: Librairie grecque-latine-allemande.

Gentilucci, M., & Gangitano, M. (1998). Influence of automatic word reading on motor control. *European Journal of Neuroscience, 10,* 752–756.

Gentilucci, M., Benuzzi, F., Bertolani, L., Daprati, E., & Gangitano, M. (2000). Language and motor control. *Experimental Brain Research,* in press.

Gibson, J. J. (1951). What is form? *Psychological Review, 58,* 403–412

Glenberg, A. M. (1997). What memory is for. *Behavioral & Brain Sciences, 20*(1), 1–55.

Glenberg, A. M., Schroeder, J. L., & Robertson, D. A. (1998). Averting the gaze disengages the environment and facilitates remembering. *Memory & Cognition, 26*(4), 651–658.

Goldstein, K. (1948). *Language and language disturbances: Aphasic symptom complexes and their significance for medicine and theory of language.* New York: Grune & Stratton.

Grodzinsky, Y. (1995). A restrictive theory of agrammatic comprehension. *Brain and Language, 50*(1), 27–51.

Grodzinsky, Y. (2000). The neurology of syntax: Language use without Broca's area. *Behavioral and Brain Sciences, 23*(1), 1–71.

Head, H. (1926). *Aphasia and kindred disorders of speech.* New York: Macmillan.

Humphries, C., Willard, K., Buchsbaum, B., & Hickok, G. (2001). Role of anterior temporal cortex in auditory sentence comprehension: an fMRI study. *Neuroreport, 12*(8), 1749–52.

James, W. (1994). The physical basis of emotion (1894). *Psychological Review, 101*(2), 205–10.

Juola, P., & Plunkett, K. (1998). Why double dissociations don't mean much. *Proceedings of the Twentieth Annual Conference of the Cognitive Science Society,* Madison, WI. (20), 561–566.

Kempler, D., Metter, E. J., Curtiss, S., Jackson, C. A., & Hanson, W. R. (1991). Grammatical comprehension, aphasic syndromes, and neuroimaging. *Journal of Neurolinguistics, 6,* 301–318.

Kempler, D., Van Lancker, D., Marchman, V., & Bates, E. (1999). Idiom comprehension in children and adults with unilateral brain damage. *Developmental Psychology, 15*(3), 327–349.

Kertesz, A. (1979) *Aphasia and Associated Disorders.* New York: (Grune & Stratton) Psychological Corporation Inc.

Koelsch, S., Gunter, T., v Cramon D., Zysset, S., Lohmann, G., & Friederici, A. (2002). Bach speaks: a cortical "language-network" serves the processing of music. *NeuroImage, 17*(2), 956–966.

Lashley, K. S. (1950). *In search of the engram* (Vol. 4). New York: Academic Press.

Lewis, J., Wightman, F., Junion Dienger, J., & DeYoe, E. (2001). fMRI activation in response to the identification of natural sounds. *Society of Neuroscience Abstracts, Vol 27,* 512.9.

MacWhinney, B. (1999). *The Emergence of Language.* Mahwah, NJ. Lawrence Erlbaum.

Mauner, G., Fromkin, V. A., & Cornell, T. L. (1993). Comprehension and acceptability judgments in agrammatism: Disruptions in the syntax of referential dependency. *Brain and Language, 45*(3), 340–370.

Mohr, J., Pessin, M., Finkelstein, S., Funkenstein, H., Duncan, G., & Davis, K. (1978). Broca aphasia: pathologic and clinical. *Neurology, 28*(4), 311–324.

Mueller, R.-A., Rothermel, R., Behen, M., Muzik, O., Chakraborty, P., & Chugani, H. (1999). Language organization in patients with early and late left-hemisphere lesion: a PET study. *Neuropsychologia, 37,* 545–557.

Mueller, R.-A., Rothermel, R., Behen, M., Muzik, O., Mangner, T., Chakraborty, P., & Chugani, H. (1998). Brain organization of language after early unilateral lesion: A PET study. *Brain and Language, 62,* 422–451.

Mueller, R.-A., Rothermel, R., Behen, M., Otto Muzik, O., Mangner, T., & Chugani, H. (1998b). Differential patterns of language and motor reorganization following early left hemisphere injury. *Archives of Neurology, 55,* 1113–1119.

Piaget, J. (1928). *Le jugement et le raisonnement chez l'enfant.* (Judgement and reasoning in the child). London, Kegan Paul Trench Trubner.

Rasmussen, T., & Milner, B. (1977). The role of early left-brain injury in determining lateralization of cerebral speech functions. *The Annals of the New York Academy of Sciences, (299),* 355–69.

Reilly, J., Bates, E., & Marchman, V. (1998). Narrative discourse in children with early focal brain injury. In M. Dennis (Ed.), Special issue, Discourse in children with anomalous brain development or acquired brain injury. *Brain and Language, 61*(3), 335–375.

Saccuman, C., Dick, F., Bates, E., Müller, R. A., Bussiere, J., Krupa-Kwiatkowski, M., & Wulfeck, B. (2002). Lexical access and sentence processing: A developmental fMRI study of language processing. Poster presented at the Meeting of the Cognitive Neuroscience Society, April, 2002.

Saccuman, M. C., Cappa, S. F., Bates, E., Danna, M., & Perani, D. (2003). The neural correlates of noun and verb processing: Semantic versus syntactic grammatical effects. Abstract of the Society for Neuroscience, New Orleans November 2003.

Saygin, A. P., Dick, F., Wilson, S., Dronkers, N., & Bates, E. (2003). Neural resources for processing language and environmental sounds: Evidence from aphasia. *Brain, 126,* 928–945.

Saygin, A. P., & Wilson, S. M. (2004). *Biological motion perception in left-hemisphere damaged patients.* Manuscript submitted for publication.

Saygin, A. P., Wilson, S. M., Dronkers, N., & Bates, E. (in press). Action comprehension in aphasia: Linguistic and non-linguistic deficits and their lesion correlates. *Neuropsychologia.*

Schlaggar, B., Brown, T. T., Lugar, H., Visscher, K., Miezin, F., Petersen, S. (2002). Functional neuroanatomical differences between adults and school-age children in the processing of single words. *Science, 296,* 1476–1479.

Shallice, T. (1988). *From neuropsychology to mental structure.* New York: Cambridge University Press.

Skipper, J. I., Nusbaum, H., & Small, S. L. (2002a). Emergence of Neural Circuits During Language Comprehension. Manuscript submitted for publication.

Skipper, J. I., Nusbaum, H. C., & Small, S. L. (2002b). Speech perception and the inferior frontal neural system for motor imitation. *Journal of Cognitive Neuroscience,* F103.

Skipper, J. I., Nusbaum, H. C., & Small, S. L. (2003). Listening to Talking Faces: Motor Cortical Activation During Audiovisual but not Auditory Language Comprehension. Manuscript submitted for publication.

Small S. L. (1997). Semantic Category Imprecision: A Connectionist Study of the Boundaries of Word Meanings. *Brain and Language, 57,* 181–194.

Small S. L. and Hoffman G. E. (1994). Neuroanatomical Lateralization of Language: Sexual Dimorphism and the Ethology of Neural Computation. *Brain and Cognition, 26,* 300–311.

Staudt, M., Lidzba, K., Grodd, W., Wildgruber, D., Erb, M., & Kraegeloh-Mann, I. (2002). Right-hemispheric organization of language following early left-sided brain lesions: Functional MRI topography. *NeuroImage, 16,* 954–967.

Stephan, K., Marshall, J., Friston, K., Rowe, J., Ritzl, A., Zilles, K., & Fink, G. (2003). Lateralized cognitive processes and lateralized task control in the human brain. *Science, 301*(5631), 384–386.

Tettamanti, M., Buccino, G., Saccuman, C., Gallese, V., Perani, D., Danna, M., Scifo, P., Cappa, S. F., Fazio, F., & Rizzolatti, G. (2002). Listening to sentences describing different motor actions activates the corresponding representations in the premotor cortex. Poster presented at the 2002 Human Brain Mapping Conference, Sendei, Japan.

Thal, D., Marchman, V., Stiles, J., Aram, D., Trauner, D., Nass, R., & Bates, E. (1991). Early lexical development in children with focal brain injury. *Brain and Language, 40,* 491–527.

Thierry, G., Giraud, A.-L., & Price, C. (2003). Hemispheric dissociation in access to the human semantic system. *Neuron, 38,* 1–20.

Todorov, E. (2000). Direct cortical control of muscle activation in voluntary arm movements: A model. *Nature Neuroscience, 3*(4), 391–8.

Ullman, M. (1999). Naming tools and using rules: Evidence that a frontal/basal-ganglia system underlies both motor skill knowledge and grammatical rule use. *Brain and Language. 69*(3), 316–318.

Van Orden, G. C., Pennington, B. F., & Stone, G. O. (in press). What do double dissociations prove? *Cognitive Science.*

Varney, N. (1980). Sound recognition in relation to aural language comprehension in aphasic patients. *Journal of Neurology, Neurosurgery, and Psychiatry, 43,* 71–75.

Vicari, S., Albertoni, A., Chilosi, A., Cipriani, P., Cioni, G., & Bates, E. (2000). Plasticity and reorganization during early language learning in children with congenital brain injury. *Cortex, 36,* 31–46.

Wang, L., & Goodglass, H. (1992). Pantomime, praxis, and aphasia. *Brain and Language, 42,* 402–418.

Wilson, S. M., & Saygin, A. P. (2004). Grammaticality judgment in aphasia: Deficits are not specific to syntactic structures, aphasic syndromes or lesion sites. *Journal of Cognitive Neuroscience, 16*(2), 238–252.

Wilson, S. M., Saygin, A. P., Schleicher, E., Dick, F., & Bates, E. (2003). Grammaticality judgment under non-optimal processing conditions: Deficits induced in normal participants resemble those observed in aphasic patients. *Brain and Language, 87*(1), 67–68.

Wright, T., Pelphrey, K., Allison, T., McKeown, M., & McCarthy, G. (2003). Polysensory interactions along lateral temporal regions evoked by audiovisual speech. *Cerebral Cortex, 13*(10), 1034–1043.

Part V

LANGUAGE PROCESSING

Chapter 10

The Lexicon, Grammar, and the Past Tense: Dissociation Revisited

William D. Marslen-Wilson
MRC Cognition and Brain Sciences Unit, Cambridge, UK

Lorraine K. Tyler
Centre for Speech and Language,
University of Cambridge, UK

In 1997 Liz Bates and Judith Goodman published an important paper entitled "*On the inseparability of grammar and the lexicon.*" This paper, which pulls together decades of work on normal and abnormal development, argues eloquently and persuasively for an "emergentist" view of language. Bates and Goodman argue against the autonomy of grammar, and, more generally, against the view that language learning depends on innate abilities that are specific to language. Instead, they put forward a unified lexicalist approach, whereby language is acquired through processes and learning mechanisms which are not grammar- or language-specific, and where lexical and grammatical development are so strongly interdependent that a modular approach to the acquisition of grammar is simply untenable.

A key part of Bates and Goodman's argument—and the focus of their discussion of language breakdown in brain-injured adults—is the claim that not only does the developmental evidence point towards a non-modular, emergentist approach to language acquisition, but also that there is no compelling evidence for modularity in the adult system (see also Dick, Bates, Wulfeck, Utman, Dronkers, & Gernsbacher, 2001). The facts of language breakdown, they argue, do not demonstrate a convincing dissociation between grammar and the lexicon, leading them to reject the view that these functions are mediated in the adult by separate, dedicated, domain-specific neural systems (Bates & Goodman, 1999, p. 71). Our goal in writing this chapter is to consider the implications of some new evidence for neural dissociations between aspects of linguistic function that also seem to separate grammatical and lexical aspects of the language system.

This evidence comes from a psycholinguistic domain which has also seen very robust debates about the issue of whether there are independent functional and neural levels of grammatical representation which are distinct from other forms of linguistic knowledge, in particular stored lexical representations. This is the continuing set of controversies surrounding the English regular and irregular past tense—its acquisition during language development, and the characterization of its representation in the adult system. Although Bates and Goodman do not discuss this controversy in their 1997 and 1999 papers, and although the rhetoric of the dispute has been somewhat different in emphasis, it shares the same fundamental contrast between domain-general processes required to learn the basic lexicon of the language—involving storage of sound/meaning relationships—and the potentially domain-specific processes required to handle regular inflectional morphology, which are argued to require algorithmic procedures manipulating syntactically organized symbols (for a recent overview see Pinker 1999). The views of Pinker and his colleagues, like the Chomskian accounts under attack by Bates and Goodman, have in common a conception of the specialness of language, where its critical features are indeed domain-specific and almost certainly innate (see also Pinker 1991; 1994). We will start with a brief summary of how the past-tense debate has evolved over the last few decades.

THE PAST-TENSE DEBATE

The English past tense has been center-stage almost from the beginnings of modern cognitivist approaches to language, going back nearly 40 years. The principal reason for this is the clarity of the contrast that it offers between a highly rule-like process—the formation of the regular past tense by adding the affix /-d/ to the verb stem (as in *jump-jumped; sigh-sighed*)—and the unpredictable and idiosyncratic processes of irregular formation (as in *think-thought; make-made*), applying to a small minority of English verbs, where each case seemingly has to be learned and represented separately. This contrast is frequently characterized—most prominently in Pinker's 1999 book—as a contrast between the domain of words (the lexicon) and the domain of rules (the grammar).

During the cognitivist upheavals of the 1960's, the acquisition of these contrasting linguistic components of the English past tense played an important role in establishing the view of mental computation as rule-based manipulation of symbol systems. Children learning English seemed to move from an early stage of rote-learning of individual past tense forms to the induction of rule-based representations, as reflected in over-regularizations such as *goed* and *bringed*. These followed an initial period when *went* and *brought* were used appropriately, and *goed* and *bringed* did not occur. It was argued that these anomalous forms could not be explained in terms of non-cognitive accounts of the acquisition process—for example, through imitation, or through Skinnerian reinforcement procedures—since the child would never be exposed to these forms in the environment. Their occurrence seemed instead to reflect the child's induction of a linguistic rule—in this case, governing the formation of the regular past tense—with the subsequent misapplication of this rule to verbs which had irregular past tenses, and where, crucially, the child had previously used these irregular and highly frequent forms correctly.

This widely accepted argument from acquisition was thrown into doubt by Rumelhart and McClelland's demonstration that a simple connectionist network could apparently simulate the crucial characteristics of the learning sequence attributed to human children (Rumelhart & McClelland, 1986). The network moved from an early period of correct generation of irregular past tense forms to a phase of over-regularization, where these irregular forms were regularized in ways analogous to the child's errors. The network could in no way be said to have learnt a symbolically stated rule. The fact that it could, nonetheless, exhibit seemingly rule-governed behavior, including apparent over-extension of these "rules," proved enormously influential in subsequent attempts to argue for (or against) a view of mental computation as rule-based and symbolic. It has also triggered an extensive and forceful debate.

Without discussing in detail the contents of this debate, it is fair to say that the controversy between connectionist and symbolic accounts of the acquisition process for the English past tense has effectively reached stalemate as far as the observable properties of the process are concerned. Early criticisms of the Rumelhart and McClelland model did pinpoint important flaws in the model, but subsequent work—for example by Plunkett & Marchman (1993)—went a long way to meeting these criticisms. Arguably, both connectionist learning models and accounts in terms of symbolic mechanisms each seem able to account for the qualitative and quantitative properties of the acquisition of the past tense by the human child.

To distinguish the two types of account it became necessary to look, in addition, at other aspects of the mental representation of English regular and irregular past tenses. Attention shifted, accordingly, to the properties of the "end state"—the manner in which regular and irregular forms are mentally represented by the adult native speaker of English. Current views of this have converged on the contrast between a *single mechanism* approach, arguing for a complete account of mental computation in terms of current multi-layer connectionist networks, and a *dual mechanism* approach, arguing that while connectionist accounts may be appropriate for the learning and representation of the irregular forms, a symbolic, rule-based system is required to explain the properties of the regular past tense, and, by extension, the properties of language and cognition in general.

In spirit, at least, these two camps map closely onto the opposing views contrasted by Bates and Goodman. The single mechanism approach shares the crucial assumptions about language function being built out of domain-general processes, the rejection of domain specific modules with specialist processing capacities, and the claim that lexical and syntactic functions are acquired together as expressions of the same general computational process. The converse of these views of course characterizes dual mechanism approaches, where the emphasis on the special computational mechanisms required for rule-based behavior is closely linked to claims about genetic specialization underlying human language (e.g., Pinker, 1994).

DISSOCIATIONS IN PAST-TENSE PERFORMANCE

The relevance of the past-tense debate to the issues discussed by Bates and Goodman is heightened by the strongly neuropsychological turn that the debate has taken over the past five years, with several results pointing to a dissociation of the underlying neural systems required for the production and perception of regular and irregular inflected forms. Patients who typically have damage involving the temporal lobe tend to show poorer performance on the irregulars compared to the regulars in elicitation and reading tasks, while deficits for the regulars are associated with damage to left inferior frontal cortex (LIFG) and underlying structures (Marslen-Wilson & Tyler, 1997; 1998; Miozzo, 2003; Patterson, Lambon Ralph, Hodges & McClelland, 2001; Tyler, de Mornay Davies, Anokhina, Longworth, Randall & Marslen-Wilson, 2002; Ullman, Corkin, Coppola, Hickok, Growdon, Koroshetz & Pinker, 1997). This has been shown in a variety of neuropsychological studies probing the comprehension and production of the regular and irregular past tense (Marslen-Wilson & Tyler, 1997; Ullman et al, 1997; Tyler et al, 2002a).

Studies of production show that patients with damage to the LIFG have difficulty in producing regularly inflected words in elicitation tasks (Ullman et al., 1997), while their performance on irregularly inflected forms is relatively normal. Studies of comprehension of the past tense have used a priming paradigm to compare the processing of regularly and irregularly inflected verbs. Patients with damage to the LIFG do not show the normal pattern of morphological priming for the regulars, in prime-target pairs like *jumped/jump*, even though the irregulars, as in pairs like *gave/give*, prime normally (Marslen-Wilson & Tyler, 1997; 1998; Tyler et al., 2002a).

Lexical access from regularly inflected forms seems generally disrupted for these patients. Pairs like *jumped/leap* fail to elicit significant semantic priming effects, even though the uninflected stems (*jump/leap*) prime normally (Longworth, Marslen-Wilson & Tyler, 2001).

These neuropsychological dissociations have been interpreted in two different ways, which again link directly to the concerns of Bates and her colleagues. Given the key assumption of single mechanism accounts, that both types of past tense forms are processed by a uniform system where different morphological types are handled by the same underlying process, the existence of plausible and replicable evidence for dissociation seems to present a serious challenge. Like Bates and Goodman (1997; 1999), single mechanism theorists in the past-tense domain regard separability of linguistic function over different neural regions as potentially damaging evidence against their theoretical position. Not surprisingly, dual mechanism theorists regard evidence for dissociation as confirmation that distinct underlying systems are engaged by regular and irregular forms (e.g., Pinker & Ullman, 2002; Ullman, 2001).

In an influential response to this challenge, Joanisse & Seidenberg (1999) have proposed a single mechanism model capable of exhibiting dissociative behavior for regular and irregular English morphology (see also McClelland & Patterson, 2002). Dissociations in past tense performance following damage to the brain are explained in terms of the differential reliance of regulars and irregulars on the contributions, respectively, of phonology and of semantics. Selective deficits for the irregulars occur as a by-product of damage to the semantic system, while selective deficits for the regulars are caused by an impairment to the phonological system.

The value of the kind of account put forward by Joannisse and Seidenberg is not only that it reminds us that differences in behavioral outcome do not necessarily reflect corresponding underlying differences in the structure of the system, but also that it puts the theoretical cards of connectionist single system accounts very firmly on the empirical table. The way in which the model explains regular/irregular dissociations makes strong empirical predictions. As we will argue below, these predictions seem to fail, with wider ramifications for the kind of approach exemplified by this type of model.

Joannisse and Seidenberg (1999) propose a multi-level connectionist learning model in which the representation and processing of regular and irregular English inflected forms is modeled in terms of their speech input, speech output, and semantics. The critical property of this model, from the perspective of explaining dissociation, is the differential reliance of the regulars and irregulars on the contribution of phonology and semantics in the learning process. The representation in the network of the mapping between stems and their regular past tense forms (e.g. *open—opened*) is primarily driven by the phonological relationship between them, since this relationship is entirely predictable. The equivalent mapping for the irregulars (e.g. *think-thought*) is more dependent on the semantic relationship between the stem and its past tense form, since the phonological relationship between them is much less uniform and predictable. This leads to the prediction that relatively selective deficits for the regulars will be caused by a phonological impairment, whereas deficits for the irregulars should be a by-product of damage to the semantic system.

To test these predictions, Joanisse & Seidenberg (1999) trained the model on simulations of speaking, hearing, repeating and generating the past tense, where all these input/output mappings pass through the same set of hidden units. They then lesioned the network in specific ways to determine whether this would have differential effects on the regulars or irregulars. When the speech output layer was lesioned, modeling an acquired phonological deficit, this affected past tense generation performance on nonwords and—at very severe levels of lesioning—on the regular past tense verbs. Lesioning the semantic layer modeled a semantic deficit, after which the model performed most poorly at generating irregular past tenses. By the same token, although this was not explicitly discussed in the 1999 paper, lesioning the speech input layer should allow the system to model deficits in speech comprehension, on the same phonological basis. Whether viewed from the perspective of comprehension or of production, in neither case is there any explicit morphological differentiation between regular and irregular forms; the differences between them reflect the relative balance between semantic and phonological factors during the acquisition phase of the network. Since the same mechanism is claimed to underlie the processing of regular and irregular verb morphology, this type of model is consistent with the broader Bates and Goodman claim that grammatical and lexical phenomena share the same substrate.

Leaving aside the question of how well the specific performance of the Joannisse & Seidenberg model actually matches observed patient performance, this type of model makes strong predictions about the basis of deficits for the regulars and irregulars in brain-damaged populations. Turning first to the predictions concerning the regulars, the model claims (a) that patients who have problems with the regular past tense will have an accompanying phonological deficit, and (b) patients who have a phonological deficit will also have problems with the regular past tense. Two studies that we have recently reported seem to conflict with both of these claims, as well as the corollary claims that the model makes about the role of phonological complexity in explaining poor performance on the regulars.

We find that patients with LIFG damage and difficulties with regular inflection do not have equivalent problems with uninflected words that are phonologically matched to regular past tense forms (Tyler et al., 2002b). In this latter study, patients were significantly impaired on same/different judgements to pairs of words containing regular past tense forms (as in *played/play*). These problems with the regulars could not be attributed to purely phonological factors, since the patients performed significantly better on pseudo-regular word-pairs (*trade/tray*) that were phonologically matched to the regular past tense pairs but were not themselves inflected forms. Furthermore, degree of impairment on the regular inflected forms, whether in this phonological judgement task or in priming tasks (Longworth et al., 2001; Marslen-Wilson & Tyler, 1997; 1998; Tyler et al., 2002b), does not seem to be correlated with degree of phonological impairment. Patients who are almost normal in standard tests of phonological performance can exhibit equivalent deficits in processing regular inflection to patients with very poor performance on these tests (Tyler et al., 2002b).

Turning now towards the claims made by single mechanism accounts for the basis of deficits for the irregulars, the critical association predicted by the Joannisse and Seidenberg model is that neuropsychological patients who have semantic deficits will necessarily have disproportionate problems with the irregulars. While it is true that many patients with semantic deficits have accompanying problems with the irregulars (Marslen-Wilson & Tyler, 1997; 1998; Tyler et al., 2002; Patterson et al., 2001), there are also patients who do not show this dissociation (Tyler et al., 2003). Using both priming tasks and elicitation tasks, we have recently shown that some semantic dementia patients (who have progressive temporal lobe damage resulting in semantic deficits) show normal priming for the irregular past tense and do not have a disproportionate problem with the irregulars in an elicitation task (Tyler et al., 2003). This is despite the fact that these are patients who have profound semantic deficits, as reflected in all standard tests of semantic function. The predicted other side of the association—that patients who have problems with the irregulars should also have a semantic deficit—appears to be disconfirmed by recent data from a patient who has a clear deficit for the irregulars, as measured by poor performance on a variety of different tests, but who has no detectable semantic deficit (Miozzo, 2003). Taken together, these sets of results demonstrate that semantic deficits do not necessarily go hand-in-hand with difficulties in producing or comprehending irregularly inflected past tense forms.

In summary, closer examination of the patient populations that exhibit regular/irregular dissociations does not come up with the critical set of linked deficits predicted by current single mechanism accounts of the source of these dissociations. Problems with the regular morphology can be dissociated from phonological impairment and phonological complexity, while there does not seem to be an obligatory causal link between semantic competency and performance with irregular past tense forms. This, in turn, suggests that the observed regular/irregular dissociations do reflect underlying differences in the functional specializations of different areas of the brain. To assess the implications of this, however, for the Bates and Goodman emergentist and lexicalist project, we need first to consider what these data are telling us about the likely structure of the cortical language system.

FRONTO-TEMPORAL INTERACTIONS
IN HUMAN LANGUAGE FUNCTION

The classic dual mechanism account, as developed by Pinker, Ullman and colleagues (Pinker, 1991; Prasada & Pinker, 1993; Ullman et al., 1997; Pinker & Ullman, 2002; Ullman, 2001), claimed that a specific rule-based system processes the regulars by adding and stripping away inflectional affixes from their stems. The irregulars, in contrast, are learned individually by rote and stored in a separate knowledge store. On this view, past tense dissociations are explained in terms of selective damage to either the rule-based system or to the store of lexical representations. In these terms, evidence for neural dissociation is clearly inconsistent both with single mechanism accounts of the English past tense and with the Bates & Goodman arguments against specialized sub-systems supporting grammatical function.

We have recently proposed a modified version of a dual route account which places less emphasis on the regularity/irregularity distinction *per se*—and its associated theoretical baggage—and more emphasis on the role of morphophonological parsing processes which allow the segmentation and identification of stems and affixes (Marslen-Wilson & Tyler, 1998; 2003; Tyler et al., 2002a; Tyler, Randall & Marslen-Wilson, 2002b). These processes, associated with LIFG, are required for the analysis of regularly inflected forms in English, with their stem + affix structure, but do not apply to English irregular past tense forms. These have no overt morphophonological structure and must be accessed as whole forms. On this account, deficits for the regulars arise when there is disruption of morphophonological parsing processes, associated with damage to the LIFG, whereas deficits for the irregulars stem from damage to temporal lobe structures supporting access from phonological input to representations of stored lexical form.

These proposals can be linked more generally to claims about the overall neural and functional architecture of the human language system, almost all of which have in common an emphasis on language-relevant processing structures in superior temporal and inferior frontal areas, and their linkage into a fronto-temporal network. The origins of these claims lie in the 19th century Broca-Wernicke-Lichtheim framework, where disorders of comprehension were associated with superior temporal lobe damage ("Wernicke's area"), while problems in language production—so-called telegraphic speech, for example—were associated with damage to Broca's area in frontal cortex. More subtle aphasic deficits were analyzed in terms of damage to connections between these areas, thought to be primarily mediated by the arcuate fasciculus, running posterior from Wernicke's area and looping round to connect to inferior frontal structures.

More recently, these types of account have been restated in a more anatomically and neurophysiologically explicit framework, deriving from work on the primate auditory system (e.g., Rauschecker & Tian, 2000). Rauschecker and colleagues have proposed an analysis of the functional organization of primate audition in terms of the dorsal/ventral distinction already established for primate vision, with a "ventral" system running anteriorly down the temporal lobe from primary auditory cortex to connect to inferior frontal areas, and a "dorsal" system running posteriorly into the temporo-parietal junction and then forward to connect to a different set of frontal lobe structures. A number of proposals have begun to emerge for the interpretation of human speech and language systems in this general framework (e.g., Hickok & Poeppel, 2000; Scott & Johnsrude, 2003). These have in common the assumption that ventral pathways in the left temporal lobe are involved in the mapping from phonology onto semantics, but put forward divergent views of the nature and function of the dorsal pathways.

In recent publications (Tyler et al., 2002a; 2002b) we have proposed a possible relationship between the global dorsal/ventral distinction and the evidence for processing and neurological dissociations involving the English regular and irregular past tenses. The ventral system, on this account, involves temporal lobe structures that mediate access (both phonological and orthographic) to stored lexical representations. The dorsal pathway links *via* the arcuate fasciculus to systems in L inferior frontal areas important for the analysis and production of complex morphophonological sequences. The language-specific properties of the English past tense would therefore map differentially onto these two systems, with irregular forms linking into ventral systems optimized for access to stored whole forms, while regular forms require in addition the involvement of frontal systems supporting processes of phonological assembly and disassembly.

In recent research we have taken forward this emerging account of the human speech and language system, using event related fMRI in the intact brain to investigate more directly the neural systems underlying the processing of regular and irregular morphology. To do this we use the same-different judgement task whose sensitivity to critical inflectional variables was previously demonstrated in research on patients with LIFG damage (Tyler et al., 2002b). The pattern of performance shown by these patients indicated that the processing of regular past tense pairs depended on brain regions that were damaged in this patient population. By running the same task on normal participants in an fMRI study, we were able to activate the full range of neural regions engaged in the processing of regular past tense inflection in the intact system, as well as illuminating their relationship to the language system as a whole.

The results confirmed, first, that regular and irregular past tenses in English differentially activate the cortical language system in the intact brain, and that these differences cannot straightforwardly be reduced to lower-level phonological factors (Tyler, Stamatakis, Post, Randall & Marslen-Wilson, 2003). The critical factor seems to be the presence of an overt inflectional affix, attached to a real-word verb stem. Second, the results make it clear that we are dealing with an extended fronto-temporal network, and that the additional demands made by regular inflected forms extend not only to LIFG structures, but also to the superior temporal lobes, and to mid-line regions in the anterior cingulate. This connected system of sites is clearly related to the classical Broca-Wernicke system in traditional neuropsychology, and to the dorsal route in more recent accounts. We now turn to a consideration of the possible functional interpretation of this fronto-temporal network, and why processes involving the regular past tense should be differentially affected when the LIFG is damaged.

Both neuropsychological and neuroimaging data associate superior temporal regions, especially on the left, with the access of lexical form and meaning from the phonological input (e.g., Kertesz, Lau & Polk, 1993). In the neuropsychological literature, the focus has been specifically on the role of 'Wernicke's area'—the posterior regions of the superior temporal gyrus (STG)—in spoken language comprehension. This region has been claimed to store 'the memory images of speech sounds' (Wernicke, 1874), with connections between Wernicke's area and other cortical regions (temporal and frontal) enabling access to both meaning and speech production Lichtheim (1885). In support of the view that this region is specifically involved in the processing of speech, neuroanatomical studies have shown that posterior STG is larger in the left hemisphere, suggesting a major role in speech processing (Geschwind & Levitsky, 1968), and patients with LH damage in this region typically have spoken language comprehension deficits (e.g., Kertesz, 1981; Damasio, 1992). It is important to note, however, as Saygin, Dick, Wilson, Dronkers, & Bates (2003) have recently reminded us, that the critical role of these structures in speech processing does not mean that they are uniquely dedicated to language functions. They also play an important role in processing and interpreting nonverbal auditory information, such as environmental sounds.

Neuroimaging studies typically find that speech processing activates broad regions of bilateral STG (Crinion et al, 2003; Davis & Johnsrude, 2003; Scott et al, 2000). In our own imaging study we found that speech (words and non-words) activates the same extensive region of STG, extending both anteriorly and posteriorly from Heschl's gyrus, as has been reported in previous studies (e.g., Scott et al, 2000; Binder et al, 2000). Within this region, the regularly inflected verbs produce significantly enhanced activation in bilateral STG compared to the irregulars. In the left hemisphere, the greater activation for the regulars compared to the irregulars is centered on Wernicke's area, with the peak activations close to those reported in other imaging studies which have explored the neural underpinnings of speech processing (e.g., Wise at al, 2001; Binder et al, 2000).

These results show that, while the exact function of the posterior STG in speech processing and spoken language comprehension is unresolved, it is clear that it plays an important role in the mapping of speech inputs onto stored representations of word meaning, and that it is particularly active during the processing of regular inflected forms. This is the basis for the first component of our analysis, which assumes that the primary process of lexical access—of mapping from acoustic-phonetic input to lexical semantic representations—is mediated by superior temporal lobe systems, possibly bilaterally, linking to other areas of the temporal lobe.

The second component of our analysis is the claim that regular inflected forms, such as *jumped*, are not well-formed inputs to this mapping process, and that the intervention of inferior frontal systems is required for the access process to flow smoothly. Although *jump*, or any other stem form, can map straightforwardly onto lexical representations, the presence of the affix (t) makes it transiently a "non-word"—in the same way, perhaps, that the addition of a (t) to the form *clan* would produce the sequence *clant* which is not a well-formed input to the access process.

To interpret *jumped* correctly, and to allow the process of lexical access to proceed normally, the past tense affix needs to be recognized, and reassigned to a different linguistic function. This process requires an intact LIFG, and intact links to left superior temporal cortex. Note that irregular past tense forms, which are never realized as an unchanged stem plus an affix, are not subject to the same additional processing requirement. They are assumed to be accessed as whole forms, exploiting the same temporal lobe systems as uninflected stems.

The clearest evidence for this functional interpretation comes from the priming results recently reported by Longworth et al (2001), showing that patients with LIFG damage, and difficulties with regular inflectional morphology, show deficits not only in morphological priming (i.e., between *jumped* and *jump*; Marslen-Wilson & Tyler, 1997; Tyler et al., 2002a) but also in semantic priming when the primes are regularly inflected forms, as in pairs like *jumped/ leap*. At the same time, critically, they show normal performance both for pairs with stems as primes, as in *jump/leap*, and for pairs where the prime is an irregular past tense form, as in *slept/doze*.

Normal semantic priming performance in these auditory-auditory paired priming tasks, where a spoken prime (e.g., *jump*) is immediately followed by a spoken target (e.g., *leap*), requires rapid access to lexical semantic representations in the processing of both prime and target. The patients' preserved performance for stem and irregular spoken primes shows that the systems supporting fast access of meaning from speech are still intact for these types of input—either through remaining functionality in left temporal lobes, or through right temporal processes. This means that, to explain the decrement in performance on the regular inflected forms, we have to attribute different properties to these inflected forms than to stem or irregular forms, and look for damage elsewhere in the brain that could be the source of these difficulties.

This brings us to the role of left inferior frontal areas, which are strongly associated with the processing of grammatical morphemes, and with syntactic function more generally (Zurif, 1995; Caplan, Alpert, & Waters, 1998; Just, Carpenter, Keller, Eddy, & Thulborn, 1996). Neuropsychological studies associate damage to inferior frontal regions, especially BA 44 and 45 (Broca's area) with both syntactic and morphological deficits (Miceli & Caramazza, 1988; Marslen-Wilson & Tyler, 1997, 1998; Tyler, 1992). A number of neuroimaging studies investigating spoken sentence comprehension have reported significant activations in BA 44 for syntactic processing, which overlap with the activations that we find in the current study for the regulars compared to the irregulars (e.g., Embick et al., 2000; Friederici, Opitz, & von Cramon, 2000). There is also evidence from a number of sources for LIFG involvement in processes of phonological segmentation (e.g., Burton et al., 2000; Zatorre et al., 1992).

Both inferior frontal and superior temporal areas will be involved in the analysis of forms like *played*, which require the simultaneous access of the lexical content associated with the stem *play* (primarily mediated by temporal lobe systems), and of the grammatical implications of the {-d} morpheme (primarily mediated by inferior frontal systems). Unless these different components of the word-form are assigned to their appropriate processing destinations, effective on-line processing of such forms is disrupted, as demonstrated in the priming studies mentioned earlier (Longworth et al., 2001; Marslen-Wilson & Tyler, 1997; Tyler et al., 2002a). In contrast, for irregular forms like *gave* or *bought*, no such on-line differentiation is either required or possible. Patients with LIFG damage do not have problems with the irregulars, suggesting that their processing does not necessitate the involvement of this region (Tyler et al., 2002a,b). Access for words like *gave* is mediated, as a whole form, through temporal lobe systems, and does not require segmentation into phonologically separate stem and affix components (Marslen-Wilson & Tyler, 1998). Thus, although irregular past tense forms will activate LIFG to some extent—for example, because of the syntactic implications of their grammatical properties—immediate access to lexical meaning does not obligatorily require LIFG phonological parsing functions in the same way as regular past tense forms.

On this emerging account, the increased activation for regulars in temporal and inferior frontal areas reflects, on the one hand, the specialized LIFG processes involved in analyzing grammatical morphemes, and on the other the continuing STG activity involved in accessing lexical representations from the stems of regular inflected forms. Although the exact nature of LIFG function is still unclear (and may be quite diverse), the area seems to be critically involved in supporting both morphophonological parsing—the segmentation of complex forms into stems and affixes—and the syntactic processes triggered by the presence of grammatical morphemes such as the past tense marker.

In a further refinement of this emerging model, we suggest that the processing relationship between L frontal and temporal regions is modulated by anterior midline structures including the anterior cingulate, which both neuroanatomical and functional neuro-imaging evidence suggest is well suited for this role. The anterior cingulate projects to or receives connections from most regions of frontal cortex (Barbas, 1995) and from superior temporal cortex (Petrides & Pandya, 1981), while recent neuro-imaging data implicate the ACC in the modulation of fronto-temporal integration (e.g., Fletcher, McKenna, Friston, Frith, & Dolan, 1999).

IMPLICATIONS

To summarize these proposals, we argue that the fronto-temporal neural system involved in language processing is critically involved in the on-line process of separating the speech input into complementary processing streams, on the one hand extracting information about meaning, conveyed by uninflected nouns and verb stems, such as *house* or *stay*, and on the other information about grammatical structure, conveyed in part by inflectional morphemes such as the past tense {-d}. These proposals point to a more specific and dynamic account of how aspects of language function are organized in the human brain, and provide a functional framework within which to interpret behavioral and neuropsychological differences in the processing of English regular and irregular past tense forms.

The core issue raised by these claims, in the current context, is the strong position they take on the differentiation of language function across different neural areas. We interpret evidence for dissociation as indeed being evidence that different areas of the brain can make different types of contribution to the functioning of the language system, and that these contributions can have a specifically linguistic character that is not reducible simply to phonological or semantic processes and their interaction. This is clearly contrary to the claims of the predominant single mechanism account in the past tense debate. However, it does not necessarily provide strong support to the converse view—the classical dual mechanism approach as stated by Pinker, Ullman, and others. The results we report, and our interpretation of them, are arguably neutral with respect to many of the most prominent theoretical issues in this domain, especially those concerning specific differences in types of mental computation, the modularity and domain-specificity of the different systems involved, and the extent to which these differences are directly genetically specified. Some or all of these may, conceivably, turn out be true of the fronto-temporal contributors to language processing, but there is little in the current data that directly addresses these issues. For example, to claim, as we and many others have done, that there is a critical role for superior temporal areas in the mapping of phonological inputs onto lexical representations, is not to exclude the possibility that these same regions also serve other cognitive functions (c.f., Saygin et al, 2003, as discussed earlier). In other words, to assign a function to a given area is not necessarily to claim domain specificity for that area.

In terms of the Bates and Goodman (1997, 1999) proposals, our analysis does seem to be inconsistent with their view that processing difficulties in aphasic patients with receptive agrammatism (Broca's aphasics) do not have any specific localization implications. Aphasic patients' deficits, for example, in the processing of grammatical morphemes, are argued not to reflect damage to specific neural subsystems, but rather the sensitivity of these morphological operations to any source of degradation in the global functioning of the relevant brain areas (Dick et al., 2001). Neurologically intact normal populations, including both elderly controls and college students, can be shown to exhibit patterns of deficit comparable to aphasic patients when required to process spoken utterances under conditions of perceptual and cognitive stress (e.g., low-pass filtering of the speech accompanied by a digit memory task). This is argued to support a distributive model of language in the brain, where language functions are distributed over several cooperating areas, rather than having any specific locus.

Our proposals, however, suggest that this view should not be taken too far. Of course language is instantiated in the brain as a distributed system, but this does not mean that specific functions may not depend on specific areas, and on the links between them, so that damage to a given subnetwork can lead to specific functional deficits. The possibility of simulating aspects of these deficits by degrading performance in unimpaired populations does not in itself, in our view, permit the inference that therefore there is no specific substrate to the performance of the linguistic processing function at issue.

More broadly, however, we see no inconsistency between our proposals here and the general emergentist and lexicalist approach to language in the brain proposed by Bates and her colleagues. As we understand current statements of this approach, it in no way excludes—and indeed seems to predict—an adult brain with highly differentiated assignments of processing functions to particular dynamic combinations of brain areas (e.g., Bates, 1999; Elman, Bates, Johnson, Karmiloff-Smith, Parisi, and Plunkett, 1996). As these authors have convincingly argued, our current understanding of the biology of neural maturation points to a process whereby cortical function differentiates during development as the result of a subtle interplay between phylogeny and ontogeny. The basic sensorimotor wiring of the brain may be genetically specified, but the way in which complex cognitive functions are recruited to different brain systems will reflect an interaction between the demands of particular kinds of processing operations and the properties of the areas being projected to.

The critical challenge for a future cognitive neuroscience of language will be to flesh out this vision of the functional and neural properties of the human language system, and of its developmental trajectory. To do this we will need to specify in detail, at multiple levels of description, what the specific functional characteristics of the system are, how they give rise to the particular, detailed properties of speech comprehension and production, and how these functional characteristics themselves flow from the properties of the neural systems underlying them. In this context, evidence for differentiation of function in the adult brain is in no way evidence *per se* against an emergentist view. Rather, it is part of the process of moving from very general questions about human language systems—modular/non-modular, domain general/domain specific, and so forth—to a specific program of investigation of the underlying scientific facts of the matter. One of the beacons that will help to guide us in this enterprise will undoubtedly be the pioneering work of Liz Bates and her colleagues.

ACKNOWLEDGMENTS

The research described here was supported by the UK Medical Research Council, including an MRC program grant held by LKT.

REFERENCES

Barbas, H. (1995). Anatomic basis of cognitive-emotional interactions in the primate prefrontal cortex. *Neuroscience and Biobehavioral Reviews, 19*(3), 499–510.

Bates, E. (1999). Plasticity, localization and language development. In S. H. Broman & J. M. Fletcher (Eds.), *The changing nervous system: Neurobehavioral consequences of early brain disorders* (pp. 214–253). New York: Oxford University Press.

Bates, E., & Goodman, J. (1997). On the inseparability of grammar and the lexicon: Evidence from acquisition, aphasia and real-time processing. *Language and Cognitive Processes, 12*(5–6), 507–584.

Bates, E., & Goodman, J. (1999). On the emergence of grammar from the lexicon. In B. MacWhinney (Ed.) *The emergence of language*. Mahwah, NJ: Lawrence Erlbaum Associates.

Binder, J. R., Frost, T. A., Hammeke, P. S. F., Bellgowan, P. S. F., Springer, J. A., Kaufman J. N., & Possing, E. T. (2000). Human temporal lobe activation by speech and nonspeech sounds. *Cerebral Cortex, 10*, 512–528.

Burton, M., Small, S., & Blumstein, S. (2000). The role of segmentation in phonological processing: An fMRI Investigation. *J Cognitive Neuroscience, 12*, 679–90.

Caplan, D., Alpert, N., & Waters, G. (1998). Effects of syntactic structure and propositional number on patterns of regional cerebral blood flow. *J Cognitive Neuroscience, 10*, 541–552.

Crinion, J., Lambon-Ralph, M. A., Warburton, E., Howard, D., & Wise, R. (2003). Temporal lobe regions engaged during normal speech comprehension. *Brain, 126*, 1193–1201.

Damasio, A. (1992) Aphasia. *New England Journal of Medicine, 326*, 531–539.

Davis, M., & Johnsrude, I. (2003). Hierarchical processing in spoken language comprehension. *J. Neuroscience, 23*(8), 3431–3423.

Dick, F., Bates, E., Wulfeck, B., Utman, J. A., Dronkers, N., & Gernsbacher, M. A. (2001). Language deficits, localization, and grammar. *Psychological Review, 108*, 759–788.

Dronkers, N., Redfern, B., & Knight, R. (2000). The neural architecture of language disorders. In MS Gazzaniga (Ed.) *The New Cognitive Neurosciences*, MIT Press.

Elman, J. L., Bates, E., Johnson, M. H., Karmiloff-Smith, A., Parisi, D., & Plunkett, K. (1996). *Rethinking innateness: A connectionist perspective on development*. Cambridge, MA: MIT Press.

Embick, D., Marantz, A., Miyashita, Y., O'Neill, W., & Sakai, K. (2000). A syntactic specialization for Broca's area. *Proceedings of the National Academy of Sciences, 97*(11), 6150–6154.

Fletcher, P. J., McKenna, K. J., Friston, C. D., Frith, & Dolan, R. J. (1999). Abnormal cingulate modulation of fronto-temporal connectivity in schizophrenia. *Neuroimage, 9*(3), 337–342.

Friederici, A., Opitz, B., & von Cramon, Y. (2000). Segregating semantic and syntactic aspects of processing in the human brain: an fMRI investigation of different word types. *Cerebral Cortex, 10*, 698–705.

Geschwind. N., & Levitsky, W (1968). Human brain: Left-right asymmetries in temporal speech region. *Science, 161*, 186–187

Hickok, G., & Poeppel, D. (2000). Towards a functional neuroanatomy of speech perception. *Trends in Cognitive Sciences, 4*(4), 131–138.

Joanisse, M., & Seidenberg, M. (1999). Impairments in verb morphology after brain injury. *Proceedings of the National Academy of Sciences, 96*, 7592–7.

Just, M., Carpenter, P. A., Keller, T. A., Eddy, W. F., & Thulborn, R. (1996). Brain Activation Modulated by Sentence Comprehension. *Science, 274*, 114–116.

Kertesz, A. (1981) Anatomy of jargon. In J. Brown (Ed.). *Jargonaphasia*. New York: Academic Press.

Kertesz, A., Lau, W. K. & Polk, M. (1993). The structural determinants of recovery in Wernicke's aphasia. *Brain & Language, 44*, 153–164.

Longworth, C. E., Randall, B., Tyler, L. K. & Marslen-Wilson, W. D. (2001). Activating Verb Semantics from the Regular and Irregular Past Tense. In J. Moore (Ed.), *Proceedings of the 23rd Annual Conference of the Cognitive Science Society* (pp. 570–575). Mahwah, NJ: Lawrence Erlbaum Associates.

Marslen-Wilson, W. D., & Tyler, L. K. (1997). Dissociating types of mental computation. *Nature, 387*, 592–594.

Marslen-Wilson, W. D., & Tyler, L. K. (1998). Rules, representations, and the English past tense. *Trends in Cognitive Science, 2*, 428–435.

McClelland, J., & Patterson, K. (2002). Rules or connections in past-tense inflections: what does the evidence rule out? *Trends in Cognitive Sciences, 6*(11), 465–472.

Miceli, G., & Caramazza, A. (1988). Dissociation of inflectional and derivational morphology. *Brain & Language, 35*, 24–65.

Miozzo, M. (2003). On the processing of regular and irregular forms of verbs and nouns: Evidence from neuropsychology. *Cognition, 87*(2), 101–127.

Petrides, M., & Pandaya, D. E. N. (1988). Association fiber pathways to the frontal cortex from the superior temporal region in the rhesus monkey. *Journal of Comparative Neurology, 273,* 52–66,

Plunkett, K., & Marchman, V. A. (1993). From rote learning to system building: Acquiring verb morphology in children and connectionist nets. *Cognition, 48,* 21–69.

Pinker, S. (1991). Rules of language. *Science, 253,* 530–535.

Pinker, S. (1994). *The language instinct.* New York: HarperCollins.

Pinker, S. (1999). *Words and rules: the ingredients of language.* New York: HarperCollins.

Pinker, S., & Ullman, M. (2002). The past and future of the past tense. *Trends in Cognitive Sciences, 6*(11), 456–463

Prasada, S., & Pinker, S. (1993). Generalizations of regular and irregular morphological patterns. *Language and Cognitive Processes, 8,* 1–56.

Rauschecker, JP & Tian, B (2000). Mechanisms and streams for processing of 'what' and 'where' in auditory cortex. *Proc Natl Acad Sci USA, 97,* 11800–11806

Rumelhart, D. E., & McClelland, J. L. (1986). On learning the past tense of English verbs. In McClelland, J. L. & Rumelhart, D. E. (Eds.), *Parallel distributed processing* (pp. 217–270). Cambridge: MIT Press.

Saygun, A. P., Dick, F., Wilson, S. W., Dronkers, N. F., & Bates, E. (2003). Neural resources for processing language and environmental sounds. *Brain, 126,* 928–945.

Scott, S., Blank, C., Rosen, S., & Wise, R. (2000). Identification of a pathway for intelligible speech in the left temporal lobe. *Brain, 123,* 2400–2406.

Scott, S., & Johnsrude, I. (2003). The organization and functional organization of speech perception. *Trends in Neurosciences, 26*(2), 100–107.

Tyler, L. K. (1992). *Spoken language comprehension: An experimental approach to normal and disordered processing.* MIT Press; Cambridge, Mass. 1992

Tyler, L. K., de Mornay Davies, P., Anokhina, R., Longworth, C., Randall, B., Marslen-Wilson, W. D. (2002a). Dissociations in processing past tense morphology: Neuropathology and behavioral studies. *Journal of Cognitive Neuroscience, 14*(1), 79–95.

Tyler, L. K., Randall, B., & Marslen-Wilson, W. D. (2002b). Phonology and neuropsychology of the English past tense. *Neuropsychologia, 40,* 1154–1166.

Tyler, L. K., Stamatakis, E. A., Post, B., Randall, B., & Marslen-Wilson, W. D. (2003). *Differentiation in the neural architecture for spoken language: An fMRI study of past tense processing.* Manuscript, Center for Speech and Language, University of Cambridge.

Ullman, M. T. (2001). The declarative/procedural model of lexicon and grammar. *Journal of Psycholinguistic Research, 30,* 37–69.

Ullman, M. T., Corkin, S., Coppola, M., Hickok, G., Growdon, J. H., Koroshetz, W. J., Pinker, S. (1997). A neural dissociation within language: Evidence that the mental dictionary is part of declarative memory and that grammatical rules are processed by the procedural system. *J Cognitive Neuroscience, 9,* 266–76.

Wernicke, C. (1874). *Der Aphasische Symptomenkomplex, eine Psychologische studie auf anatomischer basis.* Cohn & Weigert, Breslau.

Wise, R., Scott, S., Blank, C., Mummery, C., Murphy, K., & Warburton, E. (2001). Separate neural systems within "Wernicke's area." *Brain, 124,* 83–95.

Zatorre, R. J., Evans, A. C., Meyer, E., Gjedde, A. (1992). Lateralization of phonetic and pitch discrimination in speech processing. *Science, 256,* 846–849.

Zurif, E. B. (1995). In L. Gleitman & M. Liberman (Eds.), *Invitation to Cognitive Science.* Cambridge, MA: MIT Press.

Chapter 11

Perceptual and Attentional Factors in Language Comprehension: A Domain-General Approach

Jennifer Aydelott
Birkbeck College,
University of London, UK

Marta Kutas
University of California, San Diego

Kara D. Federmeier
Beckman Institute,
University of Illinois at Champaign–Urbana

INTRODUCTION

Does language possess its own distinct set of processing mechanisms, or does it share mechanisms with other cognitive processes? Traditional symbolic models of language comprehension have assumed a set of distinct processing components within a modular system (e.g., the lexicon or grammar), each subserving a language-specific function and operating on language-specific information and representations (e.g., Fodor, 1983; Grodzinsky, 1995a, 1995b, 2000; Pinker, 1994; Pinker & Ullman, 2002). According to such models, the mechanisms responsible for language comprehension are essentially separate and distinct from the mechanisms responsible for other cognitive processes, and do not share general resources with them. Further, the operation of domain-specific processing modules is thought to be impenetrable to attention and cognitive control, as well as to sources of information outside of the symbol system of that particular module (Fodor, 1983; Pylyshyn, 1980, 1984). Such models assume a static base of linguistic knowledge—i.e., linguistic competence—which is associated with distinct neural structures and may therefore be selectively disrupted by localized brain injury (Fodor, 1983). The apparent dissociations among various language impairments observed in patients with brain damage has been offered as evidence in favor of domain-specific models, in particular the frequently cited separation of lexical-semantic and grammatical processing in certain aphasic patients (e.g., Pinker & Ullman, 1994; Ullman, 2001).

Distributive models of language comprehension have offered an alternative to the domain-specific approach. According to such models, linguistic representations are acquired and modified in both the short and long term, by means of learning mechanisms that operate across all cognitive domains, not just language (Elman, Bates, Johnson, Karmiloff-Smith, Parisi, & Plunkett, 1996). As opposed to a static, localized knowledge base, under a domain-general approach, linguistic representations (which may themselves be modality-specific) are dynamic and distributed, and are routinely subject to multiple influences and to the operation of both perceptual and higher-level cognitive processes. Thus, domain-general models have called into question the utility/validity of the distinction between competence and performance in language processing, and the characterization of language disorders in terms of damage to discrete, language-specific processing modules.

This perspective makes a number of predictions about the nature of language comprehension in normal and language-impaired populations. Rather than being restricted to a set of specialized neural substrates, language comprehension processes should engage multiple distributed brain areas, which may be involved in a variety of cognitive functions that are not specific to language. Moreover, this processing network should reflect the influence of perceptual input in the formation of higher-level linguistic representations, as well as the role of domain-general processes in activating, selecting, and maintaining these representations in the process of language comprehension. It is also possible within this theoretical framework to formulate a processing account of normal language comprehension in terms of the activation of linguistic representations on the basis of sensory input, the construction of higher-level meaning from these active representations, and the integration of subsequent input with this meaning. According to this approach, then, these aspects of language comprehension draw upon processing mechanisms, shared by other cognitive functions, such as working memory and attentional control, with the nature and accessibility of the resulting higher-level representations changing over time in response to changes in the input.

Such an account of language processing allows for the characterization of language disorders in terms of disruptions or limitations in the processing resources that are necessary to access linguistic representations and to construct higher-level meanings, rather than in terms of the disintegration or loss of the representations themselves. On this account, dissociations of apparent 'language-specific' processes may emerge merely because different aspects of language comprehension critically depend upon different sources of information and different types of processing (for instance, some aspects of comprehension will be most dependent upon the assimilation of perceptual information, others upon attentional control, others upon working memory), and not because of damage to specific language modules. Indeed, detailed investigation of the nature of language disorders from a domain-general perspective reveals that such dissociations are not as specific as has been previously suggested, and in fact may be more easily accounted for in terms of a general processing model.

If this characterization of language disorders is correct, then it should be possible to induce similar 'domain-specific' language deficits in neurologically intact individuals by imposing various processing or capacity limits on normal processing. This view predicts that when unimpaired individuals are subjected to domain-general cognitive stress in the form of perceptual degradation, increased attentional demand, or reduced processing time, language processing may be disrupted in ways that mirror the various dissociations observed in language-disordered populations. In any case, investigating the effects of cognitive stress is likely to help clarify the specific role of perceptual and attentional factors in various aspects of normal language processing.

This chapter will present evidence that is compatible with a domain-general processing approach to language comprehension. To this end, we will examine one aspect of language comprehension, the processing of lexical-semantic information, in particular detail. Lexical-semantic processing is of particular significance to the present argument, as recent domain-specific models have argued for a distinct, specialized lexicon and grammar, subserved by neural structures in the posterior temporal and inferior frontal regions of the left hemisphere, respectively (Pinker & Ullman, 2002; Ullman, 2001). Having addressed the role of domain-general processes in grammatical comprehension elsewhere (Dick, Bates, Wulfeck, Aydelott Utman, & Dronkers, 2001), we will in the present chapter compare findings from behavioral studies of neurologically intact adults and patients with language disorders to explore the complex nature of the lexical impairments associated with brain injury, and discuss possible accounts of these impairments under a general processing approach. We will demonstrate that similar patterns of impairment may be induced in brain-intact individuals subjected to different types of perceptual and attentional stressors. Further, we will show that the dynamic nature of linguistic representations may be exploited to overcome disruptions produced by cognitive stress. In addition, we will present evidence from some neurophysiological studies demonstrating that language comprehension is subserved by a distributed processing network involving multiple brain areas in both the left and right hemispheres, with no clear distinction between perceptual and conceptual processing.

We dedicate this chapter to Elizabeth Bates, whose pioneering work in adult psycholinguistics, child language acquisition, cognitive development, and cognitive neuroscience has provided the theoretical framework in which this evidence is presented. Liz Bates has made an inestimable contribution to our understanding of language, cognition, and the brain through her unique perspective and rigorous approach to science. Her groundbreaking research and theoretical insights have been a source of inspiration to countless students and scholars throughout the world, and have shaped the contributions of those who have had the opportunity to train under her generous supervision. We are honored to contribute to this volume, and to offer this review of one of the many areas of language research upon which her work has made a lasting impact.

BEHAVIORAL STUDIES OF LEXICAL-SEMANTIC PROCESSING IN NORMAL AND LANGUAGE-IMPAIRED INDIVIDUALS

Language comprehension depends upon the activation of higher-level representations on the basis of sensory (auditory or visual) input. Access of word-level information is particularly important, as lexical representations include much if not all of the semantic and grammatical information necessary for the construction of sentence-level meaning. Most models of lexical access assume at least three stages of processing in the mapping from sensory information to word-level representations: the activation of a set of lexical candidates from acoustic or visual input; the selection from among these candidates of the best match with the input, which may require the suppression of incompatible candidates; and the integration of the associated lexical information with the ongoing sentence context (e.g., Faust & Gernsbacher, 1996; Gernsbacher, 1996, 1997; Marslen-Wilson, 1989, 1993; Marslen-Wilson & Warren, 1994). In this section, we will examine the role of perceptual input and attentional control on these aspects of lexical processing, and explore the possible neural mechanisms underlying these processes by evaluating the evidence from neuropsychological and neuroimaging studies.

Studies of semantic priming have provided a valuable means of examining the mapping from perception to meaning in normal adults and aphasic patients. In these studies, participants respond to a word target that is preceded by a prime word, which is either semantically related or unrelated to the target (e.g., CAT–DOG or RING–DOG). Participants are faster to respond to targets that are preceded by related primes than to targets that are preceded by unrelated primes (e.g., Meyer & Schvaneveldt, 1976; Neely, 1991). This semantic priming effect may be attributed to the spread of activation within the lexicon: when the lexical representation associated with the prime is activated by the sensory input, this activation is passed on to semantically related representations, including the upcoming target. Thus, when the target is encountered, it has already been at least partially activated ('primed') by the prior context (i.e., prime), and responses to the target are facilitated. Semantic priming thereby provides an implicit measure of the level of activation produced by an input.

Blumstein, Milberg, and colleagues have used the semantic priming effect to examine the influence of perceptual information on semantic activation in a series of recent studies. Specifically, these studies were designed to explore the role of acoustic-phonetic variation in the mapping from sound to meaning. Blumstein and Milberg set out to determine whether variations in the sensory input would directly influence lexical activation levels, by manipulating phonetic segments in a prime word and measuring the effects on responses to related targets (Milberg, Blumstein, & Dworetzky, 1988). They compared reaction times (RTs) in an auditory lexical decision task to target words preceded by related primes relative to unrelated primes (in this case, phonologically permissible nonwords), to establish a baseline measure of semantic priming (CAT–DOG vs. PLUB–DOG). In addition, they included conditions in which a phonetic segment in the prime word was replaced with another segment that differed from the original sound by one phonetic feature (e.g., GAT–DOG, a change in voicing) or by two or more features (e.g., WAT–DOG, a change in voicing, place, and manner). The results revealed that the phonetic manipulations reduced semantic priming with the size of the reduction related to the degree of phonetic distance between the intact and altered prime words (i.e., WAT produced less priming than GAT, which produced less priming than CAT). If the magnitude of the semantic priming effect is a reflection the amount of lexical activation that a sensory input produces, these findings suggest that inputs that are a partial match for a word form result in partial activation, and that the level of activation is dependent upon the degree of similarity between the input and the word form. Thus, sensory input produces a graded response at the lexical level.

This interpretation is supported by more recent studies investigating the effects of acoustic variation below the level of the phonetic segment and on semantic priming. Andruski, Blumstein, & Burton (1994), for example, manipulated voice-onset time, the primary cue to the voicing contrast in initial stop consonants (e.g., 'ka' vs. 'ga'), to produce segments that were poorer acoustic exemplars of the voiceless stop category while still being consistently identified as members of that category. They compared the amount of semantic priming produced by a prime word containing a good acoustic exemplar (CAT–DOG) with the amount of priming produced by the same word containing a poorer exemplar (C*AT–DOG), relative to an unrelated prime (RING–DOG). At a brief inter-stimulus interval (ISI) of 50 ms, the results were similar to the findings of Milberg et al. (1988): prime words containing poorer acoustic exemplars produced significantly less semantic priming than prime words containing good acoustic exemplars. Interestingly, nonwords presented in similar prime conditions (e.g., COAT–PLUB vs. C*OAT–PLUB) did not show an increase in RTs for targets following altered primes, demonstrating that the effect is not due to a general slowing in virtue of the processing of poorer acoustic exemplars. Further, the reduction in priming could not be attributed to competition at the lexical level: similar effects were produced by potentially ambiguous prime words (e.g., C*ANE–STICK, where a change in the phonetic category of the altered segment would result in a word, 'gain') and unambiguous words (e.g., C*AT–DOG, where a change in category would not result in a word). Thus, the results appear to reflect the goodness-of-fit between acoustic input and lexical form, rather than the activation of multiple lexical entries. Finally, the effects of acoustic variation on lexical activation are short-lived: no difference in priming was observed between altered and unaltered prime words at a longer ISI of 250 ms, suggesting that acoustic variation is accommodated with additional processing time. Thus, the lexical candidate that is the best match with the acoustic input will eventually become fully activated. We have since obtained similar results in our own research for a variety of acoustic cues to phonetic contrasts in initial, medial, and final position in prime words (Aydelott Utman, 1997; Aydelott Utman, Blumstein, & Sullivan, 2001).

These findings have possible implications for domain-specific models of lexical access. Specifically, the results suggest that perceptual information maps directly onto lexical representations during language comprehension, such that partial information produces partial activation. Thus, there is a direct relationship between the sensory input and the activation of word-level information. This would appear to contradict modular accounts of language comprehension, which argue for shallow information transfer between levels of processing, such that perceptual processes yield abstract outputs which serve as inputs to higher-level processing (Fodor, 1983). These results suggest that it is the sensory information itself, rather than an abstract phonetic code, that serves to activate lexical representations, and that lexical activation is graded to reflect the degree of match between sensory input and word form.

The semantic priming paradigm has also been used to explore the nature of lexical processing in patients with language disorders. Domain-specific models have assumed a strict separation between lexical processing and other aspects of language comprehension, such as grammatical processing (Grodzinsky, 1995a, 1995b, 2000; Pinker, 1994; Pinker & Ullman, 2002). Further, according to such models, lexical and grammatical processes are associated with distinct neural structures that subserve language-specific functions, which may be selectively impaired as a result of focal brain injury. The classical distinction between Broca's and Wernicke's aphasia would appear to provide compelling evidence for these claims. According to the traditional characterization of these disorders, patients with Broca's aphasia experience a loss or disruption of grammatical rules resulting from damage to left inferior frontal brain regions; this produces a deficit in syntactic comprehension ('agrammatism'). By contrast, patients with Wernicke's aphasia experience a loss or disruption in lexical-semantic representations resulting from damage to left posterior temporal brain regions; this produces a deficit in semantic comprehension (Ullman, 2001). As described above, this apparent double dissociation suggests the operation of functionally distinct, specialized neural modules for lexical and grammatical representations.

This characterization of Broca's and Wernicke's aphasia makes clear predictions about the nature of lexical comprehension in these groups. Specifically, Wernicke's aphasics should demonstrate marked impairment in all tasks requiring lexical-semantic processing, whereas performance on the same tasks should be relatively unimpaired in Broca's aphasics. Off-line measures of semantic comprehension have tended to support these predictions. Wernicke's aphasics tend to make semantic errors on word-picture matching tasks (Goodglass & Baker, 1976) and fail to demonstrate normal semantic category structure in semantic similarity judgments (Zurif, Caramazza, Myerson, & Galvin, 1974); in contrast, Broca's aphasics show relatively spared performance on these tasks. Further, when asked to judge whether two visually presented words are semantically related (e.g., CAT–DOG vs. RING–DOG), Wernicke's aphasics demonstrate poor performance relative to normal individuals, whereas Broca's aphasics are not significantly impaired (Milberg & Blumstein, 1981).

The evidence from semantic priming studies, however, reveals a more complex picture of lexical processing in these two patient populations. Blumstein, Milberg, & Shrier (1983) presented a lexical decision task to Broca's and Wernicke's aphasics, in which word targets were preceded by semantically related and unrelated primes. Similar to normal subjects, Wernicke's aphasics demonstrated significant semantic priming for targets preceded by related primes. This finding has been observed in numerous studies using various priming methodologies, including list priming, in which primes and targets are presented in a list and lexical decision responses are made to each item (e.g., DOG–CAT–RING–PLUB etc.; Milberg & Blumstein, 1981) and triplet (summation) priming, in which the target is preceded by two prime words (e.g., COIN–BANK–MONEY; Milberg, Blumstein, & Dworetzky, 1987). These results are in marked contrast to the performance of Wernicke's aphasics on explicit relatedness judgments, and demonstrate that lexical-semantic knowledge is intact in these patients.

In contrast to Wernicke's aphasics, Broca's aphasics show weak, unreliable, or absent semantic priming under the same conditions, despite their relatively spared performance on semantic judgment tasks (Milberg & Blumstein, 1981; Blumstein, Milberg, & Shrier, 1983). Interestingly, Broca's aphasics fail to show priming in paradigms in which there is no predictable relationship between the prime and the target, such as list and triplet priming (Milberg & Blumstein, 1981; Milberg, Blumstein, & Dworetzky, 1987; Prather, Zurif, Stern, & Rosen, 1992), and exhibit weak priming effects in paired priming paradigms (Blumstein, Milberg, & Shrier, 1983). This suggests that Broca's aphasics show priming only when it is possible to generate a response strategy based on semantic relatedness and/or expectancy, whereas priming in Wernicke's aphasics reflects automatic spreading activation within the semantic network (cf. Milberg & Blumstein, 2000; Milberg, Blumstein, Katz, Gershberg, & Brown, 1995). This interpretation is supported by more recent findings that Broca's aphasics are sensitive to factors that influence expectancy in paired priming tasks, such as the proportion of semantically related pairs in the stimulus set and the length of the interstimulus interval (ISI), whereas Wernicke's aphasics are not (Blumstein et al., 1995). Thus, it appears that both Broca's and Wernicke's aphasics are impaired in the processing of lexical-semantic information, but that the nature of this impairment differs markedly across the two groups: Wernicke's aphasics have difficulty making explicit judgments of semantic relatedness, but are not impaired in the automatic activation of semantically related items, whereas Broca's aphasics have no difficulty in judging relatedness, but show a pronounced deficit in automatic activation (cf. Blumstein, 1997; Blumstein & Milberg, 2000).

This contrast is further supported by studies of the mapping from sound to meaning in these patient groups. Milberg, Blumstein, & Dworetzky (1988) compared the performance of Broca's and Wernicke's aphasics on the phonetic distortion paradigm described above, in which word targets were preceded by intact and phonetically distorted related primes (e.g., DOG preceded by CAT, GAT, or WAT) as well as unrelated primes (e.g., PLUB). In contrast to normal subjects, who show a graded response to phonetic distortion, Broca's and Wernicke's aphasics demonstrate two distinct patterns of performance in response to these stimuli. Broca's aphasics show significant priming only in the phonetically intact prime condition (CAT– DOG), and show no priming for phonetically distorted primes (GAT–DOG or WAT–DOG) relative to unrelated primes. Wernicke's aphasics, on the other hand, show significant priming in both intact and distorted prime conditions, with no significant differences in priming between intact and distorted primes (i.e., CAT, GAT, and WAT all produce similar levels of priming to the

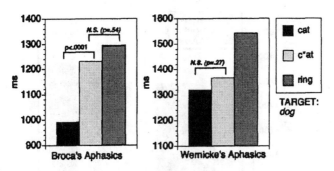

FIG. 11.1.

target DOG, relative to the unrelated prime). Thus, for Broca's aphasics, only exact overlap between sensory input and word form is sufficient to produce lexical activation, whereas for Wernicke's aphasics, any overlap between input and form is sufficient to fully activate a lexical representation.

We have since obtained similar results in studies of subphonetic variation and priming in these patient groups (Aydelott Utman, 1997; Aydelott Utman, Blumstein, & Sullivan, 2001). In these studies, targets were preceded by related primes containing phonetic segments that were either intact (e.g., CAT–DOG) or altered to produce poorer acoustic exemplars (e.g., C*AT–DOG), as well as by unrelated primes (e.g., RING–DOG). Whereas normal subjects show a graded priming effect in response to these stimuli, Broca's aphasics (Fig. 11.1, left panel) show significant semantic priming only for intact primes (CAT–DOG), and no priming for altered primes (C*AT–DOG), relative to unrelated primes. In contrast, Wernicke's aphasics (Fig. 11.1, right panel) show significant priming for both intact and altered primes relative to unrelated primes, with no significant difference in the magnitude of priming between the intact and altered conditions. Interestingly, unlike normal subjects, Broca's aphasics are influenced by both lexical competition and the locus of the acoustic distortion in the prime word (Fig. 11.2). Specifically, the effect of acoustic manipulation is most pronounced in Broca's aphasics when a change in the identity of the distorted segment would produce a real word (e.g., C*ANE– STICK, as opposed to C*AT–DOG), and when the manipulation occurs at the onset of the prime word rather than the offset (e.g., C*AT–DOG, as opposed to RUG*–FLOOR). Wernicke's aphasics show no effect of acoustic manipulation, irrespective of the locus of the manipulation in the prime word, or its potential effect on the lexical status of the prime.

Taken together, the results presented above suggest a possible account of the lexical comprehension impairments in Broca's and Wernicke's aphasia in terms of a general processing model of aphasic deficits. Blumstein and Milberg (2000) have argued that the pattern of performance observed

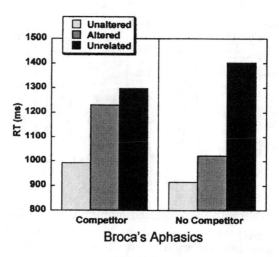

FIG. 11.2.

in these two groups reflect deficits in the activation and inhibition of lexical candidates during on-line processing. According to this view, in normal language comprehension, the sensory input activates a set of possible lexical candidates depending upon the degree of overlap between input and word form, and inhibits those lexical items that are incompatible. Broca's aphasics appear to be impaired in the activation of lexical representations, such that the sensory input fails to produce the same level of activation as in normal subjects. Thus, Broca's aphasics achieve lexical activation only when there is an exact match between input and word form. Further, Broca's patients fail to show graded activation when there is partial overlap between input and form, particularly when the input overlaps with more than one lexical representation, and they have difficulty overcoming acoustic mismatch that occurs early in a word. In contrast, Wernicke's aphasics appear to have difficulty inhibiting lexical entries that are incompatible with the acoustic input, resulting in overactivation of candidates when there is only partial overlap between input and word form.

This characterization of lexical processing in Broca's and Wernicke's aphasia is compatible with the previous observation that Broca's aphasics are spared in explicit semantic judgments and controlled processing strategies and impaired in automatic activation, whereas Wernicke's aphasics show the reverse pattern of deficit (Blumstein et al., 1995). Activation and inhibition have been associated with differing degrees of attentional load in semantic priming studies. Specifically, activation has been associated with facilitation of congruent targets in priming studies, which occurs at very brief ISIs and may be observed even when participants report no explicit awareness of the prime stimulus, as in masked priming paradigms (see

Neely, 1991, for review). In addition, as observed above, early facilitation effects are particularly sensitive to variations in the sensory input (Andruski, Blumstein, & Burton, 1994; Aydelott Utman, Blumstein, & Sullivan, 2001; Neely, 1991). On the other hand, inhibition of incongruent targets tends to emerge only at longer ISIs, and is associated with the generation of expectancies and the operation of heuristic strategies (Neely, 1991). Further, inhibition effects tend to be reduced in populations with limited attentional resources (e.g., Gernsbacher, 1997). Thus, it appears that lexical activation is a rapid, automatic process that depends on sensory information, whereas inhibition occurs later in processing and is more demanding in terms of attentional resources. The performance of Broca's and Wernicke's aphasics on tests of lexical processing may therefore be characterized in terms of general deficits in the automatic and controlled aspects of lexical access, respectively (cf. Blumstein, 1997).

The claim that facilitation and inhibition effects reflect separate processes, each with a different time course and a different degree of attentional load, suggests that these effects may respond selectively to different types of cognitive stress. Specifically, facilitation effects should be particularly vulnerable to manipulations of the perceptual input, whereas inhibition effects should be disrupted by increased attentional demand or decreased processing time. Thus, it should be possible to induce selective disruptions in the facilitation and inhibition of lexical items in neurologically intact individuals by imposing perceptual and attentional stress during language comprehension. We explored these predictions in a recent study (Aydelott & Bates, 2004; cf. Aydelott Utman & Bates, 1998) using a contextual priming paradigm. Participants made lexical decision responses to word targets (e.g., COW) which appeared in highly constraining sentence contexts (>90% cloze probability) that were congruent (e.g., *On the farm the farmer gets up early to milk the*—), incongruent (e.g., *Since everyone kept walking into my room I decided to lock the* —), or neutral (e.g., *Its name is* —) with respect to the meaning of the target word. Acoustic distortions were applied to the sentence context in each semantic bias condition, and the effects of these manipulations were evaluated relative to subjects' performance when the context was acoustically intact. Two types of distortion were applied: a perceptual distortion (low-pass filtering at 1 kHz), which was intended to interfere with the intelligibility of the acoustic signal and disrupt facilitation of congruent targets; and an attentional distortion (time compression, which speeded sentence presentation rate by 50%), which was intended to reduce processing time and disrupt inhibition of incongruent targets. Facilitation and inhibition effects were measured by comparing RTs in the biasing conditions with RTs to the same targets in the neutral condition.

The results for intact sentence contexts (Fig. 11.3) revealed that the semantic bias produced both facilitation (faster RTs for congruent targets)

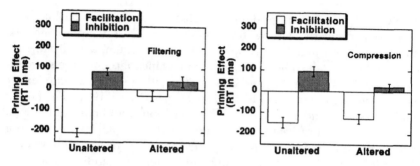

FIG. 11.3.

and inhibition (slower RTs for incongruent targets), relative to the neutral baseline. The acoustic manipulations produced different patterns of results depending upon the nature of the distortion. As predicted, perceptual distortion (filtering) reduced the facilitation effect produced by congruent contexts, whereas attentional distortion (compression) reduced the inhibition effect produced by incongruent contexts without affecting facilitation. Neither of the acoustic manipulations significantly influenced responses to targets in the neutral condition, indicating that the extent to which distortion influences priming is dependent upon the degree of semantic bias introduced by the context.

We have obtained similar findings in studies of the effects of competing speech on contextual priming (Moll, Cardillo, & Aydelott Utman, 2001; Cardillo, 2004). Interference from a competing speech signal represents a particularly complex source of cognitive stress, with a number of possible implications for language comprehension. Competing speech places an increased demand on processing resources, as the listener must selectively attend to one signal while suppressing another. Further, competing speech may also be relatively more demanding than a competing signal with no semantic content, because the speech signal will activate linguistic representations that are in conflict with the attended signal. In addition, competing speech may also affect the perceptibility of the attended signal by masking the spectral frequencies of the signal, thereby interfering with the encoding of the sensory input.

In order to separate the specific contributions of the perceptual, attentional, and semantic interference introduced by competing speech, participants were presented with a similar sentence-word priming paradigm to that described above, with four interference conditions (Moll, Cardillo, & Aydelott Utman, 2001; Cardillo, 2004). In the first condition, the sentence context (congruent, incongruent, or neutral) was presented in one ear, and a competing speech signal was presented in a different ear, so that the target signal could be isolated from the competing signal by attending selectively to one auditory channel. The second condition was identical to the first, with the exception that the competing speech signal was presented backward. Backward speech has the same spectral and temporal characteristics as forward speech, but contains no semantic content, allowing for an evaluation of the effects of selective attention in the absence of a competing semantic message. In the third and fourth conditions, the competing speech signals (forward and backward, respectively) were presented in the same ear as the target signal. In contrast to the different ear conditions, in the same ear conditions it was not possible to isolate the target signal by attending selectively to one ear. Thus, the perceptual interference from the competing signal was greater in the same ear conditions. It was predicted that, when the competing signal was presented to a different ear, attending to one auditory channel would increase the demand on processing resources, thereby disrupting the inhibition of incongruent targets, whereas in the same ear conditions, perceptual masking of the target signal by the competing signal would disrupt the facilitation of congruent targets. It was possible to determine whether the observed effects were due to the semantic content of the competing signal or to the presence of the signal itself by comparing the patterns of performance in the forward and backward speech conditions.

Results revealed that, as predicted, when forward speech is presented to a different ear from the target signal (Fig. 11.4, top panel), inhibition of congruent targets is significantly reduced, whereas facilitation is unaffected. However, when backward speech is presented to a different ear (Fig. 11.4, bottom panel), neither facilitation nor inhibition are affected, demonstrating that the interference produced by competing speech is a consequence of the semantic content of the competing signal, rather than the presence of the signal itself. When forward speech is presented to the same ear (Fig. 11.5, top panel), facilitation of congruent targets is significantly reduced. A similar pattern is observed when backward speech is presented to the same ear (Fig. 11.5, bottom panel), suggesting that the effects of perceptual masking do not depend upon the semantic content of the competing signal; however, it appears from these data that the reduction in facilitation is slightly less for backward than forward speech presented to the same ear. Nonetheless, this interaction did not reach significance and will be explored further in future research.

Taken together, the results of the behavioral studies presented above provide a picture of the component processes involved in the recognition of words in a semantic context. A set of candidate lexical representations is activated on the basis of the perceptual input, and initial activation levels are determined by the extent to which the sensory information matches a particular word form representation in the lexicon. The semantic context may also serve to activate compatible lexical entries, or to facilitate the selection of compatible entries. These represent early, automatic processes

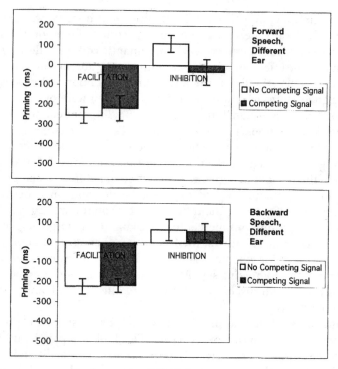

FIG. 11.4.

that place relatively few demands on processing resources. Once initial activation has occurred, the most appropriate lexical candidate must then be
selected from among the active candidates, which involves the inhibition of
candidates that are incompatible with the sensory input and/or the semantic context. The selected item must then be integrated into the overall
meaning of the sentence. Selection and integration are later-occurring,
controlled processes that are associated with increased attentional demand.

Although the behavioral studies reported above offer valuable insights
into the role of perceptual and attentional factors in lexical-semantic comprehension, the methodology requires that the underlying neural processes involved in these aspects of comprehension be inferred on the basis of
the nature of the experimental manipulations and (in the case of neuropsychological investigations) the location of the lesion that produces the
corresponding behavior. Thus, reaction time measures can tell us that perceptual and attentional factors have specific, predictable effects on behavior, but we must speculate as to the precise origins of these effects based
upon the circumstances under which they emerge. In contrast, electrophysiological methods provide a direct measure of neural activity in response to experimental manipulations, and are therefore an invaluable

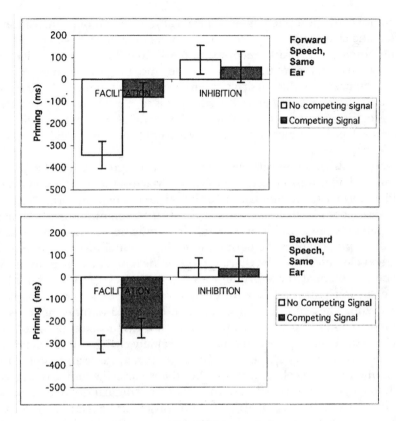

FIG. 11.5.

means of establishing in more detail the neural mechanisms responsible for expectancy generation, perceptual analysis, semantic activation, and contextual integration in language comprehension, and the extent to which these reflect language-specific processes.

ELECTROPHYSIOLOGICAL APPROACH TO THE DOMAIN-SPECIFICITY OF LANGUAGE PROCESSING

The idea that language processing, while quite special in many ways, may not rely on its own domain-specific set of specialized psychological or neural mechanisms but rather may share one or more basic mechanisms with other cognitive domains has emerged independently and in parallel from within the field of cognitive electrophysiology. Cognitive electrophysiology is a research area at the interface between cognitive/experimental psychology and neuroscience in which brain measures are used to make inferences about psychological phenomena. Specifically, its practitioners make use of systematic changes in the pattern of electrical brain activity—event-related brain potentials or ERPs—recorded at the scalp of brain intact individuals as they sense, perceive, transform, encode, and/or respond to sensory inputs. The beauty of this particular neuroimaging technique is that it is a direct measure of ongoing neural activity that is so exquisitely sensitive to sensory, cognitive, emotional, memory, and motoric factors that it would be a valuable dependent measure even if it were not generated in the brain; but, of course, it is.

Brain cells communicate via electrochemical signals, and these can be monitored noninvasively across the entire surface of the scalp as they occur. Under normal (non-stimulated) conditions, each neuron has a "resting" electrical potential that arises due to the distribution of positive and negative elements (ions) inside and outside it. Stimulation of the neuron, as by sensory input, changes the permeability of the neural membrane to these charged elements, thereby altering the electrical potential. A transient increase in potential (depolarization) at the cell body can cause an all-or-none "action potential," a wave of depolarization that moves along the cell's axon. The action potential can then be spread to other neurons via the release of chemicals (neurotransmitters) from the axon tip that travel in the extracellular space and cause permeability changes in the dendrites of nearby neurons. These permeability changes may cause an action potential in the receiving cell, or may just alter the electrical potential of that cell such that it will be more or less sensitive to other stimulation. In either case, these "post synaptic potentials" can be recorded at the scalp, thereby providing an instantaneous record of neural processing even when this activity does not lead to any overt response. Neural communication thus involves the flow of charged particles across neural membranes, which generates an electric potential in the conductive media inside and outside the cell; these current flows are the basis for electrophysiological recordings in the brain and at the scalp surface. More specifically, it is believed that much of the observed activity at the scalp emanates from cortical pyramidal cells whose organization and firing satisfies the constraints for an observable signal (see, e.g., Allison, Wood, & McCarthy, 1986; Kutas & Dale, 1997; Nunez & Katznelson, 1981 for more detail).

Researchers interested in unresolved issues within the domain of language thus tend to measure changes in the electrical brain activity as individuals read or listen to words, word pairs, sentences, or short stretches of discourse, or as they view pictures embedded in language contexts or within a series of pictorial images, and as they perform tasks ranging from reading/listening/viewing for comprehension to answering questions, making grammaticality, plausibility or categorical judgments, or performing some non-language task with language materials. From systematic changes in the pattern of electrical brain activity elicited by words and pictures under such circumstances, it has proven possible to track visual and auditory input from sensory transduction to the laying of a memory trace to the moment either makes available the knowledge to which it is linked as it enables the processes involved making sense.

Investigations of the neural basis of language processing have generally focused on the brain's response to particular events or kinds of events, such as the appearance of a word, picture, sentence or scene on a computer screen or over headphones. To examine event-related activity of this type, one typically averages the electrical signal time-locked to the event (stimulus) of interest to create an "event-related (brain) potential" or ERP—a waveform of voltage fluctuations in time, one for each recording electrode across the head. Each waveform consists of a series of positive- and negative-going voltage deflections (relative to some baseline activity prior to event onset); experimental factors, among others, are reflected in the morphology (shape) of the waveform (e.g., presence or absence of certain peaks), the latency, duration, or amplitude (size) of one or more peaks, or their amplitude distribution over the scalp.

ERPs are useful measures for the study of information processing in general, and language processing in particular, because they are a continuous, multidimensional signal. Specifically, they offer a direct estimate of what a significant part of the brain (even if we cannot infer from this measure alone precisely which part) is doing just before, during, and after an event of interest, even if it is extended in time. And they do so with millisecond resolution. This temporal sensitivity is crucial given that many important cognitive operations transpire in less time than it takes to react to a predictable sensory stimulus (i.e., a simple reaction time). At minimum, ERPs can indicate not only that two conditions differ, but reveal something about the nature of the difference—i.e., whether, for example, there is a quantitative change in the timing or size of a process or a qualitative change as reflected in a different waveform morphology or scalp distribution. To a limited extent, ERPs also can be used to examine where in the brain processes take place (via source modeling techniques and in combination with other neuroimaging techniques; for more information see review by Kutas, Federmeier, & Sereno, 1999; also Dale & Halgren, 2001), though this is not the primary aim of most ERP investigations.

Using ERP techniques, researchers have looked at language processing from early stages of word recognition through the processing of multisentence discourses, from the planning of a speech act to its articulation (e.g., Kutas & Van Petten, 1994; Osterhout, 1994; Osterhout & Holcomb, 1995). In doing so, one finds that the brain's processing of language involves many different kinds of operations taking place at different times and different temporal scales, varying in the extent to which they are general purpose. Indeed, it can be argued that one of the most remarkable findings in the cognitive electrophysiology of language processing has been that none of the ERP effects discovered to date seems to be unique to language processing. While several ERP components such as the N400 (Kutas & Hillyard, 1980), left anterior negativity (LAN), or P600 (Osterhout & Holcomb, 1992; Munte, Heinze, Matzke, Wieringa, & Johannes, 1998) have proven very useful as dependent measures that are sensitive to some important aspect of language processing, none of them seem to be language-specific (definitions aside).

The ERP technique is in fact especially amenable to looking for commonality of neural (mental) operations, because the brain's response to any given event (stimulus, response) unfolds in time as the event makes its way from the sensory receptors to the lower, intermediate, and higher-order processing areas of the brain, and back—feedforward and feedback paths. It is thus possible to catalog whether or not an event is anticipated, sensed and perceived, attended to, identified, recognized as recent, old or new, considered as (im)probable, (in)frequent, surprising, informative, congruent with the ongoing context, meaningful, and/or grammatically well-formed, among others, as well as to determine the various sensory and biological factors that influence how and when these operations are carried out. In so doing, researchers can determine just how far one can get in explaining various language phenomena in terms of basic perceptual, conceptual, and motoric processes.

Even before any stimulus or event occurs, it is possible to observe some evidence at the scalp that an individual is expecting some event—a slow growing negativity originally known as the expectancy wave or the contingent negative variation (CNV) to highlight the finding that it is the contingency between two successive events and not the processing of either event per se that is critical for its elicitation; the CNV has been analyzed into functional subcomponents (e.g., O-wave, E-wave, readiness potential, stimulus-preceding negativity). The CNV, like so many other ERP components, varies systematically in its distribution across the scalp as a function of input modality, task parameters, and response requirements—in auditory tasks the CNV is more frontal, in tasks requiring a response it is more central, in visual tasks it is more posterior, etc. In fact, it is the functional invariance and systematic sensitivity to certain stimulus and response parameters in the face of such topographical variance that has made endogenous ERP (sub)components so useful in analyzing the information processing transactions in the brain. Any warning event (overt or internally-generated) will trigger a slow rising negativity that will last until the anticipated event occurs—its presence reflects an individual's anticipation of or expectancy for some event (even when it does not always occur), its distribution reflects the nature (e.g., modality) of the anticipated event, its shape in time the duration of the interval over which the anticipation builds, and its amplitude reflects the a variety of factors such as motivation, presence of distracting stimuli, difficulty of upcoming stimulus processing (for review see Mc-Callum & Curry, 1993).

Motor anticipation is reflected in a similar slow rising negativity largest, at least for hand movements, over the contralateral motor cortex. The asymmetric portion of this brain potential, known as the lateralized readiness potential (LRP), has been used to ask many questions about the timing of information flow through the nervous system, as it reflects preparation for making a motor response even if the movement is never actually made (for review Coles, 1989). Within the domain of language, the presence or absence of the LRP on no-go trials (when in a go/no-go paradigm) has been used to infer the order of conceptual/semantic, grammatical, and phonological operations during language production (e.g., Van Turennout, Hagoort, & Brown, 1998).

Other slow negative waves have been observed in a variety of contexts, including during attention tasks (processing negativity or Nd), short term memory scanning, mental rotation, the anticipation of feedback, long term memory retrieval, and working memory use (associated with left anterior negativity or LAN), among others (for reviews see Birbaumer, Elbert, Canavan, & Rokstroh, 1990; Haider, Groll-Knapp, & Ganglberger, 1981; McCallum & Curry, 1993). These slow waves seem to have a topography that reflects stimulus content/modality—semantic with a frontal maximum, mental rotation with more parietal maximum. Like the CNV, the amplitude of these slow waves is related to task difficulty or amount of processing effort. In short term memory scanning tasks, for example, the associated slow negativity increases in amplitude with increasing memory load (Wijers, Otten, Feenstra, Mulder, & Mulder, 1989). In mental rotation tasks, the negativity increases in amplitude with the angular disparity between the objects being compared (e.g., Roesler, Schumacher, & Sojka, 1990). And, in like fashion, in language tasks the amplitude of a slow negativity varies with the number of possible co-referents for an anaphor (van Berkum, Brown, Hagoort, & Zwitserlood, 2003). Finally, it appears that the duration of these negativities reflect the duration of particular processing stages. The processing negativity (Nd) observed in selective attention tasks is maintained as long as information in the attended channel is being analyzed and discriminated from that of a channel competing for attention (e.g., Hillyard & Hansen, 1986). Roesler and colleagues have described very similar slow negative potentials that are temporally related to the process of information retrieval from long-term memory (Roesler & Heil, 1991; Roesler, Heil, & Glowalla, 1993). These negativities persisted from the appearance of a memory probe until a response indicating the search was over. The amplitudes of these negativities were related to the difficulty of the retrieval process, though they vary in their scalp distribution in a manner consonant with the functional division of the cortex according to lesion data. It is not a far stretch to characterize the slow negativities that are seen in association with certain sentence types in which some information must be held in working memory (e.g., object relatives, wh-questions, anaphoric reference) in a similar fashion (King & Kutas, 1995; Kluender & Kutas, 1993; Mueller, King & Kutas, 1997; Streb, Roesler, & Hennighausen, 1999; Vos, Gunter, Kolk, & Mulder, 2001; Weckerly & Kutas, 1999); indeed, this may explain their variable durations and varying scalp topographies across reports despite their localizing name—the left anterior negativity. On this account the LAN, though useful to examine various linguistic structures, merely reflects the use of (short-term/working) memory during language processing and not a language specific operation (e.g., Friederici, Hahne, & Mecklinger, 1996).

Anticipation, expectancy, and prediction also can be inferred from a whole host of ERP components that indicate some form of "surprise" when the expected event does not occur. There are many different ERP components that seem to reflect processes of this ilk though at different levels of the psychological and neural processing systems: the omitted stimulus potential (indexes absence of a stimulus in a temporally regular series), the mismatch negativity or MMN (reflects detection of a change in a stimulus or stimulus sequence held in auditory short term memory), P3a (indexes novelty), P3b (indexes decision making and binary categorization), N400 (reflects degree of semantic congruence), and P600 (reflects the detection of structural violations in, e.g., language and music contexts), among others. While each of these potentials could be described as indexing some aspect or type of "surprise" by virtue of a "mismatch" with or "change" from an expectation, each of them is more than simply a novelty, a surprise, or a change detector; i.e., they are not interchangeable brain events indexing interchangeable mechanisms. As such, each reveals something different about human neuromental processing. At minimum they are distinct in that the stimulus parameters and experimental setup needed to elicit them differ widely. Additionally, they reflect mental operations that differ in the extent to which they are affected by context (and what type of contexts they are sensitive to), and in the extent to which they interact with one another in space and time (see Federmeier, Kluender, & Kutas, 2002). At the same time, however, none of them is domain-specific, at least not if the domains are, say, language and non-language processing. This has practical consequences for experimental designs and is one of the primary reasons that cognitive electrophysiologists have come to the conclusion that language, though special, is *not* unique at the level of the mental operations and the brain processes that support it.

Whether or not an item is anticipated wholly or in part, once it is occurs it must be ignored or analyzed (with features extracted) to some degree, depending on how much attention it captures or has allocated to it. These sensory and attentional processes are reflected in the ERP componentry— such as the P1, N1, and P2—within the first 200 ms post-stimulus onset as the brain is determining just what it is sensing and perceiving (e.g. a letter string, a word, an object, a meaningful sound, etc.). Some aspects of (especially early) perceptual processing are likely to be similar regardless of the nature of the stimulus at least until the brain "knows" what kind of stimulus it is. Processing decisions also may be guided about what the stimulus is likely to be, based on guesses informed by frequency, recency, and predictive regularities, including the context. Whenever possible, both top-down (expectancy or context-based) and bottom-up (stimulus-based) information seem to influence brain analysis of sensory input.

The hierarchical organization of the primate visual system with its massive feedforward, lateral, and feedback connections provides the anatomical substrate for significant information/neural flow and interaction between top-down conceptual and bottom-up perceptual levels of processing. Indeed, the majority of the synaptic connections onto neurons even in primary visual cortex come from higher-order processing brain areas rather than directly from the sensory receptors per se. Presumably, this high density of "top-down" connections allows the analysis of visual input such as words and pictures to be shaped by factors such as prior experience, attention, and expectancy throughout the visual system up through the initial memory link or trace via the hippocampal formation. When, how, and how much such top-down information impacts perceptual and conceptual processes remains underspecified, especially for human visual processing. We (Federmeier & Kutas, 1999a, 1999b, 2001, 2002) have begun to examine this in a series of ERP studies designed to monitor top-down influences on the processing of pictures of familiar objects embedded in language contexts. We chose language contexts precisely because we believe that they can be used to establish expectations at various levels. In these studies, we embedded pictures in sentence contexts and manipulated a number of variables that we presumed would, to varying degrees, influence the nature and degree of top-down processing: (1) the participant's experience with a particular picture, which presumably influences the picture's perceptual familiarity and/or predictability; (2) the congruency of the picture with the prior context; and (3) the strength of that context. In one study, we also employed visual half-field presentation methods to examine issues of hemispheric involvement. For each of these studies, we also conducted a strictly word version against which the pattern of effects for pictures could be compared and contrasted in order to assess which factors were specific to language and which were not.

A total of 54 college-aged volunteers (half women) participated in the three picture studies (18 in each). All the participants were right-handed,

HIGH CONSTRAINT
Tina lined up where she thought the nail should go.
When she was satisfied, she asked Bruce to hand her the

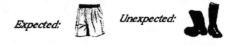

LOW CONSTRAINT
As the afternoon progressed, it got hotter and hotter.
Keith finally decided to put on a pair of

Expected: 　　　　　*Unexpected:*

FIG. 11.6.

monolingual English speakers with normal or corrected-to-normal vision and no neurological problems. The stimuli consisted of 176 sentence pairs, ending with either a congruent or an incongruent line drawing (50% each type). Approximately half of the sentence contexts were highly constraining for the final word of the second sentence in the pair (cloze probability > 78%) while the remaining half were less constraining (cloze probability 17%–78%) as shown in Fig. 11.6.

Participants read the sentence contexts word by word for comprehension while their electroencephalogram (EEGs) were collected from 26 recording sites distributed equidistantly across the scalp. Sentence-final line drawings were presented either at fixation (for 500 ms) or, in the hemi-field study, with nearest edge two degrees to the right or left of fixation (for 200 ms). Trials containing eye movements, blinks, or other artifacts were rejected off-line. In the *familiar condition*, participants were pre-exposed to the pictures (once each) prior to the experimental session, while in the *unfamiliar condition*, participants saw the pictures for the first time in the sentence contexts.

As expected, pre-exposure affected the amplitude of the early sensory components of the visual evoked potential (e.g., P1, N1, P2). In other words, a single exposure sufficed to impact the earliest sensory processing of the visual input. This can be best seen in a comparison of the ERPs to pictures viewed for the first time (unfamiliar pictures) overlapping the ERP to pre-exposed pictures being viewed a second time (familiar pictures), collapsed across congruency (expectancy), shown in Fig. 11.7. This comparison reveals that pre-exposure was associated with a reduction in the amplitude of the N1 component at recording sites over the front of the head (see left top) and the P1 and P2 components at recording sites over the back of the head (see right bottom). In a number of ERP studies of attention, the frontal N1 has been linked to allocation of visuospatial attention; more specifically, it has been hypothesized to reflect the output of a capacity-limited

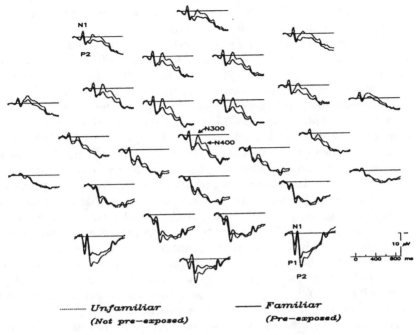

FIG. 11.7.

attentional system (e.g., Clark & Hillyard, 1996; Mangun, Hillyard, & Luck, 1993). Enhanced N1 amplitudes are observed, for example, in response to target stimuli that appear at attended relative to unattended locations in visuospatial selective attention tasks. P2 amplitudes have been linked to processes of visual feature (color, orientation, size) detection, with increased amplitudes generally observed in response to stimuli containing target features (e.g. Hillyard & Muente, 1984; Luck & Hillyard, 1994).

This familiar vs. unfamiliar comparison also provides the first sign of a remarkably fuzzy border between perceptual and conceptual processes: pre-exposure not only modulated the amplitude of early sensory-evoked and attention-sensitive components but also affected later so-called endogenous components such as the N300 and N400, known to vary with visual-semantic analyses specific to pictures (N300) and to semantic analyses more generally (N400) (see Kutas & Hillyard, 1980; Kutas & Hillyard, 1984; Ganis, Sereno, & Kutas, 1996; McPherson & Holcomb, 1999). These results thus would seem to indicate, perhaps surprisingly, that there are semantic as well as perceptual benefits to pre-exposure. The pre-exposure manipulation thus not only decreased the perceptual load associated with parsing an unfamiliar picture but also ensured that predictions, based on ongoing context, about the semantic features of likely upcoming items could also give rise to relatively accurate predictions (at least as good as participants' episodic memory based on one exposure) about the nature of the upcoming physical stimulus (as is true for words).

Examining the brain's responses to pictures that participants had seen previously once out of context further revealed that neither semantic congruence (expectancy) nor contextual constraint affected any parameter of the early sensory components evoked by these familiar pictures. By contrast, as anticipated, both these factors did modulate the amplitude of the N300/N400 components of the ERP. Consistent with prior data, the responses to (familiar) contextually congruent pictures (see Fig. 11.8) were characterized by significantly smaller N300/N400 components than those to contextually incongruent pictures. Incongruent pictures (like incongruent words) elicited large negativities between 200 and 600 ms poststimulus onset (N300/N400). And, consonant with the known characterization of the N400 congruency effect, its amplitude varied with contextual constraint, with the largest N400 responses to incongruent items when these were embedded in highly constraining contexts. These results, then, would seem to suggest that early sensory (at least low-level visual) processing, while sensitive to an existing memory trace, is much less subject, if at all, to the match between the ongoing context and/or the constraints it imposes on expectations at a semantic or visuo-semantic level.

This inference, however, must be qualified by the results of this same comparison made with pictures being viewed for the first time (i.e., unfamiliar pictures). In this case, the early sensory visual components of the ERP did show observable sensitivity to both semantic congruence and constraint (see Fig. 11.9). More specifically, the N1 components were reduced

FAMILIAR PICTURES

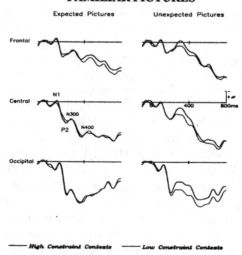

FIG. 11.8.

and P2 components to these same pictures enhanced—i.e., both these early components were relatively more positive when the sentence ending was contextually congruent and highly expected based on the preceding context. These reductions in the amplitude of the N1 and increases in the amplitude of the P2 for expected items in highly constraining contexts as compared with less constraining contexts were apparent in fourteen out of eighteen participants. Top-down information from a strong sentence context thus seems to allow for more efficient allocation of attention (N1) and more efficient extraction of visual feature information and/or reduction of visual processing load (P2). Importantly for the issues at hand, these early, perceptual effects for unfamiliar pictures were correlated with effects on later ERP components (N300/N400) linked to semantic processing. This would seem to indicate that for unfamiliar pictures strong contextual constraint not only eases the semantic processing of expected items, but also provides top-down information that can facilitate visual processing and attentional allocation as needed. The crucial point here is that for picture processing the response to expected endings in highly constraining contexts showed effects of constraint—increased positivity—in several time windows: reduced N1s and enhanced P2s, as well as greater positivity throughout the N300 and N400 time windows of the ERP.

It seems then that, at least under these circumstances, increased ease of perceptual processing and semantic analysis go hand in hand; perhaps the reduced visual processing load in highly constraining contexts frees attentional resources that would ordinarily be used up by perceptual processing to be shifted to conceptual integration processes. In any case, semantic processing is *not* isolated from perceptual factors as domain-specific theories imply. Rather, there seems to be an important link between the ease with which a stimulus can be perceptually deciphered and the nature of the semantic information subsequently derived from the stimulus and available for integration into a sentence context. This finding is especially intriguing given that these same concepts were equally easy to integrate into high as low constraint sentences when they appeared as words instead of picture; in that case, the brain responses to expected endings were unaffected by degree of contextual constraint. In short, for picture processing, there is an apparent link between perceptual and semantic processing that is not observed for word processing with the same sentence contexts and the same concepts. Of course, words as written stimuli are relatively predictable at a visual level as long as the font and size in which they appear in the experiment is fixed; words may thus be much more like familiar than unfamiliar pictures in this regard.

Perhaps somewhat surprisingly, the reduction in the amplitude of the anterior N1 that was observed for unfamiliar pictures when these were expected and embedded in highly constraining contexts was equivalent to

UNFAMILIAR PICTURES

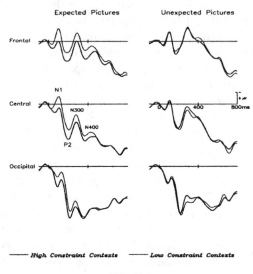

FIG. 11.9.

that for familiar pictures overall. This is an important exception to the finding that the anterior N1 is generally smaller for familiar than unfamiliar pictures. It seems, then, that perceptual difficulty/visual novelty (greater for unfamiliar than familiar pictures) can be offset by top-down information activated from semantic memory from a strong, congruent context. By about 100 ms, bottom-up factors (e.g., perceptual familiarity) and top-down factors (e.g., expectancy for an item based on prior sentence context) seem to come together to affect visual processing.

These data thus suggest that when targets are relatively easy to perceive, as in the case of words and familiar pictures, context has its primary impact on semantic integration processes. In contrast, when visual perception is more difficult (as for pictures being seen for the first time), strong contextual information, as is available in highly constraining contexts, can and does affect processing stages related to allocation of attentional resources and perceptual analysis, as well as later ones related to semantic integration.

When the results of these experiments with pictures are compared with those using words, two conclusions stand out: (1) picture and word processing in sentence contexts elicit quite similar brain responses; and (2) the time course with which pictures and words are integrated into a sentence context seem to be about the same. Thus, in these respects there is nothing domain-specific about how items from these two modalities are processed. It is thus highly unlikely that words and pictures are processed in completely independent neural systems. That said, there are circumstances under which words and pictures behave differently, and we have evidence (not presented here) that they activate different semantic featural information even in the very same sentence contexts (Federmeier & Kutas, 1999, 2001). From such data we have argued that semantic information exists in a shared distributed system with a modality-specific coding scheme. Our data and conclusions are thus consistent with those who maintain semantic information is distributed over multiple cortical areas that each preferentially process information from a particular modality. In fact, along with others, we have suggested that both hemispheres are involved in semantic (as well as more generally language) processing, although differing in how they make use of semantic information during online sentence processing.

We have examined the nature of the content and organization of semantic knowledge in the two hemispheres because we believe that this has important implications for how each might process language in particular, and make sense of sensory input more generally. We employed the visual half-field technique in normal undergraduates as they read sentences presented one word at a time, with the target (word in some experiments, picture in others) presented randomly two degrees from fixation to the right or left visual field. Here we present the data for the picture version, for exactly the same sentences as in the central vision studies discussed above; in this case, all the pictures were familiar (i.e., one exposure prior to the EEG recording).

ERP responses to pictures presented to the right visual field/left hemisphere (left) and to the left visual field/right hemisphere (right) are shown at two frontal recording sites (Fig. 11.10). With initial picture presentation to either hemisphere, semantic congruency effects were observed on the N400 (dashed boxes) component, just as they had been for lateralized word stimuli. Regardless of presentation hemifield, the ERPs to contextually expected as compared with unexpected pictures are characterized by increased positivity between 250–500 milliseconds, showing that both hemispheres differentiate items that fit the verbal context from those that do not. In fact, the ERPs to expected pictures (as was also true for words) presented in the two visual half-fields did not differ in amplitude, latency or distribution (except for slow, mirror image effects as a function of hemifield seen over medial, posterior electrodes). Semantic integration—sensitivity to semantic congruence—during sentence comprehension, as reflected in the N400, proceeds remarkably similarly in *both* cerebral hemispheres, not just the left as more standard views of language processing have maintained. Picture stimuli also show effects of semantic congruency by 300 ms post-picture onset on the N300 component regardless of visual field of presentation (dotted box), again implying a certain similarity in the two hemispheres' visuo-semantic processing.

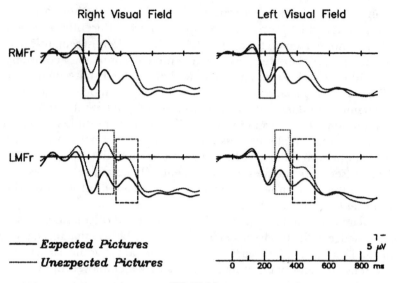

FIG. 11.10.

At the same time the two hemispheres do show some differences in the time course of their sensitivity to congruency effects: overall, the congruency effects appear earlier in the ERP responses initiated by left hemisphere processing. With initial presentation to the left hemisphere, P2 components (solid boxes, between 150–250 ms) are larger to expected than to unexpected pictures. By contrast, P2 components for expected versus unexpected pictures do not differ with presentation to the left visual field. Modulations in P2 amplitude are generally assumed to reflect detection and analysis of basic visual features such as orientation, size, color, etc. Only in the left hemisphere does processing of the individual words in the sentence context seem to provide top-down information allowing for more efficient visual feature extraction from targets (expected items) than from unexpected items. In other words, only with left-hemisphere-initiated processing is top-down contextual information used to prepare for the visual processing of upcoming stimuli. This is consistent with our hypothesis that the left hemisphere (but not the right) uses context to make predictions; importantly, here we see that these predictions can be about perceptual (and not just semantic) features of upcoming stimuli. Again, these results are remarkably similar to what we have seen with regard to the two hemispheres for words. While there are some modality-specific differences between words and pictures that stem from actual differences in the physical nature of the sensory input and the specificity of the semantic information that they render readily accessible, there is nonetheless a remarkable similarity in the timing, polarity, and morphology of semantic ERP responses for stimuli in the two modalities. Elsewhere we have suggested that pictures activate more specific semantic features than do written or spoken words, and while these influence what semantic information is available, how context is used to anticipate and integrate this information is the same regardless of the modality of the stimulus. Finally, whether for pictures or words, whereas the left hemisphere seems to use context to predict upcoming stimuli and prepare for their processing at semantic and perceptual levels, the right hemisphere's processing of a sentence context seems to provide it with less top-down information.

In sum, we find that an individual's prior experience with a visual stimulus, the fit of that stimulus to a sentence context, the strength of the context, and the hemisphere initiating processing all influence processing at both early and later stages—perceptual and conceptual. The functional specificity of the ERP waveform—including components reflecting sensory processing, feature extraction, allocation of attention, semantic analysis, etc.—has allowed us to see various effects on early ERP components that are correlated with effects on later components, suggesting a strong bidirectional link between perceptual and conceptual processing. Moreover, these effects as well as others are the same regardless of domain—at least for these mechanisms, pictures and words are the same.

Comprehending language involves a number of different kinds of brain processes including perceptual analysis, attention allocation, retrieval of information from long-term memory, storage of information into working memory, and comparisons between/transformations of information contained in working memory. Each of these processes can be examined through an electrophysiological filter—the specific ERP component that indexes a particular functional process. Here we have examined a few of these. But for lack of space, we could have detailed other ERP experiments aimed at examining the others, alone or in various combinations.

CONCLUSIONS

The evidence from normal behavior, neuropsychology, and electrophysiology reported here presents a complex picture of language as a dynamic, multidimensional cognitive system, which is highly dependent upon domain-general processes and resources. The data support an interactive model of language comprehension, in which there is no clear division or unidirectional flow of information between perceptual and conceptual processes. Instead, the evidence reveals that there is transparent information transfer between these levels of analysis, such that variations in the perceptual input directly influence the activation of conceptual information, and that active conceptual information in turn directly influences perceptual analysis. Further, both the perceptual properties of the input and the availability of attentional resources play a crucial role in language comprehension. Thus, the disruption of perceptual and attentional processes, either by distortion of the sensory input or by neurological damage, produces predictable patterns of language breakdown in normal and language-impaired individuals, indicating that disorders that have previously been considered to be language-specific may be better accounted for in terms of a domain-general processing account. Finally, the results presented here demonstrate that the neural mechanisms involved in language comprehension are also responsible for the processing of other kinds of information, including the recognition of visual objects, with no evidence for a discrete, dedicated language system.

Considering this evidence in the context of the other chapters presented in this volume, it is striking that for both comprehension and production and for language form and language meaning there is increasing evidence that the type of processing and behavior that is observed is a function, not just of the specific language level engaged or the specific language structure/representation involved, but of a complex interaction between the demands that a particular language places on the system, the demands of the specific task(s) in which the speaker/listener is engaged, and the speaker/listener's current state and prior experience, which together determine the kind and amount of various cognitive resources available to be used. In turn, it is how these resources are brought to bear that will determine the outcome, for a brain-damaged patient, a normal volunteer under stress, or even in a normal volunteer under seemingly routine processing conditions, as reflected in their brain responses. Language is thus special, not in having a dedicated set of cognitive/neural resources to draw upon, but rather in being a cognitive skill/ability that requires such efficient and intricate coordination of so many domain-general abilities, functions, and information sources.

REFERENCES

Allison, T., Wood, C. C., & McCarthy, G. (1986). The central nervous system. In M. G. Coles, E. Donchin & S. W. Porges (Eds.), *Psychophysiology: Systems, Processes, and Applications*. New York: Guilford Press.

Andruski, J. E., Blumstein, S. E., & Burton, M. W. (1994). The effect of subphonetic acoustic differences on lexical access. *Cognition, 52*, 163–187.

Aydelott, J., & Bates, E. (2004). Effects of acoustic distortion and semantic context on lexical access. *Language and Cognitive Processes, 19*(1), 29–56.

Aydelott Utman, J. (1997). *Effects of subphonetic acoustic differences on lexical access in neurologically intact adults and patients with Broca's aphasia*. Doctoral dissertation, Brown University.

Aydelott Utman, J., & Bates, E. (1998). Effects of acoustic degradation and semantic context on lexical access: Implications for aphasic deficits. *Brain and Language, 65*(1), 216–218.

Aydelott Utman, J., Blumstein, S. E., & Sullivan, K. (2001). Mapping from sound to meaning: Decreased lexical activation in Broca's aphasics. *Brain and Language, 79*(3), 444–472.

Birbaumer, N., Elbert, T., Canavan, A. G. M., & Rockstroh, B. (1990). Slow potentials of the cerebral cortex and behavior. *Physiological Reviews, 70*, 1–4.

Blumstein, S. (1997). A perspective on the neurobiology of language. *Brain and Language, 60*(3), 335–346.

Blumstein, S. E., & Milberg, W. P. (2000). Language deficits in Broca's and Wernicke's aphasia: A singular impairment. In Y. Grodzinsky, L. Shapiro, and D. Swinney (Eds.) *Language and the Brain: Representation and Processing,* pp. 167–184. Academic Press.

Blumstein, S., Milberg, W., & Shrier, R. (1983). Semantic processing in aphasia: Evidence from an auditory lexical decision task. *Brain and Language, 17*, 301–315.

Cardillo, E. (2004). Doctoral dissertation, University of Oxford. In preparation.

Clark, V. P., & Hillyard, S. A. (1996). Spatial selective attention affects early extrastriate but not striate components of the visual evoked potential. *Journal of Cognitive Neuroscience, 8*(5), 387–402.

Coles, M. G. (1989). Modern mind-brain reading: Psychophysiology, physiology, and cognition. *Psychophysiology, 26*(3), 251–269.

Dale, A. M., & Halgren, E. (2001). Spatiotemporal mapping of brain activity by integration of multiple imaging modalities. *Current Opinion in Neurobiology, 11*(2), 202–208.

Dick, F., Bates, E., Wulfeck, B., Aydelott Utman, J., Dronkers, N., & Gernsbacher, M. A. (2001). Language deficits, localization and grammar: evidence for a distributive model of language breakdown in aphasics and normals. *Psychological Review, 108*(4), 759–788.

Elman, J., Bates, E., Johnson, M., Karmiloff-Smith, A., Parisi, D., & Plunkett, K. (1996). *Rethinking Innateness: A Connectionist Perspective on Development.* Cambridge, MA: MIT Press.

Faust, M. E., & Gernsbacher, M. A. (1996). Cerebral mechanisms for suppression of inappropriate information during sentence comprehension. *Brain and Language, 53*(2), 234–259.

Federmeier, K. D., Kluender, R., & Kutas, M. (2002). Aligning linguistic and brain views on language comprehension. In A. Zani & A. M. Proverbio (Eds.), *The Cognitive Electrophysiology of Mind and Brain* (pp. 143–168). San Diego: Academic Press.

Federmeier, K. D., & Kutas, M. (1999a). Right words and left words: Electrophysiological evidence for hemispheric differences in meaning processing. *Cognitive Brain Research, 8*(3), 373–392.

Federmeier, K. D., & Kutas, M. (1999b). A rose by any other name: Long-term memory structure and sentence processing. *Journal of Memory and Language, 41*(4), 469–495.

Federmeier, K. D., & Kutas, M. (2001). Meaning and modality: Influences of context, semantic memory organization, and perceptual predictability on picture processing. *Journal of Experimental Psychology: Learning, Memory, & Cognition, 27*(1), 202–224.

Federmeier, K. D., & Kutas, M. (2002). Picture the difference: Electrophysiological investigations of picture processing in the cerebral hemispheres. *Neuropsychologia, 40*(7), 730–747.

Fodor, J. (1983). *The Modularity of Mind.* Cambridge, MA: MIT Press.

Friederici, A. D., Hahne, A., & Mecklinger, A. (1996). Temporal structure of syntactic parsing: Early and late event-related brain potential effects. *Journal of Experimental Psychology: Learning, Memory, & Cognition, 22*(5), 1219–1248.

Ganis, G., Kutas, M., & Sereno, M. I. (1996). The search for 'common sense': An electrophysiological study of the comprehension of words and pictures in reading. *Journal of Cognitive Neuroscience, 8*, 89–106.

Gernsbacher, M. A. (1996). The Structure-Building Framework: What it is, what it might also be, and why. In B. K. Britton & A. C. Graesser (Eds.), *Models of understanding text* (pp. 289–311). Mahwah, NJ: Lawrence Erlbaum.

Gernsbacher, M. A. (1997). Group differences in suppression skill. *Aging, Neuropsychology, & Cognition, 4*(3), 175–184.

Goodglass, H., & Baker, E. H. (1976). Semantic field, naming, and comprehension in aphasia. *Brain and Language, 3,* 359–374.

Grodzinsky, Y. (1995a). A restrictive theory of agrammatic comprehension. *Brain and Language, 50*(1), 27–51.

Grodzinsky, Y. (1995b). Trace deletion, theta-roles, and cognitive strategies. *Brain and Language, 51*(3), 469–497.

Grodzinsky, Y. (2000). The neurology of syntax: Language use without Broca's area. *Behavioral and Brain Sciences, 23*(1), 1–71.

Haider, M., Groll-Knapp, E., & Ganglberger, J. A. (1981). Event-related slow (DC) potentials in the human brain. *Rev Psychol, Biochem & Pharmacol, 88,* 126–197.

Hillyard, S. A., & Hansen, J. C. (1986). Attention: Electrophysiological approaches. In M. G. H. Coles, E. Donchin & S. W. Porges (Eds.), *Psychophysiology: Systems, processes and applications* (pp. 227–243). New York: Guilford Press.

Hillyard, S. A., & Muente T. F. (1984). Selective attention to color and location: An analysis with event-related brain potentials. *Perception & Psychophysics, 36,* 185–198.

King, J. W., & Kutas, M. (1995). Who did what and when? Using word- and clause-level ERPs to monitor working memory usage in reading. *Journal of Cognitive Neuroscience, 7*(3), 376–395.

Kluender, R., & Kutas, M. (1993). Bridging the gap: Evidence from ERPs on the processing of unbounded dependencies. *Journal of Cognitive Neuroscience, 5*(2), 196–214.

Kutas, M., & Dale, A. (1997). Electrical and magnetic readings of mental functions. In M. D. Rugg (Ed.), *Cognitive Neuroscience* (pp. 197–242). Hove, East Sussex: Psychology Press.

Kutas, M., & Federmeier, K. D. (2001). Electrophysiology reveals semantic memory use in language comprehension. *Trends in Cognitive Science, 4*(12), 463–470.

Kutas, M., Federmeier, K. D., & Sereno, M. I. (1999). Current approaches to mapping language in electromagnetic space. In C. M. Brown & P. Hagoort (Eds.), *The Neurocognition of Language* (pp. 359–392). Oxford: Oxford University Press.

Kutas, M., & Hillyard, S. A. (1980). Reading senseless sentences: Brain potentials reflect semantic incongruity. *Science, 207*(4427), 203–205.

Kutas, M., & Hillyard, S. A. (1984). Brain potentials during reading reflect word expectancy and semantic association. *Nature, 307*(5947), 161–163.

Kutas, M., & Van Petten, C. K. (1994). Psycholinguistics electrified: Event-related brain potential investigations. In M. A. Gernsbacher (Ed.), *Handbook of psycholinguistics* (pp. 83–143). San Diego: Academic Press.

Luck, S. J., & Hillyard, S. A. (1994). Electrophysiological correlates of feature analysis during visual search. *Psychophysiology, 31,* 291–308.

Mangun, G. R., Hillyard, S. A., & Luck, S. J. (1993). Electrocortical substrates of visual selective attention. In D. E. Meyer & S. Kornblum (Eds.), *Attention and performance 14: Synergies in experimental psychology, artificial intelligence, and cognitive neuroscience* (pp. 219–243). Cambridge, MA: MIT Press.

Marslen-Wilson, W. (1989). Access and integration: Projecting sound onto meaning. In W. Marslen-Wilson (Ed.), *Lexical representation and process.* Cambridge, MA: MIT Press.

Marslen-Wilson, W. (1993). Issues of process and representation in lexical access. In G. T. M. Altmann & R. Shillcock (Eds.), *Cognitive models of speech processing: The Second Sperlonga Meeting* (pp. 187–210). Hove, UK: Lawrence Erlbaum.

Marslen-Wilson, W., & Warren, P. (1994). Levels of perceptual representation and process in lexical access: Words, phonemes, and features. *Psychological Review, 101*(4), 653–675.

McCallum, W. C., & Curry, S. H. (Eds.). (1993). *Slow potential changes in the human brain* (Vol. 254). New York: Plenum.

McPherson, W. B., & Holcomb, P. J. (1999). Semantic priming with pictures and the N400 component. *Psychophysiology, 36,* 53–65.

Meyer, D. E., & Schvaneveldt, R. W. (1976). Meaning, memory structure, and mental processes. *Science, 192*(4234), 27–33.

Milberg, W., & Blumstein, S. E. (1981). Lexical decision and aphasia: Evidence for semantic processing. *Brain and Language, 14,* 371–385.

Milberg, W., Blumstein, S., & Dworetzky, B. (1987). Processing of lexical ambiguities in aphasia. *Brain and Language, 31,* 138–150.

Milberg, W., Blumstein, S., and Dworetzky, B. (1988). Phonological processing and lexical access in aphasia. *Brain and Language, 34,* 279–293.

Milberg, W., Blumstein, S., Katz, D., Gershberg, F., & Brown, T. (1995) Semantic facilitation in aphasia: Effects of time and expectancy. *Journal of Cognitive Neuroscience, 7,* 33–50.

Moll, K., Cardillo, E., & Aydelott Utman, J. (2001). Effects of competing speech on sentence-word priming: Semantic, perceptual, and attentional factors. In Moore, J. D. & Stenning, K. (Eds.), *Proceedings of the Twenty-third Annual Conference of the Cognitive Science Society,* 651–656. Mahwah, NJ, USA: Lawrence Erlbaum Associates, Inc.

Mueller, H. M., King, J. W., & Kutas, M. (1997). Event-related potentials elicited by spoken relative clauses. *Cognitive Brain Research, 5*(3), 193–203.

Munte, T. F., Heinze, H. J., Matzke, M., Wieringa, B. M., & Johannes, S. (1998). Brain potentials and syntactic violations revisited: no evidence for specificity of the syntactic positive shift. *Neuropsychologia, 36*(3), 217–226.

Neely, J. H. (1991). Semantic priming effects in visual word recognition: A selective review of current findings and theories. In D. Besner & G. W. Humphreys (Eds.), *Basic processes in reading: Visual word recognition* (pp. 264–336). Hillsdale, NJ: Lawrence Erlbaum.

Nunez, P. L., & Katznelson, R. D. (1981). *Electric fields of the brain: the neurophysics of EEG.* New York: Oxford University Press.

Osterhout, L. (1994). Event-related brain potentials as tools for comprehending language comprehension. In J. Charles Clifton, L. Frazier & K. Rayner (Eds.), *Perspectives on sentence processing* (pp. 15–44). Hillsdale, NJ: Lawrence Erlbaum.

Osterhout, L., & Holcomb, P. J. (1992). Event-related brain potentials elicited by syntactic anomaly. *Journal of Memory & Language, 31*(6), 785–806.

Osterhout, L., & Holcomb, P. J. (1995). Event related potentials and language comprehension. In M. D. Rugg & M. G. H. Coles (Eds.), *Electrophysiology of mind: Event-related brain potentials and cognition* (Vol. 25, pp. 171–215). Oxford: Oxford University Press.

Pinker, S. (1994). *The language instinct: How the mind creates language.* New York: William Morrow.

Pinker, S., & Ullman, M. (2002). The past tense debate: The past and future of the past tense. *Trends in Cognitive Sciences, 6*(11), 456–463.

Prather, P., Zurif, E., Stern, C., & Rosen, J. T. (1992). Slowed lexical access in nonfluent aphasia: A case study. *Brain and Language, 42,* 336–348.

Pylyshyn, Z. (1980). Computation and cognition: Issues in the foundation of cognitive science. *Behavioral and Brain Sciences, 3,* 111–132.

Pylyshyn, Z. (1984). *Computation and Cognition: Toward a Foundation for Cognitive Science.* Cambridge: MIT Press.

Roesler, F., & Heil, M. (1991). Toward a functional categorization of slow waves: taking into account past or future events? *Psychophysiology, 28,* 344–358.

Roesler, F., Heil, M., & Glowalla, U. (1993). Memory retrieval from long-term memory of slow event-related brain potential. *Psychophysiology, 30,* 170–182.

Roesler, F., Schumacher, G., & Sojka, B. (1990). What the brain tells when it thinks: Event-related potentials during mental rotation and mental arithmetic. *German Journal of Psychology, 14,* 185–203.

Streb, J., Roesler, F., & Hennighausen, E. (1999). Event-related responses to pronoun and proper name anaphors in parallel and nonparallel discourse structures. *Brain & Language, 70*(2), 273–286.

Ullman, M. (2001). The declarative/procedural model of lexicon and grammar. *Journal of Psycholinguistic Research, 30*(1), 37–69.

van Berkum, J. J. A., Brown, C. M., Hagoort, P., & Zwitserlood, P. (2003). Event-related brain potentials reflect discourse-referential ambiguity in spoken language comprehension. *Psychophysiology, 40*(2), 235–248.

Van Turennout, M., Hagoort, P., & Brown, C. M. (1998). Brain activity during speaking: From syntax to phonology in 40 milliseconds. *Science, 280*, 572–574.

Vos, S. H., Gunter, T. C., Kolk, H. H. J., & Mulder, G. (2001). Working memory constraints on syntactic processing: An electrophysiological investigation. *Psychophysiology, 38*(1), 41–63.

Weckerly, J., & Kutas, M. (1999). An electrophysiological analysis of animacy effects in the processing of objective relative sentences. *Psychophysiology, 36*(5), 559–570.

Wijers, A. A., Otten, L. J., Feenstra, S., Mulder G., & Mulder L. J. M. (1989). Brain potentials during selective attention, memory search, and mental rotation. *Psychophysiology, 26*, 452–467.

Zurif, E., Caramazza, A., Myerson, R., & Galvin, J. (1974). Semantic feature representations of normal and aphasic language. *Brain and Language, 1*, 167–187.

ADDENDUM

About Liz

When I was finishing my Ph.D. at Brown in 1996, I saw an ad for a postdoc at the Center for Research in Language at UC San Diego, under the supervision of Elizabeth Bates. I was of course very interested in the possibility of working with such an eminent scientist in such a beautiful part of the world, but I had never met Liz, and had no idea what she would be like as a supervisor. A few years earlier I had sat in on Cathy Harris's very enjoyable psycholinguistics course at Boston University, in which she spoke often and fondly of her years as a graduate student at UCSD, so I got in touch with Cathy and asked her whether she thought I should apply for the position. She replied that the only job she might find more appealing than a postdoc in San Diego with Liz would be a position as an officer on the Starship Enterprise under Captain Jean-Luc Picard. I applied for the postdoc immediately.

The following March (to my tremendous good fortune), I packed up my car, left snowy Providence, and moved to San Diego to work with Liz. Thus began one of the most important and formative experiences of my personal and professional life, a story that will be familiar to countless others who have had the opportunity to be a part of life at CRL. On my arrival in San Diego, Liz presented me with a gift: a miniature version of the Mouth of Truth, the statue into which ancient Romans placed their hands and swore to be truthful (lest the mouth close and remove all flesh below the wrist). Liz advised me to consult the statue if I were ever in doubt about the interpretation of my data, and above all else, to let truth prevail. I found that this is a standard she lives by in her own work, and that although she is known for her strong views (an understatement), she is first and foremost a seeker of truth, and a scientist of unfailing integrity. As a supervisor and mentor, Liz is as protective as a mother bear, as well as a relentlessly demanding critic who challenges her charges to live up to her own high expectations. She generously opens her home to students, postdocs, junior teaching staff, and established scientists, and she has brought about innumerable scientific collaborations (not to mention lifelong friendships and marriages) as a result of the many warm and relaxed gatherings held under her roof. She takes a sincere interest in the professional and personal lives of her students and colleagues, which in my case translated into long walks on the beach at La Jolla Shores, long drinks at sunset in the bar of the Marine Room, and long dinners at Trattoria Acqua overlooking La Jolla Cove, in which we would discuss data, dating, and how to be satisfied with both. Liz is always able to laugh at herself: when she and George decided (with great reluctance) to join a health club, she summed up her experience of the weight room orientation by saying, "Galileo recanted when they showed him *the machines.*" She shares her love of all things Italian with anyone who will listen, and those who are fortunate enough to score an invitation to the Bates-Carnevale apartment in Rome receive a crash course in the delights of Trastevere (Averna being my personal favorite). Liz brings her tireless spirit and humor to every aspect of life at CRL, and this has made it less like a research institution than an extended family. I am lucky to have been a part of this family, if only for a short time.

I suppose there is a sense in which I have Cathy Harris to thank for all of this, as it was her recommendation that convinced me to apply to work with Liz in the first place, and for this I am truly grateful. Looking back, I would disagree with Cathy on only one point: if I were back in San Diego with Liz, and I got the call from Captain Picard, I would have to turn him down.

—*Jennifer Aydelott*
London, September 2003

Author Index

Note: Page numbers in *italic* indicate bibliography references.
Those followed by "n" refer to footnotes.

A

Abrahamsen, A., 32, 34, *36*, 114, *135*
Adams, D. L., 197, *215*
Adams, R., 202, *217*, 249, *256*
Akazawa, C., 201, *217*
Akhmanova, A., 222, *235*
Akhtar, N., 154, *160*
Akhutina, T., 173, 176, 177, *188*
Albertoni, A., 245, 246, *259*
Albright, T. D., 200, *215*
Alcock, K. J., 224, *233*, *236*
Allen, J., 113, *135*
Allison, T., 251, *260*, 296, *310*
Alpert, N., 274, *278*
Altmann, G. T. M., 113, *135*
Alvarez, T. D., 230, *236*
Amyote, L., 113, *137*
Andersen, R. A., 213, *215*
Anderson, J., 92, *108*
Andonova, E., 173, *188*
Andruski, J. E., 285, 291, *310*
Anisfeld, M., 154, *160*
Anker, S., 231, *233*
Anokhina, R., 266, 270, 271, 273, 274, *279*
Ansari, D., 28, 30, *39*, 228, 230, *235*, *236*
Appelbaum, L. G., 230, *236*

Appelbaum, M., 53, 54, 76, 77, *188*, 240, 249, 252, 253, 254, *256*
Aram, D., 144, 153, *161*, *164*
Arbib, M. A., 7, 35, *39*
Arevalo, A., 171, *191*
Argaman, V., 119, *135*
Armstrong, D. F., 5, *36*
Armstrong, E., *162*
Arriaga, R. I., 47, *75*
Ashburner, J., 224, *236*
Asher, J., 103, *106*
Aslin, R., 93, *107*, 209, *218*
Atkinson, D. L., 221, *235*
Atkinson, J., 231, *233*
Atkinson, R., 101, 102, *106*
Austin, J. L., 8, *36*
Avila, L. X., 179, 180, 181, *189*
Aydelott, J., 226, *234*, 291, *310*
Aydelott Utman, J., 283, 286, 289, 291, 292, *310*, *311*, *313*

B

Bailey, D., 103, *106*
Bailey, T. M., *160*
Baird, C., 49, *76*

317

Subject Index

Note: Page numbers in *italic* refer to figures; those in **boldface** refer to tables.